Hospital Infection: From Miasmas to MRSA

This is an absorbing account of the continuing battle to control hospital infections, from the earliest days of hospital care when bad air or miasma was thought to be the cause, to the present day and the emergence of antibiotic-resistant 'superbugs' such as MRSA and necrotizing fasciitis. It succeeds on many levels: as a fascinating social history of hospital care from medieval times, when patients endured verminous conditions, to the present day; as a survey of the rise, fall and emergence of new nosocomial infections; and as a chronological account of the emergence of medical microbiology and infection control. The pivotal roles of key personalities such as Joseph Lister, Florence Nightingale, Louis Pasteur and Robert Koch are highlighted, and the history of this subject illuminates why hospitals and infections have had such an intimate and long relationship that seems destined to continue well into the future.

Graham Ayliffe has a long and distinguished career in medical microbiology and hospital infection control. His department, the Hospital Infection Research Laboratory in Birmingham, is well known around the world and he is the author of several highly regarded books on hospital infections and their control.

Mary English, formerly mycologist at the United Bristol Hospitals, is well known for her work in medical mycology and for her expertise in the epidemiology of fungal disease. She is also the author of numerous publications on medical mycology and two biographies of Victorian biologists.

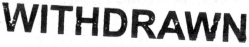

Hospital Infection

From Miasmas to MRSA

Graham A. J. Ayliffe
and Mary P. English

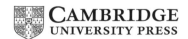

CAMBRIDGE
UNIVERSITY PRESS

PUBLISHED BY THE PRESS SYNDICATE OF THE UNIVERSITY OF CAMBRIDGE
The Pitt Building, Trumpington Street, Cambridge, United Kingdom

CAMBRIDGE UNIVERSITY PRESS
The Edinburgh Building, Cambridge CB2 2RU, UK
40 West 20th Street, New York, NY 10011-4211, USA
477 Williamstown Road, Port Melbourne, VIC 3207, Australia
Ruiz de Alarcón 13, 28014 Madrid, Spain
Dock House, The Waterfront, Cape Town 8001, South Africa

http://www.cambridge.org

First published 2003 **Coventry University**

Printed in the United Kingdom at the University Press, Cambridge

Typefaces Minion 10.5/14 pt and Formata   *System* LaTeX 2_ε [TB]

A catalogue record for this book is available from the British Library

ISBN 0 521 81935 0 hardback
ISBN 0 521 53178 0 paperback

Every effort has been made in preparing this book to provide accurate and up-to-date information which is in accord with accepted standards and practice at the time of publication. Nevertheless, the authors, editors and publisher can make no warranties that the information contained herein is totally free from error, not least because clinical standards are constantly changing through research and regulation. The authors, editors and publisher therefore disclaim all liability for direct or consequential damages resulting from the use of material contained in this book. Readers are strongly advised to pay careful attention to information provided by the manufacturer of any drugs or equipment that they plan to use.

We dedicate this book to
Professor E. J. L. Lowbury and the
late Professor Sydney Selwyn
for their encouragement.

Contents

Foreword

History tells us how we got here. However, nowadays literature is regarded as out of date after ten years, by which time journals and textbooks may have been removed from library shelves to make space for newcomers. Thus, not many people have the time or facility to look back. This is more than just a pity; it may lead to repetition of old mistakes, or extra labour in refashioning of the wheel. This book therefore fills a need. The past does need restating from time to time, although one lecturer perhaps went over the top when he said his (definitive) work was based on that of 'early English workers'. Nonetheless, my feelings when reading a recent report on hospital infection from contaminated ice, a topic I wrote up in the 1970s, were one of relief that I had got it right, and one of satisfaction that readers were being reminded of the problem.

Hospital-acquired infection is a fairly new study. It has reached maturity, and is at last properly recognized as a problem justifying the resources required for control. Why new? Well first, 'hospitals' are a recent phenomenon. Until recently, most people were nursed at home. The older hospitals such as that in Beaune (or, in a lesser but more approachable site, Higham Ferrers) were in fact charity-sponsored homes for the elderly, and contained spacious accommodation. Second, bacteria were only recognized as such during the last half of the nineteenth century. Neither Semmelweis nor Florence Nightingale knew of their existence when producing their seminal works, although the former referred to 'cadaveric particles', and the latter wished for 'cleanliness'.

This book covers early medieval times (miasmas) to the present day (MRSA), and even gives a glance into the future. Although the basics of control of hospital-acquired infection stated here are now well understood, the incidence has not decreased recently. Two factors may account for this – first, the ever-increasing complexity of medical practice allowing the survival of more susceptible patients, and second, the ability of the microbes to become resistant to antimicrobial agents. Both are discussed authoritatively herein.

The authors have an established literary track record, and fortunately have had the time and inclination to delve into and record the past. As the topic is relatively young, they have lived through a significant part of the times they describe and so can add the personal touch. Indeed, Professor Ayliffe and his coworkers in Birmingham have generated much of the literature over recent years, so it is very fitting that he should have been the senior author of this book. His work is ably complemented by Mary English with her knowledge of past times. It is an honour to be associated with them.

Bill Newsom
Cambridge May 2002

Preface

Hospital infections are infections acquired either by patients while they are in hospital or by members of the hospital staff. They are still a problem in hospitals today and in most countries 5–10% of patients in a hospital at any one time will have acquired an infection. Hospital infections are mainly of surgical wounds, the urinary tract and the respiratory tract, and are usually associated with a medical or surgical procedure. The introduction of antibiotics in the 1940s had a considerable influence on treatment, but the emergence of resistant strains of pathogens is now a major problem and some infections are already almost untreatable. Before the twentieth century, infectious diseases and infected traumatic wounds were the main hospital infections.

Wound infection must have been a problem since the earliest times. The invasion of dead tissue by bacteria in which tissue is broken down into elemental substances that can be reused by plants is one of the most important processes of nature. It is possible that in the early human wound infections, bacteria invaded gangrenous or dead tissue and found it necessary to adapt themselves to human defences or be destroyed. In order that certain species survive, it was also necessary that they should be transferred directly from one host to another. This relationship between bacteria and man and other animals has continued to develop up to the present time. Post-traumatic wound infection must have occurred from the earliest days of man's existence, and treatment to aid healing and avoid infection has been described in writings of all the great civilizations. Hippocrates in 500 BC wrote on many aspects of medicine and provided good descriptions of many diseases, including cellulitis and gangrene.[1]

Although the large armies of the ancients were afflicted by similar forms of fever, bowel diseases and pestilence as were armies in the nineteenth century, wound infection is mentioned rarely. A possible explanation for this is that few wounded survived the savage battles, and prisoners were either killed immediately or sold as captives. Although there were physicians available for treating sick and wounded soldiers, there was apparently no medical organization among the ancient Greeks and Romans corresponding to the military and civil hospitals of the eighteenth and nineteenth centuries. It was not until the fifteenth century that an attempt was made to provide some of the European armies with medical organizations.[2]

Hospitals existed in ancient civilizations, but few detailed descriptions are available. In 500 BC, there were hospitals in India, Egypt, Palestine and Greece, usually associated with temples. The most important information on medicine in ancient Egypt has been obtained from medical papyri, and the Jews described general hygiene and the isolation of infected patients in some of the books of the Old Testament.[3] The Greeks provided hospitals adjacent to the temples of Asklepios at Epidaurus and other sites, but the treatment tended to involve religious ceremonies and rites rather than surgery. The Romans at a later time built large, permanent hospitals (*valetudinaria*) for their legions, and high standards of care were provided, including trained orderlies known as *nosocomi* ('nosocomial' is a word derived from the Greek and Latin words for hospital, and hospital-acquired infection is commonly referred to as nosocomial infection).

There was little further hospital development until medieval times, when the Arabs practised high standards of medicine and built a number of hospitals. In Europe, the Hôtel Dieu was founded in the early ninth century in Paris, and in England, St Bartholomew's and St Thomas's hospitals were founded in the twelfth century; other hospitals were attached to the great European universities, such as Bologna. Most of the medieval hospitals were monastic infirmaries in which the treatment of the soul was considered more important than cures of the body. In England, there were about 500 almshouses or small hospitals by 1400.

Although hospitals were often used for the sick during epidemics, there were few major operations, apart from amputations, before 1800 and little evidence of problems of hospital infection, other than typhus in the 1700s; Pringle was one of the first men to recognize typhus as a hospital infection. From 1800 to the 1860s, there were limited healthcare resources; cities and hospitals became increasingly overcrowded, and anaesthesia allowed more adventurous surgery. Hospitals became more likely to spread disease than to check it, and reports of outbreaks of hospital infections such as pyaemia, erysipelas and gangrene were common. The term 'hospitalism' was used for hospital infection in the mid-1830s by James Simpson. The well-known reduction in mortality from postoperative infection was associated with the discovery of bacteria by Pasteur and Koch and with Lister's antiseptic treatments. The twentieth century saw the development of aseptic techniques, and from the 1940s a considerable increase in cross-infection with antibiotic-resistant bacteria has remained until today.

This book covers the period from the sixteenth and seventeenth centuries until the end of the twentieth century, and includes the development of theories on the mode of spread of infection, hygienic conditions, epidemic diseases and cross-infection and its prevention in hospitals. It commences with a discussion on magic and miasmas, and continues to the emerging diseases and epidemics of methicillin-resistant *Staphylococcus aureus* (MRSA) at the end of the twentieth century.

Although we have endeavoured to include relevant data from other countries, most of the sources are from English-language references and inevitably there is a bias towards British hospitals. The latter part of the book includes much of the work and personal experience of one of the authors (GA) and his colleagues over the years, initially in Bristol with William Gillespie and George Alder, then in Hammersmith Hospital with Mary Barber, and in Birmingham with Edward Lowbury and other colleagues at the Hospital Infection Research Laboratory. A large number of workers have made considerable contributions to infection control in the past 50 years and we regret being unable to include more of them in the book.

Most of the earlier references are from secondary sources, but primary sources or reviews are included more often for the nineteenth and twentieth centuries. The references are selective rather than comprehensive, but most of the topics are covered in the bibliography. Some of the commonly used terms are explained in the text for readers less conversant with microbes and infection.

We wish to thank the Wellcome Tust for a grant and the Wellcome, Royal Society of Medicine, Bristol University, Birmingham University, Birmingham Central Library, Manchester Library, Lincoln Library and several other town and hospital libraries for their help, and the following for their useful comments or for providing information: Dr V. G. Alder, Mr J. Hansford, Ms Lynda Taylor, Prof. Hans Kolmos, Dr Helen Glenister, Dr. A. B. Shaw and Mr J. Babb. We wish to thank the following for photographs: the Wellcome Trust (Figures 2.1, 2.2, 2.3, 2.4, 3.1, 3.2, 6.1, 6.2, 6.3, 6.4, 8.1, 8.2, 8.3, 8.4, 8.6, 9.1, 17.1 and 17.2), Prof. Manfred Rotter (Figure 5.1), Dr Michael Barnham (Figure 10.2), Mr Peter London (Figure 10.1), Mr N. Hicks (Figure 11.2) and the City Hospital Trust photographic department, Birmingham.

Theories of infection: from magic to miasmas

The management of patients with infectious diseases, the control of epidemics and the planning of hospitals have always been dependent on the contemporary theories of infection. For this reason, it may be useful to devote some space to a brief history of the development of infection theory over the centuries.

In ancient times, belief in black magic and the malevolence of witches and evil spirits was universal and, despite the rise of Christianity, had an immensely firm grip on people and their rulers right through to the Tudor period and beyond. The help of practitioners of the occult was called upon regularly in times of sickness, and even today raw beef features in a magical cure for warts. During the Great Plague in London (1664–5), some recommended the wearing of a tassel of tarred rope to ward off the disease, and a doctor who felt the symptoms coming on after he had dissected a plague victim placed a dried toad on his chest to draw off the poison. Pepys used a hare's foot to keep away the colic, but when the charm failed a friend pointed out that it did not include the joint; after it had been replaced by a complete specimen, Pepys was never troubled by colic again.[1] Perhaps the most generally accepted belief was the cure of the King's Evil (scrofula, or tuberculosis of the glands) by means of the royal touch. This piece of pagan magic was christianized by Henry VII, who invented a church ritual during which the ceremony was performed, a ceremony that was only removed from the Book of Common Prayer by George I.[2]

With the advent of Christianity, these pagan beliefs were very slowly superseded by the idea that sickness was a punishment from God for the sins of the victim or the community, and that consequently the only sure remedy was prayer and penance until His forgiveness was granted. As late as the sixteenth century, the Elizabethan Prayer Book required clergymen visiting sick parishioners to remind them of this, and it was held that the ministrations of physicians and surgeons would be successful only if they had prayed beforehand. From an early date, in times of plague, masses and prayers were addressed to holy relics, but by degrees, bitter experience and the deaths of hundreds of priests and monks showed such faith to be ineffectual; indeed, it has been suggested that one factor reducing opposition to the Reformation was disillusion with the healing power of relics.[2] Throughout the history of human thought, magic, religion and science have fought for supremacy in the explanation of disease, and it was only in medieval times that science began to get the upper hand.

At the end of the fifteenth century, the ancient Greek doctrine of the humours was still the basis of disease theory. Patients were believed to belong to one of four groups or 'complections' – choleric, melancholic, phlegmatic or sanguine – each associated with an appropriate 'humour' – yellow or green bile, black bile, phlegm and blood, respectively. Badly balanced humours predisposed to specific types of disease, but it was admitted that some diseases, mostly those known to be infectious, were exceptions.[3]

The oldest of the more 'scientific' theories of the spread of epidemic disease was that of the corruption of the air, an idea that began at least in the sixth century, and was to persist into the nineteenth century. Corruption could be induced by any extremes of weather, such as excessive dryness, heat or rain,[4] or more locally by the putrid miasmas arising from decaying organic matter, corpses, cesspools, marshes and the like. Limited public health measures were aimed at cleaning up such places; for instance, in 1488 Henry VII issued a statute regulating slaughterhouses in towns, and in 1495 he decreed that marshes near towns must be drained before they were built over. It was believed that when inhaled, miasmas (which some held to consist of poisonous particles) were absorbed in some way by the body, and then attacked the humours to cause disease. Some suggested that epidemics occurred when the process was made more virulent by a malign conjunction of the stars. There was also supposed to be a factor of individual predisposition, a concept that was combined with a stress on the importance of personal cleanliness,[5] an unexpected concept considering the general disregard for such matters at the time. As yet, no distinction was made between different infectious diseases, so that any miasma could cause any disease.

For the whole medieval period, including the terrible years of the Black Death, the main prophylactic measure against infectious diseases was fumigation by the burning of incense, herbs and aromatic essences.[6]

The belief that disease is spread by corrupted air, distinguishable from pure air by its noxious smell, is, as already discussed, a very ancient one, and over the centuries means have been sought to contain epidemics by removing evil odours. It was not until the eighteenth century that a distinction was clearly made between merely concealing the stench with aromatic scents and actually destroying it. At that time, fumigation became widely recommended as one of the measures for preventing the spread of typhus.

Fumigation usually refers to the production of smoke or a vapour, often odorous such as incense, to remove infection, pests, evil spirits or unpleasant smells. An early account of fumigation was given by Homer in the *Odyssey* in about 800 BC, in which Odysseus used sulphur dioxide to fumigate his house on his return after he had killed his wife's suitors. In early Indian writing (Sushruta 800–600 BC), the fumigation of an operating room with fumes of mustard, butter and salt might be considered an early form of 'antisepsis'[7] of the air, although it was also used to get rid of evil spirits. Sulphur fumigation was commonly used to prevent the spread of plague in the Middle Ages. In the seventeenth century, the possible connection between fermentation and disease was recognized by Robert Boyle. Francis Bacon (1663) also related gangrene to putrefaction and listed substances that would prevent putrefaction, including sulphuric acid, salts and sugars.

Despite the universal acknowledgement of the divine wrath and putrid air as the generators of disease, practical observation had forced on man since the earliest times the idea that in the case of leprosy contagion was a factor in its spread, but it was not until the Middle Ages that a turning point was reached and the ravages of the epidemic leprosy of the time, together with the plague, forced a full recognition of infection as a cause of some diseases.[8] No explanation of the phenomenon would, however, be put forward until the sixteenth century, with the result that, although stringent precautions were taken against the spread of both leprosy and plague, no attempt was made to segregate other fever patients in hospitals. For instance, in 1148 all sick people, regardless of whether they were suffering from diseases now known to be infections, were being admitted to St Bartholomew's Hospital, London.[9] By about 1300, however, Bernard Gordon of Montpellier had listed eight diseases that he recognized as infectious – bubonic plague, phthisis, epilepsy, scabies, erysipelas, anthrax, trachoma and leprosy.[8] With regard to erysipelas, Walshe records that a special order of monks was created to work in hospitals dedicated to patients suffering from St Anthony's fire, which he takes to be synonymous with erysipelas, considering that this is an early recognition of the contagiousness of the disease. But 'St Anthony's fire' was a term used indiscriminately at the time for erysipelas and the gangrene and subsequent withering of limbs that resulted from ergot poisoning, a mysterious and terrifying, though non-infectious, disease that could well have precipitated the setting up of a dedicated nursing order.

The Black Death, or bubonic plague, was probably brought to Europe by a ship trading from the Near East, which docked at Messina in Sicily in 1347. From there, the disease spread throughout the continent with devastating speed. It is estimated that one-quarter to one-half of the entire population of Europe was wiped out between 1348 and 1359, and at least half the population of Britain succumbed.[6]

The causal bacterium, *Yersinia*, formerly *Pasteurella, pestis* (see Chapter 9), was carried by its vectors, the black rat and its flea *Pulex irritans*. The black rat, the common species of the age, lives and breeds in houses, unlike the brown rat that has now replaced it and prefers outhouses and sewers to domestic premises. The association of rats with the disease was unrecognized for several centuries after the Middle Ages, although there are two intriguing biblical references to mice in conjunction with epidemics, which are now considered to have been plague – the 'emerods' with which Ashod smote the Hebrews (1 Samuel: v), and the plague visited by the Lord on the army of Sennacherib (2 Kings: xix, 36).[6]

Monasteries were decimated by the plague early, the first casualties being those of the Dominicans and Friars Minor of Messina, who were left behind to attend to the first European victims after the rest of the population of the city had fled. In England, the communities of St Albans, Glastonbury and Bath abbeys were halved.[10] Lepers were particularly vulnerable, both because of their concentration in lazar houses and because of their lack of immunity due to their underlying disease.[9]

The obvious infectivity of the Black Death not only reinforced the idea of the segregation of victims to protect the rest of the community, but also the panic it created resulted in the introduction for the first time in history of two further forms of prophylaxis. The possibility of spread through patients' clothing, bedding, etc. led to the disinfection or burning of fomites, and the use of quarantine began as a means of safeguarding whole communities. Municipal authorities placed the homes of plague victims under a ban; they and all their contacts were also banned, and their food was provided for them. The dead were passed out of houses and removed in carts for burial outside the city, and their houses were fumigated (although only with the usual incense and aromatic herbs), and their effects burned. Occasionally, a group of people, knowing they harboured plague cases, made the heroic decision to immolate themselves so as to prevent the disease from spreading further. Perhaps the most famous case, in 1666, is the village of Eyam in the Derbyshire Peak District, the inhabitants of which, after a few wealthy families had fled, drew a cordon sanitaire about half a mile around the village. Food was brought to the boundary, but no person crossed it, neither entering nor leaving the village. The inhabitants were decimated, 259 of them dying before the end of the outbreak.[3]

In Europe, Venice was the chief port for trade with the Orient, and it was here that quarantine was practised for the first time. In 1348, a committee of three prominent citizens was set up with powers to isolate suspected ships, goods and people, a practice that spread throughout Europe. Then in 1377, the municipal Council of Ragusa (Dubrovnik) ordered that ships be held in isolation for a period of 30 days (later extended to 40 days, this being the origin of the word 'quarantine'). In 1383, citizens of Marseilles erected the first quarantine station, where all incoming vessels and their contents were rigorously inspected and exposed to air and sunshine, and their crews isolated in special lazar houses.[5] Such isolation hospitals might also be built outside towns at the beginning of an outbreak in the hope of controlling it.

Although by the Middle Ages contagion had been recognized as a factor in the spread of disease, its cure was still the preserve of the Church and even residual pagan beliefs. Doctors could offer little more in the way of treatment than blood-letting and purification of the air. The intercession of the saints was therefore of extreme importance, and one saint in particular was associated with the Black Death. St Roche was born in Montpellier in the south of France in about 1350, and spent his life going on pilgrimages and working among the sick. While on a pilgrimage to Rome, he fell victim to the plague and fled to a neighbouring forest to die, but he was brought a daily supply of bread by the dog of a local landowner, recovered, and was eventually pronounced cured by an angel. This is why he is accompanied by a dog, an angel or both in the statues that grace his many shrines in France and Italy. After his recovery, the saint set out on his last pilgrimage to Angera, but was accused of being a spy and thrown into prison, where he died, leaving a scribbled message on the wall of his cell saying, 'He who is seized of the plague and seeks refuge in Roche will gain relief in the disease.' From that time on, plague victims sought St Roche's intercession, and many hospitals in Europe were dedicated to him. His cult reached England, where his statue used to stand in a number of churches. In Exeter, in the early sixteenth century, there were a chapel and hospital dedicated to the saint, which were commemorated until very recent times by a small roadway called Rock Lane, but even this has now disappeared. It is perhaps of interest that statues of St Roche usually show him pointing to a lump a little above one of his knees, clearly a bubo. In fact, the bubo would have been situated in his groin, but this was an awkward site to display in a statue!

In the first half of the sixteenth century, Girolamo Fracastoro (1483–1553), working in Venice, gradually reasoned his way to an astonishingly modern theory of infection. His initial interest was syphilis, recently introduced into Europe and by then reaching epidemic proportions, but his work gradually extended to include all epidemic diseases. In the 1530s, he considered, like others, that corrupted air was the cause of epidemics, but he suggested that the source of the corruption was astrological, different conjunctions of the planets causing different diseases in different hosts. Here we have the first mention of the specific nature of diseases and their causes, an idea which, with remarkable prescience, he particularly emphasized.

But it was his essay on contagion, published in 1546, that anticipated the science of bacteriology by 300 years. First, he was clear that infection was the cause, of which epidemics were the consequence; second, he suggested that contagion was caused by infective 'seeds' – he called them 'seminaria' – which were too small to be visible to the naked eye; third, he stated that these seeds were specific for specific diseases; and finally, he suggested that the seeds were self-propagating and acted on the humours and vital spirits of the body, although careful reading of the text makes it clear that there is no suggestion that 'seeds' are living organisms.[8] He also recognized that infection could take place in three ways: by direct contact between people, by fomites (a term he introduced), and at a distance through the air. However, he continued to believe implicitly in astrology and the power of the conjunction of the stars as the source of the phenomena that he described. For a while, his ideas were widely accepted, but gradually they were forgotten and supplanted once again by the old, erroneous miasmatic theory,[11] together with a continued belief in witchcraft, sorcery and alchemy.

No further advances were made until the seventeenth century, but by then the repeated outbreaks of plague were crying out for an explanation. In 1658, Athenasius Kircher (1602–88), a Jesuit priest, published a tract on plague entitled 'Scrutinium Pestis'. Although he did not cite Fracastoro, he did in fact follow him in believing that both God and the stars had a hand in the occurrence of epidemics, but that 'natural causes were also important, and that these included self-propagating seminaria specific to each disease'. But Kircher had the advantage over Fracastoro in that he possessed a 'very delicate' microscope. Though he could not possibly have seen bacteria with this instrument, he could see small moving objects, and when he made observations – 'experiments' he called them – on rotting meat, decaying wood, soil and such materials, he could describe the living 'worms' and 'creeping things' that he saw, some of which turned into winged forms. He concluded from his observations that the bodies of those who died from plague generated corpuscles, which might be living or non-living, and which could infect bread, wood and other porous substances as well as the air, and so spread the disease by finger contact or inhalation. Among the 12 different ways in which contagion might take place, he lists the physician attending plague cases since the 'virulent corpuscles which have been breathed out or transferred by manual contact will adhere to the innermost recesses of the pores so that contagion may readily be communicated to those not already infected with the disease'.[8] Perhaps this is the first mention of iatrogenic disease. Kircher emphasizes throughout that the 'seeds' specific to plague are the essential cause of the disease and are always present, and that the living seeds reproduce themselves in vast numbers in the victim's body, to be given off eventually through all body openings to infect new hosts and fomites.[8]

Despite Kircher's continuing belief in the deity and the stars as additional causes of epidemics, his 'Scrutinium Pestis' was the first effective recognition that living, multiplying organisms specific to a disease are the primary cause of that disease, a recognition that he backed up with 'experiments', however inadequate to modern eyes, to prove it. His theory immediately attracted attention throughout Europe, including England, but here, one otherwise extremely advanced and influential clinician, Thomas Sydenham (1624–89), continued to insist that it was the 'epidemic constitution' of the atmosphere that was responsible for epidemics.[8] At the end of his life, however, Sydenham broadened his theory somewhat. The outbreak of 'fever' in 1658–60 did not appear to be related in the usual way to the weather or the season, so he suggested that there must have been 'some secret and remarkable change in the bowels of the earth', rather than in the air, to account for it, an idea that was expanded by his friend Robert Boyle. Sydenham believed that the poisonous effluvia were mineral particles that originated in the earth's crust, where they could, in some undefined way, spread or multiply, and from which they were liberated by eruptions or slower movements of the crust.[12]

Meanwhile, from Italy emerged yet another brilliant scientist, Francesco Redi (1620–98), a medical man, philosopher and naturalist.[13] As a doctor, he advocated observation as opposed to theory, and hygiene rather than therapy. As a naturalist, he was particularly interested in insects, and it was this interest that led to his major contribution to science, the first experimental refutation of the theory of spontaneous generation, at least so far as it applied to insects and larger organisms. He did this by exposing pieces of meat in jars to the warm summer air, some with the jars uncovered and some with their mouths covered by pieces of gauze. While the meat putrefied under both conditions, maggots were generated only from the unprotected pieces, those covered with gauze remaining maggot free, although blowflies were attracted to the jars and maggots hatched from the eggs they laid on the gauze. Redi's conclusion – that in all cases where living things had apparently been produced by dead matter, the 'seeds' of the life form had in fact been introduced from outside – was readily accepted by others. But this brilliant deduction could not, of course, be applied to the as yet undiscovered micro-organisms. Another discovery by Bonomo in 1687 was that of the scabies mite, which some considered a turning point in medicine in that it made doctors think of exogenous pathogenic agents rather than disturbed humans. Nevertheless, it was not until the nineteenth century that the theory of spontaneous generation was finally laid to rest for both putrefaction and disease.

The century's advances were completed by a Dutchman, Anthony van Leeuwenhoek (1632–1723), whose brilliant observations with the simple microscopes of his day first disclosed to man the protozoa and the bacteria.[14] He described cocci, rods and filaments in rainwater and saliva, and although he did not relate these to disease he was the first to describe them. He even noted that his 'animalcules' died in the presence of pepper and wine vinegar and was probably the first to describe the effects of chemicals on actual micro-organisms.[7] We can see now that by then science was sufficiently advanced to have made it possible to have put together a theory of infectious disease approaching that of modern times, but then the medical world failed to marshal the new facts into a cohesive whole and draw the necessary conclusions.

During the period under review, the theories held by the medical profession on the manifestations and relationships of the fevers were changing in line with those on infection. At the beginning of the period, fevers were thought to be a continuum: they were considered to be a single disease with different malignancies, taking different courses. Thus different types of rash were regarded as indications of the relative severity of the fevers rather than distinguishing one fever from another. But by the later seventeenth century, this view was changing as a number of new theories were put forward.[15] The humoral theory of disease was gradually replaced by a more mechanistic approach emphasizing malfunctions of the body fluids and the vessels through which they flowed. For instance, it was suggested that normal blood contained particles natural to it, but in a disease it became clogged by foreign particles emanating from the disease process; for recovery, these foreign particles had to be removed by the body itself or, failing that, with the intervention of the doctor. Another suggestion was that the fever process was a fermentation. These theories, even if untenable in the light of modern knowledge, represented a totally new outlook on fevers, the symptoms could be assigned to specific material causes, and the whole approach to them and their management, not only clinical but social, was open to change.[16] For instance, Thomas Sydenham, in the first edition of his book on fever therapy, written in 1666, clearly regarded all fevers as a unity, but by the third edition (1676) careful observation had caused him to acknowledge some clear distinctions, especially in the cases of smallpox and plague.[17] Other authors at this time increasingly began to write about smallpox and measles, in particular, as distinct from other fevers.[15]

Except for a widespread outbreak in 1603, little is heard about bubonic plague in Britain between the time of the Black Death and London's Great Plague in 1665, but in fact there were limited but lethal outbreaks, all over the country and especially in London, and throughout Europe too, between the two major outbreaks. As in earlier years, outbreaks were at first attributed to the divine wrath, but this theory became less and less tenable as it dawned on the populace that priests and monks were as likely to succumb as the most disreputable layman. The miasmatic theory as expounded by the medical profession then began to come into its own. Various sources for the corruption of the air were suggested, including stagnant water, carrion, overcrowding and, as ever, the conjunction of the stars.[2,6] In Italy, the hypothesis was put forward that the corruption consisted of venomous atoms generated from any of the above sources as well as from infected people. Not only were the atoms poisonous but they were also exceptionally sticky, so that they adhered to any solid body, and if they were inhaled or absorbed through the pores of the skin, they would poison the body causing the death of the infected person: hence followed the practice of some doctors of washing the face, neck and hands in vinegar before seeing patients, in order to close the pores.[18] The atoms could also be passed from person to person, and from an animal or an inanimate object to a person, a theory that led naturally to the use of isolation procedures and quarantine to control the spread of the disease. The waxed cotton robes worn by doctors as personal protection against the plague were based on the theory that the slipperiness prevented the venomous particles from sticking to them, an example of a successful preventive measure based on a hopelessly incorrect theory; for of course, the waxy surface did prevent the fleas with which the patients were infected from transferring themselves to the doctor. In fact, in 1657, Father Antero Maria de San Bonaventura, the administrator of the pest house at Genoa, unaware of the prescience of his words, remarked: 'The waxed robe in a pest house is good *only* [our italics] to protect one from the fleas, which cannot nest in it.' Father Antero was driven to this remark by his experiences in the lazaretto:

I have to change my clothes frequently if I do not want to be devoured by fleas, armies of which nest in my gown, nor have I force enough to resist them, and I need great strength of mind to keep still at the altar. If I want to rest for an hour in bed, I have to use a sheet, otherwise the lice would feed on my flesh; they vie with the fleas – the latter suck, the former bite.[19]

The Middle Ages to the seventeenth century: hospitals and infection

In the Middle Ages, medicine in Arabia, in common with many other aspects of Arabic culture, was far in advance of that practised in Europe. Its roots lay in Greek thought, and it owed its achievements largely to the encouragement and philanthropy of the rulers, the caliphs, thus differing sharply from Western medicine, which was dominated almost entirely by the Church. The Koranic insistence on cleanliness of the body, which was carried through into everyday life, was in marked contrast to the Christian emphasis on purity of the soul, with scant attention being paid to personal hygiene. The infectivity of some diseases was recognized to the extent that in times of epidemics, movement out of the infected country was prohibited.[1] Lepers were first segregated in the year AD707.[2] Smallpox had been reported from both Arabia and the West in the sixth century, when it was first thought to be caused by miasmas, an idea that was still current in the ninth century when Rhazes (born AD850) wrote his brilliant treatise on the disease.

The glory of Arabic medicine was its hospitals, founded and endowed by rulers and the nobility who were inspired by Islamic teaching. Most cities had their own hospitals, the earliest being founded in Baghdad in the ninth century.[1] The founder of a later hospital there, the Adude, selected its site most carefully for its healthy aspect by hanging up pieces of meat in different parts of the city and building on the site where putrefaction set in most slowly. Cairo's oldest hospital was founded in 873, but its most important one was the great hospital of Al-Mansur, founded in 1284. It was open to all, rich and poor, freemen and slaves, men and women. Conditions were luxurious: there were separate wards for fever patients, ophthalmic cases, surgical cases and dysentery, and water was laid on throughout.[2]

In Christian Europe, hospitals began as clerical rather than secular institutions and remained as such for many centuries. Monasteries had, of necessity, to have an infirmary where sick brothers and sisters could be tended, and gradually these were opened, first to passing pilgrims, then to other travellers, and finally to local people in need of succour. By the fifteenth century, several religious orders had been founded specifically to heal the sick and needy, and there were several thousand monastic infirmaries in Europe, 750 in England alone.[3] The principle on which the treatment of the sick was based was that disease was ordained by God for the punishment of sin, the cure of the soul always taking precedence over the cure of the body.

Lepers were a special case. They had been excluded from society since ancient times, condemned to living outside the walls of the towns in the utmost poverty and distress, and to warning the healthy of their approach by ringing a warning bell. In Europe, leprosy was prevalent in the eleventh century and it was probably introduced into England at the time of the Norman Conquest, reaching its peak there by the twelfth century; by 1400 it had practically disappeared. It was the Church, following the precepts set out in the Book of Leviticus, that first undertook the task of combating the disease.[4] Special leper hospitals are first mentioned by Gregory of Tours in the sixth century, but the fear of infection was such in the medieval period that by the thirteenth and fourteenth centuries, there were 220 lazar houses (lazarettos, leprosaria) in England and Scotland alone, and 2000 in France. Following the example of the Church, wealthy private benefactors then began to found lazar houses, some endowing them, others relying on public charity to keep them running. One such hospital in London was St Giles' Hospital, founded in 1100 by Queen Matilda, the wife of Henry I.[5] When municipal hospitals began to appear in the thirteenth century, some leprosaria were transferred to their charge,[6] and it was thus that the idea of the control of communicable disease as a public health measure began.

The design of most monastic infirmaries was based on the Gothic hall, which fortuitously allowed patients maximum light and air. The lofty wards that resulted had ventilators in the roof, and windows along each side, which could be opened and closed by a system of pulleys. The lines of well-spaced beds projected from each long wall, as they do today. This arrangement may have been found draughty, because in later infirmaries, wooden or stone cubicles were built around each bed. The larger infirmaries had their own water supplies and kitchens.

Apart from monastic infirmaries, idealistic men had, from very early times, been founding charitable houses where widows, orphans, the old, the poor and the sick could receive shelter and care. These institutions gradually came under the protection of the Church and were often the special responsibility of the bishops. In fact, ecclesiastical legislation from the fourth century onwards had been concerned with these matters, and by the eighth century the obligation to provide physicians for the sick housed in these institutions was specifically imposed.[3] Many of them were what we would now consider to be almshouses rather than hospitals, but of the true hospitals, the best known in England are St Thomas's, founded in 1106, and St Bartholomew's, founded in 1123, although York had a hospital as early as 936, Rochester in 1078, and Worcester in 1085. There were probably 10 to 20 such hospitals in the period between 1066 and 1100, but the numbers had risen to 300 or 400 by the end of the thirteenth century, although some had only short lives.[5] The general decline that set in at this time was due largely to falling financial support from patrons.

On the Continent, in contrast, the provision of hospitals was almost continuous from the time the great Hôtel Dieu was founded in Paris in the ninth century. In Paris, in addition to the monastic hospitals and those supported by the Church, many hospitals were founded during and after the Crusades by the Knights Hospitallers of St John; at first, these were usually rough and simple buildings with straw-strewn floors for beds.

In the Middle Ages, living conditions for rich and poor alike were hardly conducive to good health. With the advent of Christianity and its emphasis on the cleanliness of the soul rather than of the body, the excellent hygienic standards of Roman times began to decline rapidly. In towns, drainage consisted of an open sewer running down the middle of the street, with privies draining into cesspools under the house or, in riverside houses, projecting from walls and emptying straight into the river, from which most of the town's drinking water was obtained. Into the river too was dumped all sorts of garbage and slaughterhouse refuse.

Bathing was an infrequent event among the rich, and probably never indulged in at all by the poor, although in the late Middle Ages some public baths were built for them. However, these baths soon became insanitary centres for debauchery and the spread of disease, especially syphilis, and were gradually disappearing by the end of the fifteenth century.[7] The poor lived in grossly overcrowded conditions and consequently in a state of indescribable filth, and even the wealthy preferred to live in huge, gregarious households. A pointer to the conditions reigning at the time is the very large number of recipes for the eradication of lice and fleas found in twelfth-century documents, while contemporary medical treatises are full of descriptions of patients' motions, indicating that dysentery due to bad hygiene must have been common.[5] From time to time, proclamations from the authorities led to the removal of some particular nuisance, but in the absence of any organized public health system, there was little general improvement over the whole period of 500 years.

At the beginning of the Middle Ages, the hygiene of monastic hospitals was probably little different from that of domestic premises, for it is recorded that as far back as the seventh century, epidemics of 'pestilence' broke out in monasteries, which, before the growth of towns, were comparatively large communities. It is likely that this pestilence (probably plague) was carried from monastery to monastery by travelling monks, who would have infected the inhabitants of villages where they lodged on their way, thus being not unimportant in spreading the disease.[8]

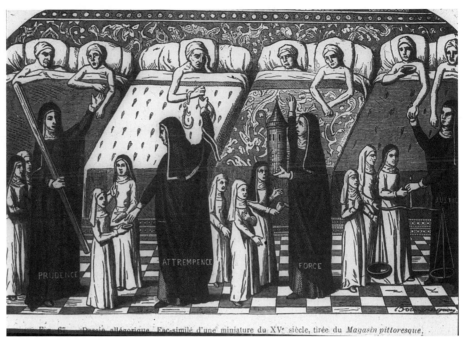

Figure 2.1   A ward in the Hôtel Dieu, Paris, in the fifteenth century, showing overcrowding and sharing of beds. Reproduced from an original engraving by Tollet (1892). Wellcome Library, London.

From the start of the twelfth century, however, hygiene began to improve. In Cistercian monasteries, clean water was regarded as essential. All those built in the countryside at this time were close to a river, and kitchens, lavatories and infirmaries were supplied with clean running water by means of a dam upstream from the buildings and pipes running under them. The sewerage was passed back to the river by means of sluices downstream from the monastery. In town monasteries and their hospitals, this arrangement was less easy; nevertheless, most monasteries were close to running water and were equipped with pipes and drains, and eventually even the smaller hospitals had some kind of water supply.[3]

Unfortunately, almost all records of conditions in English hospitals of the early Middle Ages, together with their daily routines, have been lost, but those of the great Hôtel Dieu in Paris survive and were probably very similar to other European hospitals. For that early date, they were exemplary and as yet showed no signs of the deterioration that would eventually render the hospital the byword for horror that it would become during the next few centuries.

The Hôtel Dieu was founded in about 800, consisting then of a single ward adjacent to the west end of the original building of the Cathedral of Notre Dame on the Ile de la Cité (Figure 2.1). The present cathedral was erected in the twelfth century on the site of the original building, but its greater size displaced the hospital, which had to be rebuilt. By the thirteenth century, the hospital had three large, open wards,[9] which were kept spotlessly clean, as is shown by the accounts of the period, which record that 1300 brooms were used annually and that the walls were lime-washed every year. The windows in the high walls could be opened and closed by a system of pulleys, and the number of beds per ward was strictly controlled by their width and by the dimensions of the ward. On admission, the patients' clothes were taken from them, washed, and stored until they left. The custom that appals us today is that of allocating two or three patients to each bed, but this was the accepted practice in ordinary households of the time, and beds were deliberately built wide enough for multiple occupation. The patients lay on straw mattresses and were covered by linen sheets and counterpanes made of heavy grey cloth. The sheets were washed once a week by a staff of 15 laundresses in the river outside the hospital. There was a plentiful supply of water within the hospital, and patients' hands and faces were washed daily, as were the floors of the wards.[3] There was no new building for nearly 300 years; then, in 1532, a 100-bed ward was added for contagious cases, particularly plague victims.

A rare English record suggesting attention to hygiene at St Thomas's Hospital, Canterbury notes a payment of 46s 8d to the warden's wife for 'wasshyng the bedds for poure people'. Included in an enquiry in 1535 into the Savoy Hospital, London was the question of whether any patient had been required to lie in the unwashed sheets of a previous inmate.[10] A century or two later, such standards would have declined badly.

For obvious reasons, ordinary hospitals did not normally take in plague victims.[10] For instance, in the sixteenth century, St Thomas's Hospital, London, had a 'night-layers' ward where homeless vagabonds could stay overnight, but this was closed for a year from May 1563, evidently because of an outbreak of plague. Again, written 'orders' for the hospital for the year 1700 include instructions that no plague victims were to be admitted.[11] St Bartholomew's Hospital, in September 1665, during the Great Plague, asked the King to ensure that no sick or wounded seamen were sent there 'during these contageous times' for fear they might bring the disease. Only some of the hospital's doctors remained at their posts during the outbreak; the others fled London.

To cope with plague victims, pest houses and convalescent homes were set up all over Europe to which sick citizens were dispatched. There were at least five pest houses in the London area, each under the charge of a physician whose job was only part time, for in practice there was little he could do. At the 90-bed pest house at St Martin-in-the-Fields, Dr Tristan received a fee of £170 during the Great Plague, in addition to which he had a private practice from which he sold a nostrum against the plague invented by himself.[12]

Pest houses were often set up as a last-minute panic measure. An example comes from Italy, where, during the summer of 1630, plague was approaching the town of Pistoia, north-west of Florence. On 27 September, a pest house or lazaretto was set up outside the town walls, under the charge of a physician and a surgeon who were given strict instructions not to venture into the city. The outbreak began, and the first patients were admitted on 8 October, but the doctors reported that there was nothing in the pest house that they needed and no attendants. By 23 October, there were so many patients that 'there is no room in it [the pest house] for all of them'. By 1 December, patients were sleeping five to a bed, and there were no sheets and few blankets. Meanwhile in a convalescent home in another town, 21 patients were sleeping in six beds and the food supply was so meagre that they were starving. It seems clear that this state of affairs was brought about not by lack of will or understanding, but by the health deputies' lack of funds.[13]

In the periods when plague reached epidemic proportions, the provision of adequate accommodation for victims in pest houses was totally impractical, and it was in these fearful times that the practice of sealing up victims in their own homes, together with their families, was resorted to.

In the sixteenth and seventeenth centuries, the evolution of hospitals took a rather different course in England from that on the Continent. In England, when Henry VIII ascended the throne in 1527, he began the feud with the Pope that eventually led to the King's break from the Catholic Church. Due to the Church's near monopoly in health matters, the ensuing Reformation, including the dissolution of the monasteries and the sequestration of their wealth, resulted in Henry VIII coincidentally sweeping away the entire English hospital system. Even the few lay hospitals mostly ceased to function because of either bad management or insufficient financial support from their founders. In 1544, the situation in London became so desperate that, following a petition from the citizens, the King allowed the reopening of St Bartholomew's and St Thomas's hospitals as lay institutions; however, for many years, they were almost the only large, general hospitals in the country. The old hospitals at York and Winchester were refounded at a fairly early date, but 23 of the principal English counties had no hospital until the eighteenth century.[14] The few small hospitals or converted lazar houses that survived probably did more harm than good, for they were hardly ever cleaned, sharing beds was common, and the nurses were rough and ignorant.

London had always been blessed with some good water, but outside the capital, supplies of clean water were almost nonexistent, and sanitation was still unknown anywhere in the country. It is to Tudor times and Sir Thomas More that we can trace the first public health administration. More was made Commissioner for Sewers in 1514 and during his tenure of the post he made enormous improvements in

London's drainage and in the quality and quantity of its water supply. That he was an enlightened health reformer is shown in his great book *Utopia*, in which he advocated public hospitals treating rich and poor alike, together with isolation hospitals and a municipal nursing service.[15] Under More, the Corporation of London issued many regulations concerning infectious diseases, scavenging and sanitation.[14] But despite these advances, only the well off had a privy over a cesspit in the garden to supplement the ubiquitous chamber pot in the bedroom. Chamber pots were emptied into the street, and those who had not even that lowly convenience simply relieved themselves in the open.

As in the Middle Ages, a varied and active insect population subsisting on the person was accepted as normal, even by the well off, so it is hardly surprising that nothing was done to suppress such fauna in hospitals. Sheets were used only by the rich; in general, beds were covered with sheepskins and fur rugs, excellent domiciles for fleas, which also inhabited in droves the rushes with which the floors were strewn. A form of disinfestation used when winter clothes and bedding were stored for the summer was to roll them up very tightly, bind them with straps, and stuff them into deep chests. The resulting deprivation of light and air was supposed to be fatal to fleas. As to the bugs that lived unmolested in the wooden bedposts and panelling, the Tudors regarded them as part of normal life, and the lice that shared their clothing suffered little more disturbance than the occasional use of a backscratcher.[14]

In hospitals, until they disappeared at the Reformation, it was hardly surprising that little interest was taken in matters of hygiene, for the connection between public filth and disease had yet to be understood. But already in the sixteenth century, some attempt was being made to segregate diseases, in addition to the plague, known by observation to be infectious. The sweating sickness, an infectious disease that has now disappeared entirely, was prevalent at the time, and to cope with this St Thomas's had a special 'sweat ward' in the churchyard in which patients with this condition were isolated.[11] Conditions within the hospital were poor, however: water was obtained from polluted wells, although at that time Thames water was comparatively pure; patients lay several to a bed in unventilated wards; and until well into the seventeenth century, linen was still washed with wood ashes – it was not until 1635–6 that six pounds of soap a week was allotted for this purpose. Soap was apparently not introduced into St Bartholomew's until 1558.[10]

Throughout the first half of the seventeenth century, the need for hospital services in London continued to increase and overcrowding became a serious problem, until the Civil War (1642–9), when, due to inadequate funding, the turnover of patient numbers fell dramatically in St Thomas's and St Bartholomew's and did not return to pre-war levels until the 1650s. Meanwhile, London's needs remained unmet. The recovery was helped by a series of Acts of Parliament that absolved hospitals from taxes and attempted to divert to them money taken from estates confiscated in the war. But on the whole, the high ideals of the Puritan reformers, the victors in the war, made little difference to public medicine in England, and the Restoration extinguished their efforts.[16]

Towards the end of the seventeenth century, St Thomas's was rebuilt around a series of courtyards, which improved ventilation on the upper floors, but on the ground floor an arcade ran round the court, making the wards small and dark. Ventilation and light suffered further when the window tax was imposed in 1696 and every other window was bricked up.[9] By 1700, conditions in the hospital had improved somewhat. Typhus, enteric infection and scarlatina had been recognized as fevers, the value of fresh air was understood, and patients had a bed each. Water was now obtained from the river rather than tainted wells.[11] The hospital's written 'orders' for 1700, which had changed only gradually over the years, include the following points, which summarize the situation regarding hygiene at the time:

- No patient suffering from an infectious disease was to be admitted.
- Sisters had to clean their wards by 6 a.m., to keep their yards clean, and to not allow hens in the yards.
- Every tenth bed had to be left empty to air, and only one patient might be allocated to each bed.
- Old sheets had to be washed and given to surgeons for dressings.

On the Continent, in contrast to events in England, there was very little interruption in social and political life attributable to religious conflict, with the result that the evolution of hospitals progressed far more steadily. Leprosy persisted rather longer there than here, so that lazarettos were still in active use into the seventeenth century. In France, lazarettos were finally abolished by Louis XIV in 1662, their funds being devoted to general hospitals and to charity.[6] Also in France, in addition to the monk-controlled infirmaries, the Hôtel Dieu hospitals in Paris and other cities, e.g. Lyons, not only remained active, but expanded their work. Numerous great hospitals sprang up in Italian cities too, most notably those of the Knights Hospitallers of St John, who, having set up so many small, primitive hospitals throughout Europe in the Middle Ages, now began to build magnificent, specially designed establishments in a number of European countries. In Valetta, they founded a magnificent infirmary in 1540. Its huge main ward measured 185 × 35 feet (56 × 11 m) and had an arched roof 31 feet (9 m) high designed especially to mitigate as far as possible Malta's high summer temperatures, but incidentally allowing a large volume of air to each patient (Figure 2.2). The iron bedsteads had white coverlets and were surrounded by white curtains, and the whole was 'extremely neate, and kept cleane and sweete'. At first, for reasons of hygiene, food was served on silver plates instead of in the usual wooden vessels, but later silver was replaced by pewter.[17]

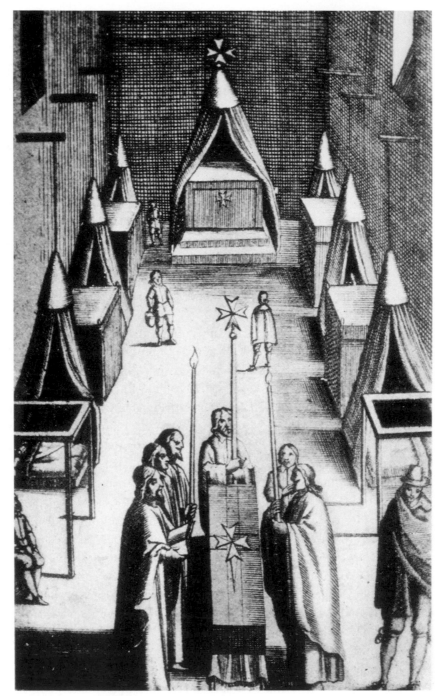

Figure 2.2   The great ward of the Hospital of the Knights of St John in Valetta as it appeared in the seventeenth century. (N.A. Nutting and L.L. Dock (1937). *A History of Nursing.* London: Putnam. Wellcome Library, London.)

In Italy, the design of hospitals was receiving great attention, as exemplified by the Ospedale Maggiore in Milan. Its plan had been prepared in 1456 and its cornerstone was laid soon after. It consisted of one large, square court on each side of an oblong central court in which stood the chapel. The square courts were each subdivided into four smaller courts, on to which the wards opened. The ceilings of the wards were 33 feet (10 m) high, and a real effort was made to sleep only one patient to a bed, an ideal that was exceeded only in times of crisis and if it was impossible to send contagious cases to other hospitals. Sanitary facilities were remarkable, for between every two beds there was a door leading to a privy in the thickness of the huge wall; under the privy corridor ran a sewer feeding into the canal next to which the hospital was built. Some aspects of this hospital were, however, less satisfactory. The basement beneath the wards was used for storage and services, the latter including the slaughtering and butchering of animals. The original burial arrangements for the hospital begger belief. The dead were laid out on gratings in the cellar of the chapel, just above the waterline of the canal, and simply allowed to rot. Not surprisingly, the resulting stench eventually drove the authorities to buy land for a burial ground away from the hospital.[9]

In Florence, four great hospitals had been founded in the fourteenth and fifteenth centuries, and by the sixteenth century, their prime concern was the acutely ill. In 1500, Santa Maria Nuova had both male and female wards, the former with 100 double beds with a full complement of bedclothes. In this ward between 1503 and 1512, the death rate was 10.5%, but between 1518 and 1522 it had fallen to 8.6%, the average length of stay being 11–15 days.[18,19] Little is known about the diseases from which the patients in this hospital suffered, but extraordinarily detailed records remain for San Paolo Hospital for a short period in the sixteenth century, which throw some light on the management of infectious disease.

Between October 1567 and September 1568, 364 patients were admitted to San Paolo Hospital, the diagnoses of 346 of which are stated in the surviving records.[20] Patients with diseases that could be considered potentially infectious include:

- 220 with 'fever', the type rarely being specified; the heaviest influx of these patients was in May, July and August;
- 46 with skin diseases, comprising 42 cases of scabies, two of smallpox, one of herpes and one of erysipelas; for scabies, April and May were the peak months;
- 14 with boils, ulcers and 'drainings';
- two with typhus;
- one with dysentery.

The hospital was furnished with large wooden beds, which were often shared – four specific instances of sharing are recorded, but sharing of beds was seldom due to overcrowding. Although these events were taking place over 20 years after Fracastoro published his great work in 1546 (see Chapter 1), no attempt seems to

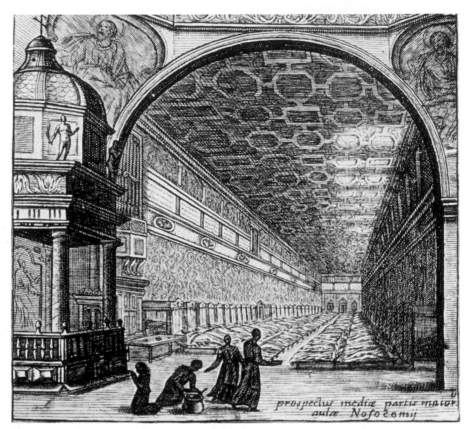

Figure 2.3   A ward in the Santo Spirito Hospital of Rome in the seventeenth century, showing a large, overcrowded ward. (A. Castiglione (1947). *History of Medicine*, (2 vol). New York: A. Kopf. Wellcome Library, London.)

have been made to isolate infectious diseases, but the existence of a small upstairs ward known as the 'fractured head room', where accident cases were often put, may have helped to control the incidence of erysipelas and gangrene in these patients. Only 3.5% of patients died in hospital, five of them of fever, and there is no mention in any of these very detailed records of any disease spreading within the hospital. Of the patients discharged, 20 were readmitted, 14 for reasons related to their original diagnosis. All those suffering from erysipelas or boils were discharged as cured.[20] It would seem that, despite the shared beds, other conditions in this hospital were excellent and certainly not obviously conducive to cross-infection.

However, such high standards were not universal by the seventeenth century. In Santo Spirito in Rome, although the large wards were very lofty, they had four rows of closely packed beds running their entire length, and in no hospital was any attempt made to limit the uses to which each ward was put (Figure 2.3). Contemporary pictures show operations being carried out in the middle of surgical wards, and the dead were sewn into their shrouds on the spot. However, in a few hospitals, notably the Hôtel Dieu in Paris, conditions were without doubt atrocious, and far worse than in the general run of such institutions.[21]

The exemplary conditions in the three large wards of the Hôtel Dieu in the thirteenth century were described in the previous chapter. In 1532, further expansion took place, a 100-bed ward being added for contagious cases, particularly plague victims. Expansion continued of the Ile de la Cité until no more room was available, when permission was given to throw a new bridge over the Seine; on this was built a two-storey ward for lying-in patients. Now that the hospital had access to the Left Bank, expansion proceeded apace. Large, four-storey wards were built, and as at first crowding was not a serious problem, it was possible to transfer most patients from the old wards to the new and to reserve the old buildings on the Ile as service areas. But by 1666, the situation had changed. One of the four-storey wards contained 110 *grands lits*, each holding from three to six patients lying head to foot across the bed, together with nine *petits lits* for single patients. As the wards had windows on only one side, there could be no through-ventilation. Conditions were similar in other wards and much worse in periods of pestilence,[9] despite the fact that the Hôpital St Louis, which had been built specifically to take infectious cases from the Hôtel Dieu, had been completed in 1612.

The horrors of the Hôtel Dieu were in no way attributable to any deliberate policy of neglect or to evil intent. On the contrary, the hospital's problems arose from blind adherence to the Christian principle that succour must be given to all who requested it, regardless of cost. The Hôtel Dieu refused to abandon this principle of universal charity, although other, similar institutions had long ago discarded it as unworkable, and it was this that led to the appalling conditions for which it was infamous.[9,21]

The emergence of gunpowder in the Middle Ages and larger numbers taking part in battles increased the number and severity of wounds. From 1515 to the end of the century, cruel civil, religious and foreign wars were associated with many casualties. Military surgeons have always been faced with major problems, and amputations were probably the commonest of the operations carried out. These were usually followed by infection and amputations particularly by hospital gangrene (hospitalism).

In the sixteenth century, gunshot wound infections were commonly treated with boiling oil to overcome 'their poisonous nature'. Ambrose Paré, a French military surgeon, described in 1536 his experiences on one night when the supply of boiling oil ran out.[22] He dressed the wounds with a 'digestive of egg yolks, oil of roses and turpentine'. After a sleepless night, he was surprised to find that the wounds healed with less pain and fever complications. Some of Paré's recipes were rather less impressive, for instance newborn puppy dogs boiled in oil of lilies, and mixed with earthworms prepared with oil from Venice. Paré wrote little on hospitals and

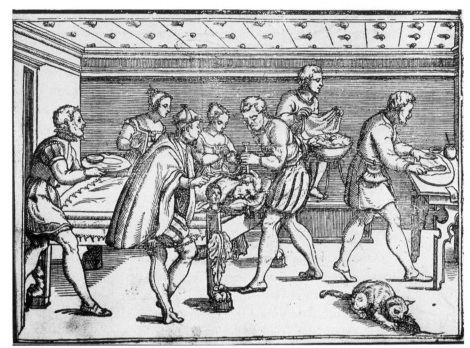

Figure 2.4   A surgeon operating with a trephine for a skull fracture in the sixteenth century. (Giovanni Andrea Della Croce (1583). *Cirugia universale a perfetta*. Venice: Ziletti. Wellcome Library, London.)

did not describe gangrene or other wound infections in his treatise, although they were obviously common. He does refer to an autopsy finding of metastatic abscesses in the lungs following wound infection, due to corruption of the blood. Paré also used immediate debridement (removal of dead or infected tissue) and ligature of blood vessels rather than cautery after amputation. At the battle at Metz in 1552, Paré thought the great mortality of the wounded was due to the severity of wounds from 'great strokes of cutlasses and arquebusses' and the extreme cold rather than poisoning with gunpowder in the air. In 1562 at the sieges of Bourges and Rouen, the mortality from 'gangrenous' wounds was very high and Paré accepted the common belief of the time that this was due to the poisonous air. He stated that 'such was the malignity of the air, and so putrid were all the wounds, that the surgeons could scarcely look upon the sores, or endure the smell; and if they neglected them for a single day, they found them full of worms'. Nevertheless, he believed in good nutrition and hygiene. For instance, he complained in one instance of rags used for dressing wounds being rewashed only once a day.

In addition to Paré, there were other conservative military surgeons in the sixteenth and seventeenth centuries. John Woodall was the first surgeon-general appointed to the East India Company in 1612. He wrote one of the first treatises on naval medicine, *The Surgeon's Mate*.[23] He also never used cautery when carrying out an amputation and suggested the use of ligatures of blood vessels. He apparently carried out large numbers of amputations with a relatively low infection rate.

Although miasmas were still considered to be the main route of infection of wounds, many surgeons, such as Theodoric and later Pringle, Lind and others, accepted that infection was contagious (see Chapters 3 and 4).

The eighteenth century: hospitals and infection

The cataclysmic religious and political events in sixteenth-century England had, as we have seen, destroyed the country's entire hospital system, with the exception of the two royal hospitals in London. As virtually none were built in the seventeenth century, England was effectively without hospitals for 100 years. When building did begin again in the eighteenth century, it took place all over the country on a huge scale. But, as the Church of England failed to replace its Roman Catholic predecessor in charitable provision for the sick, all the new foundations were voluntary hospitals, endowed and supported by the wealthier members of the local population for the benefit of their own citizenry. In London, as well as the two hospitals that survived the holocaust, five new voluntary hospitals were founded, while in the provinces, 28 hospitals opened their doors during the century. The first was Winchester, which reopened its original foundation in 1736, to be followed in 1737 by the Bristol Royal Infirmary; Newcastle Infirmary opened in 1751, Chester General Infirmary in 1755, Lincoln County Hospital in 1769, the Norfolk and Norwich Hospital in 1771, and others on to Sheffield Royal Infirmary in 1797. The story was similar for the five large Scottish cities.[1] Thus an accident of history meant that Britain had an unprecedented opportunity to set up a countrywide network of hospitals that would incorporate all the most modern ideas on the prevention of the spread of infections within them. Unfortunately, the opportunity was not always taken.[2]

Europe, on the contrary, was already well endowed with hospitals at the beginning of the eighteenth century, supported as we have seen from a variety of sources, and differing greatly in the quality of care offered: some were models of salubrity, while others killed nearly as many patients as they cured. Hospital building on the Continent was more often a matter of enlarging or adapting old foundations than of building anew. Nevertheless, considerable thought was often given to the incorporation of new ideas when additions were undertaken.

British hospitals

Advances in hospital hygiene in eighteenth-century Britain were nearly all pioneered in the armed forces, most particularly by John Pringle in the army and James Lind in the navy, but these advances took a long time to filter through to the civilian hospitals. As this chapter is concerned mainly with the latter, the work of Pringle and Lind will be discussed later (see Chapter 4).

Standards of hygiene and ventilation among the general population at the time were not high. Among the urban poor in towns, overcrowding and filth were rife and would have been taken as the normal state of affairs by all. Even well-to-do homes were seldom furnished with privies, and standards of personal cleanliness were low. Consequently, although the newly built hospitals would have started clean and freshly painted, hygiene would not necessarily have been considered a top priority. Indeed, it would not have been surprising if little attention was paid to it, as age and overcrowding caused the gradual deterioration of the buildings.[1] Buildings constructed early in the century often had no clean water supply or means of drainage, and the majority, like private houses, had neither toilet facilities nor ablutions until near the end of the century. When these were first installed, they were mainly curtained off from the wards, but this proved so unsatisfactory that better arrangements had to be made eventually. Even at the end of the century, new hospitals were still being built with windows only at the narrow ends of the long wards, and the wards themselves might be divided in half longitudinally, allowing them to accommodate four rows of beds. Again, it was not until the end of the century that bug-ridden wooden bedsteads were replaced entirely by iron ones in which the insects could find no refuge. This delay was despite the fact that Pringle's first publication on hygiene in military hospitals had appeared in 1750.[3,4]

Pringle was taken seriously by one far-sighted physician in Dublin. In 1768, Edward Foster published a small book with the lengthy title, *An Essay on Hospitals, or, Succinct Directions for the Situation, Construction and Administration of Country Hospitals.*[5] In it, he laid down that:

Hospitals ought to be single houses with numerous windows to each side, opposite to each other; by which means a renovation of fresh air is in our power, at any time, in a manner much preferable to any ventilators, whereas, were the houses double, from the necessary partitions running along their middles, or were the windows to be placed all in one of their sides, this circulation could not be procured, and the imperfect aid of ventilators must become necessary.

He continued with further admirable instructions. Rooms, windows and doors must be lofty and, despite his aversion to ventilators, he advocated one or two chimneys in every ward, as much for purposes of ventilation as for the warmth of

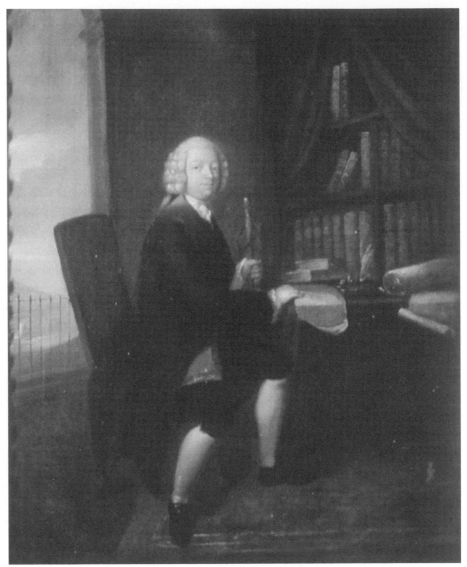

Figure 3.1   Sir John Pringle (1707–82). (Oil painting, Wellcome Trust Museum.)

the fire. The ground floor of the building, he said, would usually be damp, and should therefore be used for domestic and administrative purposes only. Wards could hold up to 20 beds, but five of them must be in single cubicles, as much to isolate infectious patients as to give privacy to those who were critically ill. He laid great emphasis on the cleanliness of bedding and clothing, and on the training of nurses who, 'above all things … ought to pay the most strict and attentive observance to the cleanliness and regularity of their patients, as on these depends a very great part of the cure'. In only one aspect of Foster's *Directions* did he unwittingly court disaster. The operation room, which should be on the top floor so that it could be lit by a skylight, could, he suggested, double as a chapel; and the dead-house could, for convenience, be located next door to it. The reason given for keeping the dead-house away from the patients was to save their feelings!

In England, there were hints that it was not always the conservative outlook of the medical profession that prevented advances in hospital design. John Aikin of Manchester, friend and collaborator of John Howard, wrote in 1771 of the conflict between architect and physician, the former insisting on squeezing the greatest possible number of beds into the smallest possible space, while the latter demanded all the space that could be procured.[1,6] The architect, Aikin noted, always won, with the result that:

as far as diet, nursing and medical assistance are concerned, they are of eminent use and comfort to the poor; but the grand necessity of life, air, is never to be had in salutary degrees of purity, and frequently is vitiated so as to become a poison. Every hospital, I fear, without exception, may in some measure be considered as a lazaretto, having its own peculiar disease within it.

This 'peculiar disease' referred to 'hospital fever' (typhus) and 'hospitalism' (gangrene and wound infection). Aikin stated that his main purpose in writing was to warn against overcrowded hospitals at all costs. Even when there were insufficient beds to accommodate all the sick, it was preferable to refuse some patients admission rather than to overcrowd the hospital. He opposed large wards and advocated as the ideal small rooms opening on to airy galleries.[6]

Despite Aikin's strictures and all the faults of the hospital system, there were remarkably few accounts of outbreaks of infection in the annual reports of the institutions over this period, especially in country hospitals. Blizzard, in 1779, did support Aikin in stating unambiguously that 'animal effluvia produce contagion', remarking particularly on the evil effect of such effluvia on compound fractures and fractured skulls. But country hospitals on the whole appear to have had a good record; the faults seem mainly to have arisen in city hospitals serving large populations of poor and overcrowded slum dwellers.[1]

Most early hospitals were purpose built, but a few were not, and problems could arise. The Bristol Royal Infirmary, for instance, on its foundation in 1737 was housed in a converted brewery on a cramped city site and had only 34 beds. Despite the lack of space, wings were added in 1740 and 1750, converting it to an H-shape and increasing its complement of beds to 132. By 1774, outbreaks of 'hospital fever' had begun to take their toll and complete rebuilding was necessary.[7] The story of Leeds General Infirmary, although also a city hospital, was very different. It did not open until 1770, much later than the Bristol Royal Infirmary, but it was purpose built on a good site, and members of the medical staff served on its Building Committee throughout the planning stages.[7] The Norfolk and Norwich Hospital (1771) was another highly successful, purpose-built hospital. Its H-shape allowed through-ventilation, its wards were 15 feet (4.6 m) high with plenty of space between the beds, and its large sash windows on both long sides of the wards were opened daily. The wards were washed down every week, although in 1788 the matron was given permission to defer this for one week if the weather was damp or wet. That the hospital board was aware of the danger of cross-infection is shown by its decree that patients with head lice must be shaved before admission.[8] When John Howard, the philanthropic Quaker and prison reformer, visited Norwich towards the end of the century, he was well pleased with its hospital.[9]

Manchester Royal Infirmary was opened in 1752 and developed improved standards of cleanliness under the influence of John Aiken,[6] although conditions were not ideal. In 1771, orders were given that 'every patient has clean sheets on their first admission, that clean sheets are supplied at least once every three weeks and that two patients be not suffered in the same bed except that there is no spare bed in the house'. Despite these limited measures, in 1788 many patients were discharged with slight fever and the medical officers recommended:

Proper openings for the admission of air were needed.
Ceilings should be raised.
Iron beds should replace wooden ones.
Floors should be washed with soap and water and no sand should be allowed to remain on them.
Five more nurses should be engaged.

All of this points to a probable outbreak of hospital gangrene, due to overcrowding, deficient ventilation, and perhaps choked drainage.

Most new hospitals, like those described above, were built on an H-plan so as to allow good ventilation, but some larger ones, such as St Bartholomew's in London (reconstructed in 1729), consisted of four large ward blocks surrounding a central courtyard. The Royal Naval Hospital at Plymouth was unique and much admired by hospital planners in France, in consisting of separate pavilions arranged around a huge courtyard, so allowing maximum circulation of fresh air.[10] In fact, the object of all the designs was good circulation of air in conformity with the then current miasmatic theory of infection, and Howard, in his 1789 report on hospitals, was on the whole satisfied with what he saw.[7] The successful practices that had been pioneered by Pringle and Lind nearly 50 years earlier had at last filtered through to civilian hospitals. By the end of the century, however, the rapidly growing urban population was making ever greater demands on the limited hospital space. More beds were being packed into the existing wards until there were sometimes four rows in long wards designed for only two. The overcrowding led to poor hygiene, and standards of ventilation inevitably fell, until finally, despite the fact that known

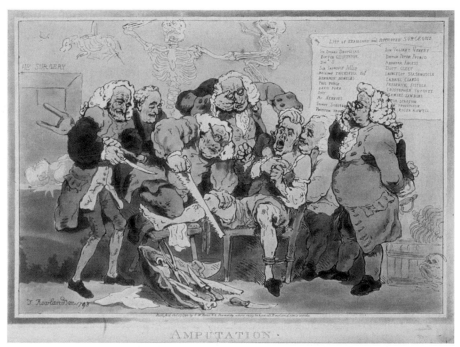

Figure 3.2   Five surgeons participating in the amputation of a man's lower leg in the eighteenth century. (Aquatint by T. Rowlandson, 1793.) (Wellcome Library, London.)

fever cases were deliberately excluded by most management, infections of all sorts again became rife.[3]

Newcastle Infirmary is a case in point. It had been built in 1751, but conditions were beginning to deteriorate by 1774; by the end of the century, all the wards contained 20 or more beds, and small rooms that should have been used for isolation purposes had all been taken over as storerooms. The crowded wards led to a foul atmosphere, and the death rate was one in 16. Gangrene was a major problem, with nine out of 59 fracture cases and five out of six skull fractures proving fatal. In 1774, Dr John Clark, Medical Director of Newcastle Infirmary, started a determined campaign to persuade his Court to take matters in hand.[11] The Court was deaf to his pleas, but he showered members relentlessly with facts and figures from other, more successful institutions until rebuilding was finally authorized in 1801. Over that period, Clark had carried on a vast correspondence with experts on hospital infections, including both Lind and Howard, and had read and quoted from their works and submitted a code to his Court listing the improvements that should be made. Comparing Newcastle Infirmary with the Royal Hospital at Woolwich, Clark noted that the latter was thoroughly and carefully ventilated, and that although it accepted patients with infectious diseases, each disease type was segregated and surgical patients were kept apart from all others. The result was that fevers never spread within the hospital and surgery had a high success rate: in 4 years, only one fracture patient out of 27, and two amputees out of 22, had died, with the overall death rate, at one in 35, being half that at Newcastle. In Northampton Infirmary, a newly built institution, every patient undergoing a major operation was put into a small ward with only one other occupant, and that a convalescent, resulting again in a low overall death rate of one in 31. Clark noted especially that there was only one death among eight patients with skull fractures. He also commended Glasgow. There, cross-infection had been prevented by reserving the small rooms off the main wards for infectious diseases, and surgical death rates were similar to those in Woolwich and Northampton. There was 'unremitting cleanliness', the wards being examined daily, and weekly reports being made to the hospital committee. No wonder Clark wrote to the court in 1801:

> Having frequently observed many of my patients, whose cases would probably have admitted of a speedy cure in a quiet and pure ward, became suddenly worse when placed in crowded apartments, especially among patients labouring under violent contusions, malignant ulcers, mortifications and gangrenes ... it was proposed that the medical and surgical patients should be separated from each other; that they should be arranged according to the similarity of their diseases; and that effectual measures should be adopted for securing the most successful elements of a hospital, viz. cleanliness and ventilation.

Clark then went on to propose that compound fractures, amputations and skull fractures should be used as yardsticks of a hospital's success, for they are 'a criterion for ascertaining the salubrity of the air, and the nature of the accommodation for the sick ... and that whenever mortality is great in these, in internal diseases it will be proportionately so'.

Edinburgh Infirmary, like Northampton, had adopted the practice of isolating fever patients in small rooms from the time it was built in 1738, the managers stipulating that each room should contain two beds and that the patient be moved from one to the other, the empty one being completely remade between occupancies.[10] But towards the end of the century, typhus outbreaks throughout the country had become so severe that whole wards, usually with separate access from the rest of the hospital, were being taken over as dedicated fever wards (see Chapter 4). However, the idea of building separate fever hospitals adjacent to the main buildings as a permanent measure, although often discussed, met with strong opposition, for despite the obvious success of fever wards, it was still considered that fevers were spread by poisonous particles dispersed in the air, so that the proximity of the main hospital to a fever hospital would be dangerous. For instance when, in 1780, the Board of the Norfolk and Norwich Hospital proposed the erection of an isolation hospital 'at the extremity of the hospital grounds', the medical staff objected because of its danger, and the plan was shelved. Some years later, it was a more enlightened physician, another Dr Clark, who fought a long battle with his Court before it finally agreed to build a fever house along with the new hospital. He was forced to give example after example of the success of fever wards before the members of the Court would accept that 'hospital fever' was contagious, not airborne, and allow the fever house to be built. In fact, the first fever hospital was opened in Waterford, Ireland in 1799 to cope with the terrible epidemics of typhus that had been devastating that country for years. The story of the fever hospitals is told in Chapter 4.

European hospitals

Many medieval hospitals were still in use on the Continent at the beginning of the eighteenth century. In Vienna, for instance, Howard described, as late as 1789, a number of convent hospitals each consisting of the original, characteristic, large single ward with its lofty roof. He reported that the sisters who ran these hospitals were devoted nurses who tended their patients well and kept them very clean, his only criticism being that the wards were usually insufficiently ventilated.[9]

The original high standards of some of the old hospitals had, however, been allowed to fall dramatically. The model hospital for men, built by the Knights of St John in Valetta in 1550, could hardly have been recognizable to Howard if he had read the original description of it before his visit. It took up to 530 patients, and its only redeeming features seem to have been that each patient had their own bed, and that of the three wards, one was reserved for the very sick, one was for middle-class patients and had two rows of beds, and one was for the poor and had beds in four rows. The stench was so overpowering that the beds had to be perfumed, and the doctors held perfumed handkerchiefs to their noses while on their rounds. Even the 'dark and damp arched cellar' had been pressed into service as a ward for skin patients and pensioners. The kitchens adjoined this cellar and were 'even darker and more offensive'. In the courtyard, there was a bowl for a fountain, but there was no running water either there or in the hospital. There was a staff of 22 to serve the whole hospital, many of the staff being convicts on the run. Howard contrasted all of this with the facilities that he found in the adjacent Grand Master's stables, where 52 horses were attended by 40 servants and there were two functioning fountains in the courtyard. His comment, 'the hospital fever [typhus] (the inevitable consequence of closeness, uncleanliness and dirt) prevails here' is hardly surprising. Of the women's hospital, he wrote: 'a more offensive and dirty hospital for women I never visited'.[9]

In Paris at the beginning of the eighteenth century, there were many old, established hospitals with very different reputations. The Charité, for instance, had spacious, uncrowded wards with only one patient per bed; it was very clean and care of the patients was excellent.[10, 12] At the opposite extreme stood the Hôtel Dieu, where conditions had continued to deteriorate even below those prevailing in the previous century, and which was now vilified throughout Europe as a charnel house for the sick poor. Both Tenon[13] and Howard[9] reported vividly on its horrors, and visiting Frenchmen and foreigners alike published dreadful descriptions of their visits. There was little more space available than there had been in 1660, and apart from the inbuilt lack of ventilation, overcrowding was still the greatest evil. One visitor reported that there were 1219 large and small beds in the hospital, crammed in wherever space could be found, and in these beds lay up to 3500 patients at any one time; each *grand lit* held up to six adults or eight children. Little attempt was made to separate infectious from non-infectious diseases, or the dying and dead from the living. The inevitable result was that scabies and vermin were universal, and no attempt was made to treat either. In fact, treatment would have been wasted effort for the bedding was seldom changed and new patients were put straight into the beds just vacated by the previous patients. The only major infectious disease for which any attempt at isolation was made was smallpox; typhus, tuberculosis and dysentery patients were mixed indiscriminately with each other, and with all the other patients. Filthy feather beds were beaten occasionally, and straw from the palliasses of incontinent patients was piled in the middle of the ward until it was collected for burning. The River Seine provided both water supply and drainage.

Patients in the surgical wards usually had the luxury of sleeping only three to a bed, but even so the mortality was hideous. Operations took place in the middle of the ward, as in medieval times. Postmortems were carried out in a separate room, but it was very close to the surgical wards. Inevitably, wound infections and gangrene were rife and even moderately serious operations proved fatal, while patients almost never survived the more difficult ones such as trepanning (removing a piece of the skull). Conditions in the maternity wards were equally terrifying. Three or four patients in all stages of childbirth, both before and after delivery, were placed in the same bed, together with their infants if they had arrived, so interchange of infections was assured and babies were often smothered by their sleeping mothers. The average length of stay in hospital of a maternity patient was 35 days, mostly spent in recovering from hospital infections. Caesarean births were, of course, particularly hazardous: out of 3445 carried out since 1500, only 79 mothers had survived. At the time that Tenon visited the hospital, an epidemic of puerperal fever had been raging for 12 years.[13]

It is not possible to give accurate mortality rates for the Hôtel Dieu as admissions were recorded only for the first day of each month and the official registers of deaths are untrustworthy. At the time when the official rate was given as 13%, Tenon estimated from his own notes that it was nearer 22%, a figure that was confirmed during the French Revolution by the Comité de Mendicité, which put it at 20%, much higher than the other Parisian hospitals. In fact, an anonymous investigator wrote in 1787 that in 52 years the Hôtel Dieu had taken in 1 000 741 patients, of whom 254 523 (25%) had died. If these patients, he calculated, had been sent to the Charité instead, 99 000 (39%) would have been saved.

Attempts to reform the Hôtel Dieu had been made as early as 1757, when the Maître Ordinaire of the Chambres des Comptes de Paris pointed out the appalling conditions and put forward ideas for their improvement. Even the disastrous fire of 1772, in which many patients lost their lives, failed to jolt the authorities into action. Plans were put forward to move the hospital, to split it up, to build ever more magnificent edifices with little attention to the use for which they were intended. But the King (Louis XV), the religious orders and Parlement de Paris could not agree, and eventually the new hospital was rebuilt in the burnt-out shell of the old, conditions in it remaining much the same as before. In 1777, these had become so bad that the new King, Louis XVI, set up a Royal Commission to investigate, but still nothing was done.

Until this time, the agitation for better hospital facilities for Paris in general, and at the Hôtel Dieu in particular, had been led by architects and philanthropists, but now the scientists and physicians began to take a hand. Tenon had already started work on his major investigation, the results of which he would publish in 1788, and Dulaurans, a military physician, published an essay in 1787 based on his own observations. He discussed the whole hospital problem – their location, size, ventilation, administration, medical and nursing staff, inspections, and even a plan for improved clinical records. Eventually, the activity of the reform movement forced Louis XVI into action, and he asked the Academy of Sciences to appoint a committee to examine the situation and make recommendations. The distinguished group did not complete its work unimpeded. It needed to obtain an overall picture of hospital facilities in Paris, and to this end it visited four other major hospitals in the city, examined them in all their aspects, and approved them. But when it came to seek entry to the Hôtel Dieu, having obtained permission from the Archbishop of Paris and the First President of the Council, the management, presumably fearing the worst, refused it entry. It was Tenon who came to the rescue, supplying the committee with the facts and figures he had collected over the years. Not surprisingly, the committee came to the conclusion, when it reported in 1786, that the Hôtel Dieu was dangerous to patients and that it provided insufficient accommodation for the needs of the city. It recommended that three existing hospitals should be enlarged, a new one be built, and the Hôtel Dieu be kept exclusively for accidents and emergencies.

After some delay, Louis XVI accepted the Rapport and 1 200 000 *livres* were raised for the building works by means of subscriptions and a lottery. However, the government used most of the money for other purposes, and the only tangible result of the committee's deliberations was the enlargement of one of the three hospitals that it had selected for action. At the Hôtel Dieu in 1787, 2500 single beds and 500 double beds were provided to replace the *grands lits*, and the maternity wards were transferred from the second to the third floor, although this was of doubtful benefit as the mothers were now in the ward next to the smallpox patients. It was not until after the 1789 revolution and the overthrow of the monarchy that real reform of the French hospital system, and in particular the Hôtel Dieu, took place.[14]

In addition to the continued use of old hospitals, new ones were being founded all over Europe, of which two will serve as examples here: one a disastrous new building and the other a brilliant adaptation of an old building. One of the first hospitals to be planned specifically for curable patients was the Fredericks Hospital in Copenhagen, built in 1758. It was planned around an open square with two additional service blocks on either side, blocks that also contained the private rooms for paying patients. Unfortunately, the hospital was built on filled land over sea water, and to save money, the single-storey wards had no basements. They already stank when the hospital opened, as did the privies, which the workmen had been using for 3 years. The floors were laid and relaid and the privies built and rebuilt to every new design the experts could produce, but still the stink remained. Clean water was, of course, not to be found locally, and the town water supply, brought into the city through pipes of hollowed-out fir-tree trunks, contained an interesting variety of wildlife from mosquito larvae to eels, and smelled of rotten fish, as a consequence of which patients were allowed to drink only tea, beer or ale. Medical and surgical patients were segregated, but the internal planning of the hospital was not entirely satisfactory, as the mortuary and dissecting room were across the corridor from one of the wards.[10]

The Vienna General Hospital (the Allgemeines Krankenhaus), although founded 25 years later, instead of being built anew was housed in a huge and architecturally magnificent seventeenth-century building arranged around several squares and planned as an almshouse for soldiers and the poor. Despite the age of the edifice he had chosen, it was the avowed intention of the Emperor Joseph II, in 1784, to found a completely modern and scientific hospital, but by using the almshouse, he missed the opportunity of dividing it into small, specialized wards and so easing the sanitary problems that had led to the horrors of the Hôtel Dieu. The new hospital was to house 2000 patients. So that the wards could have windows on both sides, the existing corridors were eliminated, the windows being high enough to allow cross-ventilation above the patients' heads. There were also numerous ventilators, even including some under the patients' beds. Beds were at least 3 feet (1 m) apart and had no curtains, and the rule of one patient to each bed was strictly adhered to. The night stools in niches in the walls were designed most carefully to prevent the escape of smells. Normally, there were about 20 beds to a ward, but in some wards there were 40 or even 50, and the design of the old building meant that some wards could be entered only by passing through others. Risks of cross-infection were reduced greatly by grouping patients according to their disease and by separating convalescents from all others.[10]

By the end of the century, there was a great deal of discussion, both in England and on the Continent, about the design of hospitals. Although theories of infection were still based on miasmas, and the idea of contagion was by no means accepted universally, there was widespread recognition that good hygiene, ventilation and space were prerequisites for the health of both patients and staff. It was the widely publicized horror stories of conditions in the Hôtel Dieu that spurred on other authorities to take preventive action in their own domains. It was also realized that the sheer size of the Hôtel Dieu magnified the scale of any outbreaks that did occur. Indeed, Joseph II was fully aware, when setting up his new Allgemeines Krankenhaus, that he was flouting all modern ideas by adapting the huge old almshouses, and he took what steps he could to counteract the problems of size.[10]

In 1788, 4 years after the Allgemeines Krankenhaus was opened, an extraordinary exchange of views, in pamphlet form, took place between two hospital planners in Mainz about the relative merits of small, ten-bed wards as against single rooms, an exchange that clearly demonstrates the conflicts within infection theory at the time.

Dr Hoffman, the Elector's private physician, championed single rooms, while Dr Strack, a university authority on hospital science, strongly recommended ten-bed wards. The argument ranged over many aspects of the problem and by the end became farcical, to say the least; however, on the subject of infection it was serious. Strack admitted that the possibility of infection was the chief objection to his wards, and he defined it as occurring 'when a totally unknown substance emitted from a sick body enters into a healthy body and there causes the same disease'. Hoffman countered with a clear description of contagion – that 'infectious material' of a certain disease could infect a body and 'bring forth the same disease.' Strack replied that although this was true, direct contact was not needed for all diseases; that some have a general cause that can affect several bodies simultaneously. Also, diseases infectious in some circumstances are not so in others; for instance, observation had taught him that typhus was far more infectious amongst the poor, and that some diseases, for instance smallpox, scabies and some forms of dysentery, would remain infectious despite all precautions. Patients with these conditions he would transfer to special, spacious wards, but he considered that most ordinary infections could be driven out by proper ventilation. Hoffman contradicted him flatly on this matter, pointing out that typhus and dysentery continued to spread in army hospitals despite their excellent ventilation. When Strack then remarked that Hoffman himself had written that smallpox could be spread on any object and that even private rooms were no safeguard, Hoffman had to agree that such rooms would not prevent infection, but emphasized that they would lessen it. It is clear from this polemic that although there was as yet no general agreement on the process of infectivity, it was recognized that there was more than one way in which an infection could be spread, that the route by which a given disease proliferated was constant and specific to that disease, and that, in consequence, precautionary measures would vary from disease to disease.[10]

Johann Peter Frank was one of the foremost authorities on hospitals and hospital infection at the time and became director of the Allgemeines Krankenhaus from 1795 to 1804. Although he recognized the hazards of hospital infection and the importance of fresh air, he was still unable to keep the hospital free of putrid and nerve fever (typhoid), and his own son died from an infectious fever.[15]

The eighteenth and nineteenth centuries: typhus in military and civilian hospitals

The worst depredations of typhus had been conquered many years before the discovery of its vector, the body louse, *Pediculus humanus*, in 1909. Over the centuries, attempts to control the disease had, of course, been based on the then current theory of infection, notably on the idea of a miasma in which the poisonous particles causing the disease were dispersed. It was only as this theory was gradually adapted and finally found wanting by the detailed observations and epidemiological studies of men like James Pringle and John Lind that typhus was finally defeated.

Its causal organism, *Rickettsia prowazeki* (see Chapters 7 and 9), not only produces disease, sometimes fatal, in man, but is also inevitably fatal to its vector 11–12 days after the insect becomes infected. It is, therefore, a prerequisite to the onset of a human epidemic that the infected louse should be able to reach a new host in this comparatively short period of time; overcrowded conditions are ideal for the purpose. In addition, the louse must be able to feed and multiply unmolested, and to find temporary refuge should it be unable to transfer directly to a new host. Unwashed bodies, filthy clothing and communal bedding offer such conditions. To overcrowding and filth must be added poverty, together with the ignorance or callousness of authority that allows such conditions to exist, and famine, which lowers natural resistance to disease, and we have a picture of the environments in which typhus flourishes. In the past, such conditions were especially likely to occur in army camps, ships, prisons and hospitals, as well as among the poor in famine-stricken lands.

The first description of an epidemic that is recognizable as typhus is probably that at the Monastery of La Cava, near Salerno, in 1038. The next undoubted outbreak occurred during the siege of Granada in 1489–90, when six times as many of Ferdinand and Isabella's troops died of typhus as were killed in the battle.[1] The disease ravaged Italy in the sixteenth century and was described accurately by Fracastoro in 1546. Typhus also entered Europe through Turkey, where it was rife in the sixteenth century and from whence the Turkish conquerors brought it to Hungary, so that by the seventeenth century the infection was endemic in most of Europe. In the first half of the Thirty Years War, from 1618 to 1630, the armies of both sides were decimated by typhus and battles; marches then spread typhus through Alsace to Bohemia, South Germany and France.[2]

In England, typhus caused a huge mortality among overcrowded, filthy and half-starved prisoners in our jails, from which one of its names, jail fever, arose. Further, when the prisoners were brought to trial, the disease-bearing insects, being no respecters of persons, were wont to move on to pastures new in the court officials and judges. A number of outbreaks at such 'Black Assizes' are recorded:[1] perhaps the best known is that at Oxford in 1577, but one also occurred at Exeter in 1730, and the last occurred at the Old Bailey in 1750.[3]

In Ireland, typhus was so persistent and devastating that it became known in some circles as the Irish ague. A severe outbreak followed a famine in 1740, but the worst onslaught was associated with the great potato famine of 1846, when there were over 1 000 000 cases, 40 000 of them in Dublin alone.[4] On the American continent, Cortés probably bought typhus to South America in the sixteenth century; in North America, it never became a scourge, playing little part even in the Civil War.

It was not until about 1670 that it began to be recognized that all the different forms of 'fever' then known were in fact different diseases, not different manifestations of the same disease; that measles, for instance, could not transmute into smallpox (see Chapter 7). Conversely, all the fevers, including typhus, were still known by a bewildering variety of names based on some characteristic of the particular outbreak: hence 'jail fever', 'camp fever' and 'hospital fever', all typhus, were considered to be distinct diseases, as were 'pestilential', 'spotted', 'petechial', 'putrid' and 'malignant' fevers. Murchison, in his *A Treatise on the Continued Fevers of Great Britain*,[3] (which included typhus, relapsing and enteric fevers, and 'febricula') devoted two closely printed pages to names that had been used for typhus in the past in various European countries. In view of this massive confusion, it is not to be wondered at that there were numerous contradictory theories about the origin and spread of typhus, and that it was long before reasoned steps would be taken to contain it.

Typhus and the military in the eighteenth century

Despite the devastation wrought by epidemics of typhus among civilians in the first half of the eighteenth century, it was in the armies of Europe, in almost continuous conflict over wide areas of the Continent, that its attack was most concentrated, and also where the first steps were taken to study its behaviour and so to control its relentless spread. It was the work of John Pringle (1707–82), a British army surgeon, that at last began to show the way towards the prevention of the worst depredations of typhus in military hospitals.[5,6,7]

The War of the Austrian Succession began in 1740 and raged through central and western Europe for 8 years, spreading disease and terror wherever the armies trod. England was drawn into the struggle, fighting in Germany in 1743, and Pringle's account of events makes horrifying reading. After the Battle of Dettingen, which took place in June, the nearby village of Feckenheim was used as a hospital both for the wounded and for 1500 sick men from the line, most of whom were suffering from dysentery and fever. They were billeted in the homes of villagers, in barns and in any other buildings that could be commandeered. Brocklesbury, in 1764, described a typical cottage, too small for a family of eight, which was used to house up to 80 sick soldiers 'lying heel to head, so closely confined together within their own stinking cloaths, foul linen, etc. that it was enough to suffocate the patients, as well as others, who were obliged to approach them'.[8]

'The conditions', he wrote, converted the 'simplest inflammatory fever' into a 'most dangerous putrid, or jail fever'. The inevitable result of such conditions was that most of the villagers, as well as the medical and auxiliary staff, went down with dysentery, typhus or both, with a terrible mortality among both soldiers and villagers. However, as far as the army was concerned, typhus was confined to the village and those billeted there; the men with dysentery who had remained in the camps did not contract the second disease.

At Feckenheim, however, the situation had become much worse by the end of October. Pringle reports that of '14 mates employed about the sick', five died and all the rest became seriously ill with hospital fever, while the village lost half its patients to the disease and the villagers were almost wiped out. The general hospital at Newied, to which the patients from Feckenheim and other village hospitals were transferred, was initially affected less badly by typhus, but although the Feckenheim patients themselves improved there, they infected those from elsewhere. Then, as the army moved on into Flanders during the winter and all the patients had to be transferred there by water, half died of hospital fever on the way in the filthy, overcrowded boats. Once in Flanders, hospital fever died away and the 'remittent fevers' again became dominant.

In 1745, while heavily engaged in the European war, England's attention was forcefully diverted to a new danger on her own doorstep, namely the rising of the Scots in the Forty-five Rebellion. Men had to be brought back from Europe to confront this, but Pringle's account of events shows that now he was able to use the knowledge he had gained in Europe to attempt to control typhus in the army hospitals for which he was responsible. In December 1745, a large number of sick soldiers were brought home from the European battlefield and had to be found quarters in which to recover before being sent to Scotland, for which purpose a workhouse at Litchfield was fitted up as a hospital. At this time, when it was almost universally held that epidemics were caused by miasmas, of which foul air was a manifestation, Pringle's comment – 'too many [patients] being admitted, the air was corrupted, and the common inflammatory fever changed into one of the jail kind, of which several died' – was entirely logical. His further observation that 'at all other places where the soldiers were taken ill, and where there was no common hospital, hospital – or jail fever was unknown', presages the action he was about to take further north.

Both in northern England and in Scotland, Pringle took great care to see that in both camp and hospital the men had well-ventilated, clean quarters, and that overcrowding was prevented; very little infection occurred. But at Inverness, in May 1746, a sudden influx of wounded meant that the jails had to be pressed into service as hospitals, and the small town became crowded and filthy with the army's presence. Pringle tackled the conditions in the hospital/jails energetically. He ensured that they were cleaned every day and that the wards received special attention; he separated the different diseases; and he relieved overcrowding by transferring some patients to ships anchored in the harbour. Unfortunately, his excellent arrangements were foiled by an unforeseeable event which, nevertheless, gave him the opportunity for a classic epidemiological study.

Some deserters who had been imprisoned on the Continent were shipped to England and jailed there. They were then sent to Inverness for trial, guarded by a contingent of troops, who quickly caught jail fever from their charges and introduced it into the town. It was this incident that enabled Pringle to write to a fellow physician, Richard Mead, in 1750, that the 'spotted hospital fever' was the same disease as 'jail', 'camp' and 'ship' fevers, and so to become the first person to understand this. Later, in the first edition of his *Observations on the Diseases of the Army*, in his account of the above incident, Pringle put the matter even more forthrightly: 'The symptoms of the jail-fever were in every point so like those of the hospital fever, that, as they were formerly only conjectured to be the same distemper, they were now proved to be.' The arrival of the deserters at Inverness proved disastrous, for from February 1746, after the defeat of the rising at the Battle of Culloden, until August, upwards of 2000 men, including the wounded, passed through the hospitals; nearly 300 of these men died, mostly of hospital fever.

Meanwhile, the European war was drawing to a close, but in the last months, although typhus continued to wreak havoc, dysentery appears to have been the worst killer both among the troops and in the villages where they were billeted. The British army was then in the Dutch Brabant, and when, in November 1747, the time came to ship them home, they were embarked at Willemstad, bound for the East Anglian ports. Unfortunately, bad weather kept the men crowded together below decks and contrary winds caused long delays, with the inevitable result that typhus broke out. The situation was worst on a ship bringing 400 patients from the general hospital at Oosterhout to Ipswich Hospital, most of whom had hospital fever on arrival. At first, the death rate was high, but good ventilation and the dispersal of patients by billeting them in the town reduced it rapidly. Pringle does not mention the fate of the citizens of Ipswich, on whom the soldiers were billeted.

In his letter to Dr Mead, which he wrote before he returned to civilian life and published in 1750 under the title *Observations on the Nature and Cure of Hospital and Jayl-fevers*, Pringle suggested that the disease could be prevented by enforcing certain regulations:[6]

First, to allow no prisoner, upon enlargement, to carry out his cloaths; which should be burnt, and supplied by others at the publick expense; secondly, to order, that the cloaths of malefactors, after execution, should also be burnt, but above all, that before prisoners are brought into court, they should be cleaned and put in cloaths to be kept for that purpose, and washed from time to time.

Pringle could hardly have improved on these instructions if he had propounded them in the twentieth century after the louse-borne nature of typhus was finally discovered.

The importance of Pringle's pioneering work on the prevention of hospital infections in general, and on the control of typhus in particular, cannot be overemphasized; it was, after all, he who had first enunciated the idea of hospitals as dangerous places for the sick to be in, and all his work was directed towards changing this. Nevertheless, he still considered ventilation to be the most essential means of preventing the spread of typhus, as is clear from his book on diseases of the army first published in 1752. In this book, he advocated placing patients in well-separated beds in large, airy rooms with open windows, as well as regularly fumigating the wards. As we know now, apart from the spacing of the beds, these precautions would have had little direct effect on the spread of typhus, although indirectly the changed attitude they must have generated in the staff would surely have led to something that was indeed essential – improved general cleanliness. Although Pringle considered air purification by improved ventilation to be of first importance, he recommended burning incense, wood or juniper berries, sulphur and gunpowder, or the use of 'steams' of vinegar as additional measures.[7]

Pringle is particularly recognized as the founder of disinfectant tests before germs were discovered, but he gave the credit for these tests to suggestions made by Francis Bacon. Pringle used a putrefied substance, such as beef or the yolk of an egg, as the contaminant. In one test, he dipped a thread into egg yolk already putrefied and transferred it to a phial containing half the yolk of a new-laid egg diluted with clean water. The other half of the fresh egg yolk was put into another phial with clean water only and was used as a control. The egg with the contaminated thread putrefied more quickly. Putrefaction was assessed by smell. Pringle used this test to measure substances that prevented putrefaction and developed a coefficient for assessing disinfectants. Sea salt was used as the control. He tested mainly salts but found that acids and alkalis were the most effective.[9,10]

It was Pringle's slightly younger contemporary, James Lind, who would realize that hygiene pre-empted ventilation as the most vital preventive measure.

James Lind and 'ship fever'

James Lind (1716–94), who was physician to the Haslar Naval Hospital near Portsmouth, is best known for his pioneering work on scurvy, but his *Essay on the Most Effectual Means of Preserving the Health of Seamen,* written in 1757, was a second landmark, with Pringle's work, in the history of the conquest of typhus.[11] It was Lind who first stated clearly that typhus does *not* appear to be spread through the air. For instance, he noticed that ventilators did not stop the spread of typhus in jails, although nowhere did he contradict Pringle's advocacy of uncrowded, well-aired conditions: he held that although fresh air in itself would not prevent the spread of typhus, it might 'abate its malignity'. He went on to state categorically that the disease was associated with dirt, giving as one example the huge incidence of typhus in convict ships as against its virtual absence from slavers. The filthy clothes and bedding in the crammed convict ships were the undoubted sources of the outbreaks there; but the slaves, although even more crowded than the convicts, were almost naked and were provided with no bedding, and among them typhus was virtually unknown. With hindsight, we can see that this is not the whole story: some of the convicts would have been infected with typhus-bearing lice when they boarded the ships, whereas the Africans would have been infection-free when they were herded aboard, so that they carried no inoculum to start an outbreak. However, it is highly unlikely that the crews of sailors were always free from 'ship fever' and that their infected lice never reached the unhappy slaves, so that it is probable that the appalling conditions in which the tragic cargo was kept at least saved its members from contracting typhus.

From such observations, Lind concluded that filthy clothes and bedding 'contain a more certain, a more concentrated, and contagious poison, than the newly emitted *effluvia* [his italics] or excretions from the sick'. In further evidence, he pointed out that at the Haslar hospital, the labourers, who carried the sick to the wards and bundled up and removed their infected clothes, repeatedly contracted typhus themselves, whereas the nurses, who attended washed patients in clean wards, were affected much less often. His instructions to sick-berth attendants on ships show the horrific conditions in which the seamen of the time lived: 'Filthiness being a chief source of infection', he wrote, 'patients must be kept clean. Their hands and feet should be washed with soap or vinegar', and 'when their linen becomes foul and stiff with sweating [and apparently only when it reaches this state!] it must be fumigated with brimstone, soaked in vinegar and washed'. The beds of jail fever patients were to be destroyed on the patient's recovery 'because they strongly retain and communicate the contagion'. It had become perfectly clear to Lind that miasmas and effluvia were unimportant in the spread of typhus: the disease was propagated, he considered, by materials that were capable of 'imbibing or retaining infection', a very reasonable conclusion one and a half centuries before the discovery of the true mode of propagation of the disease, but it was long before Lind's theory was universally accepted.

Like adherents to the miasma theory, Lind recommended fumigation both of the air and of fomites by the (largely ineffectual) methods then current, including that all wards should be regularly fumigated or smoked, and that clothes and bedding should be exposed to air. He suggested fumigation should be carried out with sulphur sprinkled on charcoal fires, but he also used wood smoke and burning gunpowder, and he particularly stressed the importance of protecting the medical and nursing staff against infection both on board ship and in hospital. This was to be done by the wearing of waxed linen outer clothing, as had been recommended to plague doctors in medieval times, by pushing rolls of lint soaked in camphorated spirits up the nostrils, and by mouthwashes, frequent spitting, and disinfection of the hands before and after touching the patients. Finally, a major concern was to minimize the risk of transferring infection from ship to shore and vice versa, to which end Lind ordered that hospitals should be warned if a ship intended to send infected seamen to them, and that ships should be very careful if they proposed to take on men straight from hospital.

He cited the terrible examples of Gibraltar and Mahon, where seamen landed for hospitalization had introduced the disease both to the garrisons and to the civilian populations. On re-embarking in Gibraltar, the seamen spread the disease to the entire fleet. Through his firm and logical policy, Lind succeeded in almost abolishing typhus from the navy. In the army, lessons taught by Pringle and Lind were well learned. Monro, writing in 1780 on the health of soldiers and the conduct of military hospitals, emphasized the absolute necessity of clean, well-aired wards with daily fumigation, the washing of each man and his clothes on arrival, the isolation of fever patients in separate wards, and the provision for them of frequent changes of linen.[12] Lind's instructions for the protection of medical staff were followed to the letter. A hospital ship docked at Sheerness in 1795 and received ill sailors from Russian ships. Smyth described the conditions: 'the sick of all description lay in cradles, promiscuously arranged, to the number of nearly 200 patients which about 150 were in different stages of a malignant fever, and extremely contagious, as appeared evident from its rapid progress and fatal effects amongst the attendants on the sick and the ship's company'. The fever was variously described later as 'putrid, petechial fever' or 'malignant fever'. Fuming was carried out twice daily with concentrated vitriolic acid and powdered nitric acid, mixed in teacups. The teacups were immersed in pots of hot sand and carried round the wards. This caused some 'coughing', but surprisingly no other ill effects! The patients' clothes and linen were exposed to the vapour, then dirty linen was removed, rinsed, dried and again exposed to the vapour. Cleanliness and ventilation were also attended to. Infected Russians continued to be brought in, and the effects of fuming were reported as excellent. The fever (probably typhus) was finally eradicated. It is likely that the good response was due more to the treatment of clothes and bedding and general cleaning than to room fumigation.[13,14]

Similar results with a variety of fumigants were reported for jail distemper, which Pringle had recognized as being probably the same disease as hospital fever.

Guyton-Morveau published his 'Treatise on the means of purifying infected air' in 1802 in France.[15] He described the successful prevention of an outbreak of 'hospital fever' by fumigation with mineral acids at the earlier date of 1773, and many other outbreaks. He probably originated the use of hydrochloric acid for fumigation and its subsequent use in England and elsewhere. He assumed that epidemic diseases were carried in the air and must be controlled by fumigation, which destroys odours of putrefaction.

Due to problems of rampant fever, especially among the wounded in military hospitals, instructions for maintaining cleanliness and purifying the air of wards were also produced by the French Council of Health in 1795.[16] These stated that 'cleanliness which is so essential in all circumstances of life . . . ought . . . to constitute the principal object of the attention of all hospital agents'. The directions were as follows:

On admission, hands and feet of patients to be washed in warm water.

Utensils to be washed frequently.

Foul linen to be hung out of doors until washed.

Blankets to be beaten from time to time, and fumigated with burning sulphur.

Woollen mattress stuffing to be beaten and carded every 6 months and straw and wool mattress covers washed in lye [a strong alkaline solution].

Wooden bath tubs to be painted and varnished.

Vinegar which it has been the practice to bestow uselessly on fumigations, should be mixed with water and employed in gargles or for sprinkling the floors of wards before they are swept.

Walls and ceilings to be whitewashed once a year and bedsteads, window frames, tables etc. to be washed in lime water or lye.

Number of beds per ward to be fixed and not exceeded. To be 2ft apart in high wards, but 2ft 6in apart in 9ft high wards. No beds in centre of ward.

Patients must not enter or leave wards containing contagious diseases.

Detailed instructions about position and mechanics of 'necessaries' were made: 'Their seats to be washed daily and this article of cleanliness should be made a very strict regulation of policy.'

Ventilation and means of achieving it were discussed in detail.

Although it is uncertain whether these instructions were followed, some are remarkably similar in general principle to instructions on cleanliness in the late twentieth century, bearing in mind that germs had not been identified and miasmas were considered responsible for spread of disease.[17]

Fumigation with these agents continued until the twentieth century, when they were replaced with formaldehyde gas (see Chapter 11).

In 1798, nearly 50 years after Pringle's first publication, the Regulations of the Army Medical Board codified the same instructions.

Typhus in civilian hospitals in the eighteenth and nineteenth centuries

Fever hospitals

On the Continent, typhus cases, like all other fever patients, were admitted freely into general hospitals, no attempt being made to segregate them from other patients. Some hospitals, such as the Hôtel Dieu in Paris, even mixed their typhus cases with others in beds sleeping up to eight people. In consequence, there were frequent outbreaks of 'hospital fever', as John Howard had cause to note in his journey around Europe inspecting hospitals and prisons, an account of which he published in 1789.[18] Despite the cleanliness of Avignon Hospital compared with the appalling conditions he had found at Lyons, he reported: 'the surgeon complained that the slow fever [typhus] was produced by the infectious air of the house'. It may be noted that in France, miasmas rather than dirt were still being blamed for the spread of typhus. Again, Howard compared the conditions in the hospital for men at Valetta, Malta, very unfavourably with those in the Grand Master's stables. The smell in the hospital has already been commented on, and 'the slow hospital fever (the inevitable consequence of closeness, uncleanliness and dirt) prevails here'. Howard's report is a terrible indictment of the deterioration that had taken place in the hospital since it was founded 250 years earlier (see Chapter 3). In 1808, typhus was prevalent even in the Hospice de la Maternité in Paris.[19]

Paris had had a hospital for infectious diseases, the Hôpital St Louis, from an early date (1612), but its existence did not, as we have seen in the case of the Hôtel Dieu, prevent the admission of fever patients to general hospitals as well, with the inevitable dire consequences. The disastrous fire at the Hôtel Dieu in 1772, which necessitated its almost total rebuilding, led to a reconsideration of hospital provision of all types in the city, an exercise to which Tenon, in 1788, made a major contribution through his book *Les Hôpitaux de Paris*.[19,20] In this book, Tenon argued the case for specialist hospitals, as well as for a general hospital for each section of the city. For infectious diseases, he considered that there should be two types of hospital: one, such as the Hôpital St Louis, would be for use in large outbreaks of a single disease when all the patients were suffering from the same affliction and there was no need to isolate patient from patient or ward from ward; the other would be for small outbreaks of different diseases, where each disease needed to be strictly isolated from the others, thus eliminating the risk to the patients of cross-infection. The Hôpital St Louis, which had recently been used for non-infectious diseases, must, he argued, be kept open as a fever hospital in addition to any new hospitals that might be built for the purpose.

In British civil hospitals, almost all of which excluded fever patients, leaving them to die either in their own homes or in overcrowded workhouses, it was some time before the lessons learned in military and naval hospitals began to be applied. The miasma theory was so persistent and ingrained that there was considerable hesitation in accepting Lind's demonstration that, in the case of typhus at least, the disease could be spread not through the air but only by close contact with the foul clothing, bedding or bodies of infected people. But slowly and tentatively, patients began to be admitted, first to designated fever wards either adjacent to or even within general hospitals, and later to specially built fever hospitals. The fever, or isolation, hospital movement in England owes its origin to the typhus epidemics of the late eighteenth century.

Chester was probably the first town to build dedicated fever wards for its hospital. Dr John Haygarth[18,21] was so alarmed by the outbreak of typhus in the city in 1784 that in order not only to save the lives of existing victims but also to prevent the spread of infection by removing them from their crowded homes, he had two wards on the top floor of the hospital fitted up as fever wards. They could be entered without passing through any other part of the building, and very strict rules about access were applied to both staff and patients. 'No fever patients, nor their nurses, are suffered to go into other parts of the house. No other patient is allowed to visit the fever wards; nor any stranger unless accompanied by the apothecary or his assistant.'[22] Later, Haygarth had new wards built 13 yards (12 m) from the main hospital. When the next typhus outbreak occurred 10 years on, it was effectively suppressed, and Haygarth was able to state that in 12 years the disease never spread from the hospital.

The usual practice in Manchester Infirmary when there was an outbreak of hospital fever was to dismiss the affected patients back into the community. However, when an outbreak started in 1795, the infirmary changed its usual practice and transferred the victims to special wards set aside for the purpose. The outbreak was contained. Three years later, the disease broke out in the city's cotton mills, whose operatives lived in disgusting conditions in cellars and common lodging houses. The situation became so serious that the Board of Health was forced to set up a fever hospital, or House of Recovery as it was called, so as not to frighten away prospective patients. Like the Chester fever wards, the hospital was dedicated to preventing the spread of typhus as well as to saving the lives of those already affected. The building itself was clean and airy, with iron bedsteads, straw mattresses that were changed frequently, and no curtains. The heads of local families were given instructions for the prevention of infection in the home, and rewarded for keeping to the rules. The mere existence of the House of Recovery encouraged the mill owners to improve conditions in their factories and to attend to their workers' health.

In Liverpool, events at first followed a similar course. An outbreak of typhus occurred in the infirmary in 1787 following a breakdown in discipline and a failure to attend to ventilation and cleanliness. Two wards in the hospital were promptly fitted up as fever wards, the fever patients were transferred to them, and the outbreak was contained. But then, contrary to the infirmary's rules, fever patients began to be admitted to these wards from outside the hospital, and still the disease remained confined there. It was not unusual for typhus to break out in the city's 1200-bed workhouse, but in 1793 the onslaught was more serious than usual and it was impossible to find room for so many patients in the infirmary's fever wards, so two wards were set aside for typhus patients in the workhouse itself. This proved so successful that the infirmary was able to cease altogether from admitting patients from the town and port and to send them to the workhouse fever wards instead. So Liverpool had no House of Recovery until 1806, but when one was finally built it was supported entirely by the rates, rather than by patronage as were the earlier institutions. Other cities had followed Manchester's example earlier than Liverpool; for example London's House of Recovery opened in 1801.[22]

Scotland was slower than England to take up the idea of fever wards and fever hospitals in the fight against typhus for, unlike those in England, its hospitals had never refused admittance to fever patients. In the 5 years after the opening of Glasgow Royal Infirmary in 1794, 14% of all admissions were of patients suffering from 'fever', and in 1816, there was a severe outbreak of typhus in the city, and the multitudes who flocked into the infirmary 'exceeded all precedent'. There was a similar situation at the Edinburgh Royal Infirmary during the 1818 outbreak in the city, and at the Aberdeen Royal Infirmary the same year. The action taken included extra care over cleanliness and ventilation, and the conversion of barracks, factories and other suitable buildings into temporary fever hospitals to ease overcrowding.[22]

In Ireland, typhus was always associated with the famines to which that country was especially prone, and when the mass migrations to England, particularly to Liverpool, began, it was said that the Irish were the source of the outbreaks there.[21] Originally, fever patients in Ireland were admitted to general hospitals, but as a result of the prevalence of the disease, the trend towards fever hospitals began early. Waterford opened the first in the country and the second in the British Empire in 1799, followed by Kilkenny in 1803, Cork Street, Dublin in 1806, and others. In 1818, an Act was passed at Westminster giving official status to Irish fever hospitals, which had up to then been strictly voluntary establishments. Many new hospitals opened at around the same time. But although these hospitals offered an essential refuge for the sick, they took a hideous toll of their staff. In 1817, 'no clinical clerk, apothecary, unseasoned nurse or servant' escaped infection at the Cork Street Hospital; in all, 198 attendants on the sick were affected.

Epidemiological theory and segregation policy

Despite James Lind's definitive studies in the middle of the eighteenth century on the epidemiology of typhus, the medical profession still did not speak with one voice a century later on the most effective means of controlling the disease; on whether ventilation and the generous spacing of beds, or scrupulous cleanliness was the most important measure. The difficulty arose from the tenacity with which the medical profession clung to the two historic theories: the miasma theory, and the idea of the identity of all, or most, fevers. The miasma theory would, in fact, remain popular until well past the middle of the nineteenth century, and its complementary idea of 'effluvia', which could only transfer the poison over short distances, accounted well enough for most cases of typhus. As to the identity of the fevers, smallpox, measles and plague were recognized as distinct as early as the seventeenth century, but others, such as typhoid and typhus, were not distinguished until well into the nineteenth century. It was demonstrable that adequate ventilation and space controlled some fevers and benefited all, supposedly by diluting the poisonous particles in the miasma, so that it was easy to conclude that ventilation was the all-important factor. It was only as, one by one, the medical men of the time came to realize the errors of these two ancient beliefs, and to accept Lind's brilliant deductions, that the complete control of typhus in hospitals could become a reality.

However, the conversion of the medical profession was both slow and erratic, some eighteenth-century workers being far in advance of others towards the end of the nineteenth century. Monro, for instance, although, as we have seen, insisted in 1788 that hospital wards must be kept well aired and free from offensive smells, also emphasized the absolute necessity of scrupulous cleanliness.[12] Good, in 1795, went even further in his discussion of conditions in prisons and poorhouses.[23] In such establishments, clean linen was rarely, if ever, allowed, and this was 'not only a cause of fever, but a cause of aggravating that fever when produced'. 'No medicine', he wrote, 'is much more advantageous than the daily change of linen'. Thomas Beddoes, an enthusiastic proponent of fever hospitals, writing in 1803, noted that the occasional case of apparent infection over a distance, which some doctors would ascribe to poisonous miasmas, could always be traced to contact with infected sheets or other fomites.[24] But 60 years later, an Irishman, Hudson (1868), would state his belief that typhus was generated by 'an animal miasm', which might either arise spontaneously in conditions of overcrowding, or be introduced and spread by infection.[25] He called this poison 'ochlesis', and considered that it was both 'a powerful predisposing cause requiring extraneous infection to produce typhus', and that it could generate the disease *de novo*. In Vienna, Hildebrand had held precisely the same views, couched in different terminology, as far back as 1810. Murchison, in his magnificent tome on the 'continued fevers', written in 1873, reviewed all the then existing literature, described his own experiences at the London Fever Hospital, and drew conclusions similar to, but more precise than, those of Hudson.[3] In the light of 'the known facts relating to the etiology of the disease', he considered that:

1 Typhus is due to a specific poison.
2 This poison is communicated from the sick to the healthy, through the atmosphere, or by fomites, but is rendered inert by free ventilation.
3 The poison is also generated *de novo*, in the exhalation of living human beings, by overcrowding and bad ventilation. [Exhalations seems to include all bodily secretions, not only breath.]

Murchison particularly specified that:

it is highly improbable that so contagious a poison as that of typhus is a mere chemical compound of ammonia; but even the view that it consists of minute particles of living matter is not incompatible with its having an independent origin in overcrowding.

As late as 1887, no less an authority than John Simon, in his *Public Health Reports*, considered that ventilation was by far the most important means of controlling typhus in hospitals.[26] He rashly took the cleanliness of hospitals for granted, so that when 'patients who have come to hospital to be treated for perhaps some comparatively trifling ailment, will contract a fever which may well kill them outright and this not withstanding that the ward discipline has been strict', it could only have been due to poor ventilation.

Just when it seemed that the benefits of fever wards and fever hospitals had been firmly established, doubts as to their efficiency began to be voiced, based mainly on the large numbers of medical and nursing staff who contracted the fever from their patients. In 1842, Dr Graham of Edinburgh started a correspondence on the subject with many leading physicians in London and the provinces, and all who replied were in favour of placing fever patients in general wards provided the proportion of fever cases was kept low,[22] a proviso based on extension of the miasma theory. It was held that the more concentrated the poison in the miasma, or the stronger the offensive smell, the greater the likelihood of the transfer of infection. It was therefore logical to deduce that a ward devoted entirely to fever patients was much more dangerous to the attendant staff than a general ward containing only a few fever patients, and that for the same reason there was little danger of the other patients contracting the disease.

In 1860, Murchison carried out his survey of 69 London and provincial hospitals, enquiring into their practice with regard to the admission of fever patients into general wards; 40 hospitals replied.[3] Eight of the 11 London hospitals admitted fever patients in small numbers for teaching purposes, five of the 20 English provincial hospitals also did so, but in Scotland only Edinburgh admitted two fever patients to each 19-bed ward for teaching purposes. In London, he noted, most of the fever cases were of enteric fever, and were of little danger to other patients. When typhus patients were admitted, the disease could spread. Murchison gave as illustration an outbreak at Guy's Hospital in 1862, when one or two typhus cases had been admitted to a ward containing 50 patients, of whom seven contracted the disease and five died. Murchison went on to collect the mortality figures for general hospitals with and without fever wards, and for fever hospitals discriminating between typhus and enteric fever, concluding that:

Cases of typhus (and of relapsing fever) ought never to be treated in a ward with other patients; even in no larger a proportion than 1 in 6, there is a danger of these diseases spreading. There is no evidence that in a well ventilated Fever Hospital the mortality from continued fevers is greater than in a general hospital. In proportion to the number of cases treated, the danger of the disease spreading is much less on the plan of isolation, than on that of mixing.

Within a fever hospital, Murchison advocated the segregation of different types of fever in different wards, as Tenon had done in Paris 100 years earlier. As to the danger to attendants of catching typhus, Murchison suggested that fever hospitals should select their staff from those who were immune to the disease by virtue of having had a previous attack or being of an age when an attack was unlikely to prove fatal.

In 1864, a Report on Hospitals was presented to the Privy Council with figures on infection reflecting closely those produced by Murchison, but despite its findings the government recommended that cases of typhus and scarlatina should be admitted to general wards in a proportion of not more than one in six and was severely criticized by a number of medical authorities for so doing. In 1866, over 40 years after the Fever Hospital Act had been passed for Ireland, a Sanitary Act for the mainland allowed local authorities to provide and maintain hospitals for infectious diseases here, but little was, in fact, done. Then the 1875 Public Health Act enabled local authorities to provide for patients with infectious diseases, but even at this late date the Superintendant of Guy's Hospital was warning that 'it is still very doubtful whether the concentration of large numbers of persons suffering from similar maladies has not an evil influence in intensifying the virulence of the disease'.[22]

In Britain and on the Continent, despite continued outbreaks in cities, usually precipitated by famine, typhus began to decline rapidly during the second half of the nineteenth century, due largely to the massive public health campaigns that had finally been forced on the governments of the day. But the disease continued to cause havoc in famine-stricken Ireland and in eastern Europe, where it had its roots both in poverty and in continued warfare, armies in the field being an ideal breeding ground. At the beginning of the Crimean War, in 1854–5, of all the armies engaged in fighting, the English suffered most from typhus, being the victims of the most indescribably sordid conditions both in camp and hospital. But under the drastic sanitary reforms instigated by Florence Nightingale, the disease apparently became less of a problem, although dysentery and cholera were severe in the hospitals.[27] The French, however, lost half their army of 12 000 men to typhus, despite having infinitely better hospital conditions than the British.[3] In an effort to control the disease, typhus patients were placed in tents with the lower flap turned up all round to provide ventilation, and the tents were moved regularly to new, clean sites.[27] The discovery of the louse as a vector in 1909 led to improved control measures in the twentieth century (see Chapter 9).

The eighteenth and nineteenth centuries: lying-in hospitals and puerperal fever

There have been reliable records of puerperal fever as a complication of childbirth since ancient times. The first known mention of the problem is that by Hippocrates, who gave a clear description of five cases in his book on epidemics (c. 400–380 BC).[1] Avicenna discussed the disease, and cases were recorded and described all over Europe in the seventeenth century. In Germany, especially in Leipzig, the numbers of cases in the middle of the century suggest the possibility of epidemics in the general population: if so, these would be the first on record.[2] Only in France is a hospital outbreak recorded at this early date, because only in France was there a hospital with a lying-in ward, the Hôtel Dieu in Paris. In 1626, the new, two-storey ward on a bridge over the Seine (see Chapter 2) was opened,[3] but by 1646, the first outbreak of puerperal fever had occurred, accompanied by a huge death rate. It seems that by this time, the lower floor of the ward was being used for patients with open wounds. De Lamoignon, the 'Premier President' of the hospital, blamed the outbreak of puerperal fever on foul air rising from that ward and infecting the lying-in women.[4] In the light of modern knowledge, he may well have been right about the source of the infection if not about the means of transfer.

The eighteenth century saw the rise throughout Europe of special hospital services for lying-in women. These were almost exclusively for the poor, for the better-off preferred to have their babies delivered at home. In the British Isles, the first hospital to designate a ward specifically for lying-in women was St James's, Westminster, in 1739, and the first hospital built for the purpose was the Dublin Lying-in Hospital (later known as the Rotunda), which opened in 1745. By 1747, the Middlesex Hospital had allocated special beds in general wards for the purpose,[5] but William Hunter, the hospital's obstetrician at the time, felt very strongly that there should have been a separate maternity ward. When, in 1749, this was finally refused, he and some associates resigned and founded the first lying-in hospital in England, the British Lying-in. It is ironic that it was here that the first hospital outbreak of puerperal fever in England occurred 11 years later.[6]

Table 5.1. Outbreaks of puerperal fever and 'ulcerous sore throat' in London in the eighteenth century

Puerperal fever	Sore throat	
City	Hospital	City
—	—	1755
1760	1760	—
1769–71	1769–71	1770
—	—	1772–3
—	—	1777–8
1787–8	1787–8	1785–94

Source: Adapted from DeLacy.[6]

In 1752, the General Lying-in in Grosvenor Square opened its doors and, after several moves, eventually became Queen Charlotte's, Goldhawk Road. A few years later, in 1757, the Middlesex at last opened its own maternity wing in a new building;[5] the City of London Lying-in was in use in 1772. The provinces were slower than London in opening special lying-in hospitals. Newcastle upon Tyne, in 1760, was the first, but it was not until 1790 that Charles White founded the Manchester Institution, followed by Edinburgh in 1803, although Edinburgh had had designated maternity wards in its Royal Infirmary for many years. All these hospitals were run by voluntary bodies; the first local authority maternity hospital was that at Rochdale, which opened in 1918. In all, there were ten lying-in hospitals in England by the end of the eighteenth century[5] and doubtless, in addition, many designated beds and wards in general hospitals.

Lying-in hospitals, by their nature, offered huge opportunities for outbreaks of infection, but were hospital outbreaks of puerperal fever in any way precipitated by events in the communities served by them? Hospitals could certainly suffer severe outbreaks when there were no problems in the community. For instance, Professor Young, when reporting in 1773 the recent devastating outbreak in the lying-in wards of the Edinburgh Infirmary in which almost every woman contracted the disease and the mortality rate was 100%, commented that there were no cases in the city.[7] However, there is no doubt that many hospital outbreaks did coincide with a community epidemic. For instance, Nightingale in 1871 gives 'prevalence of puerperal fever as an epidemic outside the hospital' as one of a number of causes of a hospital outbreak.[8] That in Paris, associated with the terrible outbreak in the Hôtel Dieu, is probably the best known, but Table 5.1 shows that all three hospital outbreaks in lying-in hospitals in eighteenth-century London coincided with community outbreaks. In addition, two out of three outbreaks in the Rotunda were associated with epidemics in Dublin.[6] It is not possible to determine whether the infection spread from the community to the hospitals or from the hospitals to the community.

The streptococci that cause puerperal fever are also responsible for other diseases, notably the 'ulcerous sore throat' that was very prevalent at the time, scarlet fever and erysipelas. Even at that time, doctors were connecting epidemics of these diseases with outbreaks of puerperal fever, although they attributed all but erysipelas to unfavourable weather conditions. John Clark, discussing an outbreak of puerperal fever in London in 1787, stated that 'the ulcerous sore throat...had been very general...in London'. He went on to note that it was 'a curious circumstance, that before the attack of the epidemic of lying-in women in Paris in the year 1746...there had been an epidemic of low fever with an ulcerous sore throat'.[9] A recent study of the interrelationship of the two diseases in the eighteenth century has emphasized the extreme difficulty of drawing meaningful conclusions from the haphazard statistics of variable quality, which are all that are available. Nevertheless, it is clear that two of the three London community outbreaks of puerperal fever coincided with community epidemics of sore throat, and that the third puerperal fever outbreak in both the community and hospitals occurred in the middle of a prolonged sore throat epidemic, although three other sore throat epidemics were not associated with puerperal fever (see Table 5.1). Ulcerous sore throat may well have been one precipitating cause of puerperal fever, but it was by no means the only one.

It has been suggested (see Chapter 6) that eighteenth-century hospitals have been given an undeservedly bad name by twentieth-century commentators who, instead of using such eighteenth-century information as is available, have taken the appalling figures of the nineteenth century and concluded that the earlier period, with its less advanced medical knowledge, must have been worse. The same misrepresentation has been inflicted on lying-in hospitals. In fact, there were only three major epidemics in the few hospitals that had been built in London up to the end of that century (see Table 5.1), although a single hospital might have an outbreak in a year when others were having few problems. DeLacy[6] has scrutinized in detail the figures for individual hospitals used by McKeown and Brown,[10] and has pointed out that these authors averaged the mortality rate over long periods, thus masking the epidemic years and raising the average mortality over the period. For instance, if the annual figures for the British Lying-in[6] are averaged over 25-year periods, as done by McKeown and Brown, the mortality in the first quarter (1750–74) is 20.7/1000, but in the second quarter (1775–89) it is almost halved, being 10.7/1000. If the two epidemic years of 1760 and 1770, with mortalities of 59.9/1000 and 59.1/1000, respectively, are excluded from the first quarter, then the mortality drops by over 3/1000 to 17.3/1000. More revealing, if the figures are averaged over 10-year rather than 25-year periods, then the gradual improvement over the first 40 years, and the

Table 5.2. Mortality per 1000 births at the British Lying-in Hospital

Years	Mortality	Worst year	Mortality
1749–58	23.8	1754	36.8
1759–68	20.3	1760	59.9
1969–78	18.8	1770	59.1
1779–88	16.6	1781	26.4
1789–98	3.4	1790	11.1

Source: Adapted from DeLacy.[6]

Table 5.3. Maternal mortality from all causes per 1000 births at the Rotunda Lying-in Hospital

Years	Mortality
1745–60	11.5
1761–70	14.8
1771–80	10.6
1781–90	9.6
1791–1800	8.8
1801–10	9.7
1811–20	15.0
1821–30	13.3
1831–40	13.1
1841–50	13.6
1851–60	15.6
1861–70	32.7
1871–5	21.7

Source: From Steele.[11]

dramatic fall in the last 10 years, is evident (see Table 5.2). In 1799 and 1800, years not included in Table 5.2, the figures were 1.9/1000 and 0/1000, respectively. Figures for the Rotunda in Dublin, quoted by Steele in his 1877 study of the mortality of hospitals, tell a similar story (see Table 5.3),[11] but he could only conclude that because of the excellent reputation of the hospital both for its sanitary arrangements and for teaching, there must be some 'hidden' cause for the inexorable rise in the death rate in the nineteenth century. Figures for other individual hospitals tell a similar story, and it seems probable that an unduly dark picture has been painted of British lying-in hospitals in the first 50 years of their existence.

The rapid spread of puerperal fever once inside a lying-in hospital or ward was a matter of grave concern to the medical profession. Up to the end of the 1770s, the miasmatists' theory of infection held almost universal sway, inauspicious weather conditions being blamed as the main cause of epidemics. For instance, Leake, the obstetrician at the Westminster Lying-in Hospital, begins an account of the cases seen from October 1769 to May 1770 with a detailed description of the weather over that period.[12] To purify the air in his wards, Leake relied heavily on fumigation by burning wood, brimstone or gunpowder, as advocated by James Lind (see Chapter 4). In France at the time, many lying-in women were delivered in general wards among patients with open wounds; Peu, a Paris obstetrician, had recognized that the hideous death rate among the women was associated with the infected wounds of the other patients. In England, Leake agreed with Peu that this was due to 'the putrid effluvia continually exhaling from the wounds of the sick', and deduced from this that beds must be well spaced and the wards 'kept exceeding clean' and 'ventilated by a stream of fresh air passing through them, as they become empty by succession'.[12] By similar means, Professor Young of Edinburgh brought the devastating outbreak of puerperal fever at the Royal Infirmary under control. Young's successor, William Hamilton, also recognized the contagiousness of puerperal fever and its resemblance to erysipelas.

Charles White, the pioneering physician and obstetrician of Manchester, who had trained under William Hunter, a member of the Scottish group that played down the importance of the weather in cross-infection (see page 57), held similar but even more stringent views:[7] he advocated not only widely spaced beds but also small wards, single-bed wards being the best of all. White advised on the design of the Rotunda Hospital in Dublin, and it may have been for this reason that no ward at the Rotunda held more than seven beds, with some having only two. White also suggested two other sources of infection: the filthy river water drunk by so many of his patients, and the nurses attending them. He described the nurses as a powerful body of women who made no attempt to change their practices, even if ordered to do so by the doctors. It has to be remarked, however, that neither White nor any of his contemporaries make any mention of the personal hygiene of midwives or other attendants.

The emphasis laid on space, ventilation and cleanliness by the medical profession towards the end of the eighteenth century, although based on an incorrect theory, did much to control puerperal fever in British hospitals at the time. On the Continent, however, the importance of atmospheric conditions beyond the control of man held sway for much longer, leading to a laissez-faire attitude that resulted in dirt and overcrowding being tolerated for longer, to the great detriment of women in labour.

Dr Alexander Gordon of Aberdeen, in 1795, was the first person to discard completely the idea of any form of miasma, whether atmospheric or purely local, as a cause of the spread of disease. He was born in 1752 and, having completed his medical training at Aberdeen and Edinburgh, he joined the navy as a surgeon. After 5 years' service, he left and began to train in midwifery at various London establishments, including the Middlesex Dispensary and Westminster Hospital. He returned to Aberdeen in 1785, where he settled down into general practice, and was also appointed physician to the Middlesex Dispensary, devoting himself to midwifery.[13] It was his work at the Middlesex Dispensary that formed the basis for his *Treatise on the Epidemic of Puerperal Fever of Aberdeen* (1795) in which he demonstrated unequivocally the contagious nature of the disease nearly 50 years before the better-known work of Simpson, Semmelweiss and Holmes.

Edinburgh, where Gordon had received part of his initial medical training, was the centre of a distinctive circle of physicians and obstetricians who were not acceptable to the Universities of Oxford or Cambridge or to the Royal College of Physicians because of their dissenting religion or their despised speciality. They held a number of distinctive views, one of which was the importance of contagion in infectious disease. William Hunter, who had been one of the group of men to break away from the Middlesex Hospital to found the British Lying-In, was a leading member of the group, as was Thomas Young, Professor of Midwifery at Edinburgh. It was Gordon who took their ideas to their logical conclusion.[6] The epidemic he described in his *Treatise* began in Aberdeen and its surroundings in December 1789 and continued until March 1792. Gordon, having seen puerperal fever in London, was the only practitioner in the district who was familiar with it, for the last local outbreak had been 30 years earlier. Like White, Gordon says that he noted 'the state of the atmosphere' throughout his other observations; however, in contrast to White, he deliberately gave no details in his report, for he discovered at an early stage that it was irrelevant to his enquiry. He listed, in chronological order of the onset of the illness, all 77 lying-in women for whom he was responsible over the period, giving their age, the street or village in which they lived, the outcome of the illness, and the name of the midwife in attendance; in 12 cases he delivered the patient himself. He then traced the movements of the midwives and himself from patient to patient, coming to an unequivocal conclusion:

This disease siezed such women only as were visited or delivered by a practitioner, or taken care of by a nurse, who had previously attended patients affected with the disease . . . The midwife who delivered No. 1 in the table, carried the infection to No. 2, the next woman whom she delivered. The physician who attended Nos. 1 and 2, carried the infection to Nos. 5 and 6, who were delivered by him, and to many others . . . It is a disagreeable declaration for me to mention, that I myself was the means of carrying the infection to a great number of women.

So sure was he of the accuracy of his results that he wrote:

> I arrived at that certainty in the matter, that I could venture to foretell what women would be affected with the disease, upon hearing by what midwife they were delivered or by what nurse they were attended during their lying-in; and in almost every instance my prediction was verified.

He went on to state that 'the nurses and physicians, who have attended patients affected with the puerperal fever, ought carefully to wash themselves, and get their apparel properly fumigated, before it be put on again'. Although he laid little emphasis on the personal hygiene of the attendants, he was one of the first people to mention the matter specifically.

Gordon, like Peu in France and Leake in England, drew attention to the association between erysipelas and puerperal fever, and indeed went some way towards explaining it, pointing out that women only contract puerperal fever after they have given birth because before then 'there is no inlet open to receive the matter which produces the disease. But after delivery the matter is readily and copiously admitted by the numerous patulous orifices, which are open to imbibe it, by the separation of the placenta from the uterus'.[13]

Sadly, the publication of Gordon's *Treatise*, blaming himself and named midwives for the puerperal fever epidemic, 'raised against him such strong prejudices in the public mind as materially to damage his professional prospects in Aberdeen' and he was forced to rejoin the navy. In 1799, he contracted tuberculosis and died at the early age of 48.

Another physician who realized the contagiousness of puerperal fever was John Armstrong (1784–1829) of Sunderland. He wrote a book, *Facts and Observations Relative to the Fever Commonly Called Puerperal*, in 1814, and stated: 'I am now well convinced, that when puerperal fever is once generated, there is almost always cause to apprehend its being communicated to other puerperal women, especially by accoucheurs and nurses who have previously waited upon affected persons'.[15]

It might have been expected that the low incidence of puerperal fever achieved in England by the end of the eighteenth century thanks to the work of White, Gordon and Armstrong would have continued into the nineteenth century, but this was not to be. Most doctors still refused to accept that their own personal hygiene could possibly be the cause of the death of their patients, and childbirth was still considered by the Royal Colleges to be a natural function for which no special medical training was needed. Attempts were made by select committees in 1834, 1878–9 and 1892 to increase the time spent by medical students on midwifery, but all were stubbornly opposed by the teaching bodies,[16] and mortality in childbirth, both inside and outside hospitals, continued to rise inexorably. In London, in the British Lying-In, the overall death rate in 1799–1800 was 3.2/1000 births, but in 1865–75 it was 19.4/1000.[12] The City of London Lying-In showed a similar increase from

4.3/1000 in 1800–10 to 14.3/1000 in 1865–76. In Dublin, where White's teaching had had considerable influence in the eighteenth century, the average death rate had been between 9/1000 and 14/1000 but it reached 33/1000 between 1861 and 1870.

These high death rates may have been one reason why only 15 new lying-in hospitals were built in Britain during the nineteenth century despite the large increase in population over the period. It was not until Lister's antiseptic techniques were introduced into midwifery, together with Dettol and other chlorine antiseptics, that maternal mortality in hospitals finally began to drop.

It fell to another Scot, James Young Simpson (1811–70), to rediscover and extend Gordon's work, and to attempt to overcome the wilful blindness of the obstetricians concerning their own part in causing the fearful mortality of the middle years of the nineteenth century.[17] In 1836, when Simpson was only 25, there was an outbreak of puerperal fever in his Edinburgh practice, followed closely by another in the practice of a friend. Immediately before this, Simpson had helped with the dissection of two fatal cases of the same disease and, in light of this experience and of his knowledge of Gordon's work, he immediately accepted the communicability of the disease. In 1840, he began to express these views in his lectures, 3 years before O. W. Holmes's paper on the subject appeared. Also in 1840, Simpson was appointed to the Chair of Midwifery at Edinburgh at the early age of 29. He did not publish his own views on the infective nature of puerperal fever until 1850, by which time Semmelweiss's first paper on the subject had appeared, duly acknowledged by Simpson (he does not seem to have known of Holmes's work). Simpson disagreed strongly with Semmelweiss's view that the infection was transmitted by animal matter in a state of putrefaction, preferring to blame 'an inflammatory secretion, just as the inoculable matter of smallpox, cowpox, syphilis'. Although he never accepted the germ theory of disease, this was a remarkably clear statement for its time of the specificity of infective agents.

Gordon's *Treatise*, as well as establishing the communicability of puerperal fever, had demonstrated the relationship of the disease to erysipelas. Simpson took up this subject in another paper in 1850, establishing the similarity of the two diseases and reinforcing the idea of their intercommunicability, but some refused to accept this as late as 1875. Even after Simpson's methods for reducing the onslaught of puerperal fever had been published, many obstetricians failed to act on his recommendations, especially the more fashionable doctors, who regarded it as an insult that they should be accused of spreading infection.[14,17,18] As late as 1865, no less a journal than the *Lancet*, renowned for its aggressive backing for medical reform, published a violent attack on Dr James Edmunds, a cofounder of the Ladies' Medical College and follower of Semmelweiss, for accusing his own profession of spreading puerperal fever, although it eventually apologized.[19]

Simpson's interests now began to broaden and his idea of 'hospitalism' (see Chapter 6) and the means of preventing it were increasingly emphasized. His statements on the dangers of size and overcrowding in general hospitals applied equally to lying-in hospitals, and he campaigned vigorously for change.[18]

Although no attempt was made to put Gordon's and Simpson's ideas into practice in Europe or America, and very little in Britain, a few obstetricians did heed their message and advance ideas of their own. The contagiousness of the disease and the part played by attendants in spreading it were emphasized further in 1825, when a Frenchman, A.G. Labarraque, made the first chlorine solution specifically for disinfection purposes,[2] and the avoidance of unnecessary interference by attendants during childbirth was emphasized.

Robert Collins was the most distinguished Master of the Rotunda in the nineteenth century. When he became Master in 1826, he found the hospital in a very unhealthy condition. At that time, more women died in childbirth from puerperal fever than from any other cause. To combat this, he attempted to reduce admissions and instituted a strict routine of fumigation and disinfection with chloride of lime. When a ward was full, it was emptied before admitting new patients (i.e. cohort nursing, which is still a measure for controlling the spread of hospital infection). Each ward was washed every 10–12 days with chloride of lime. Midwives and patients were forbidden to move from ward to ward, and febrile patients were separated from healthy women. This he considered of major importance. He did not accept that puerperal fever was due mainly to miasmas, but thought that it derived from some local cause. As a result of these efforts, he had no deaths from puerperal fever in the last 4 years of his Mastership.[20] His book, *Practical Treatise in Midwifery*, published in 1835, came to the notice of Semmelweiss, who hoped to travel to Dublin but was forced to change his plans. Nevertheless, the book probably influenced his work. Table 5.3 shows once again that averaging mortality over periods of years masks very significant fluctuations within those periods.

Next to try to break through the barrier of professional opposition was an American, Oliver Wendell Holmes (1809–94), who had studied in both Britain and France, and who became Professor of Anatomy at Harvard in 1847. In 1843, he published a pamphlet entitled *The Contagiousness of Puerperal Fever*,[21] in which he laid much emphasis on Gordon's work and stated categorically that 'the disease known as puerperal fever is so far contagious as to be frequently carried from patient to patient by doctors and nurses', stressing also the relationship between puerperal fever and erysipelas. He made seven recommendations for preventing its spread. These included avoiding being present at postmortems on cases of puerperal fever, erysipelas and peritonitis; if it were essential to be present at a postmortem, the doctor should wash thoroughly afterwards and make a complete change of clothing; he must accept that if a single case of puerperal fever were to occur in his practice,

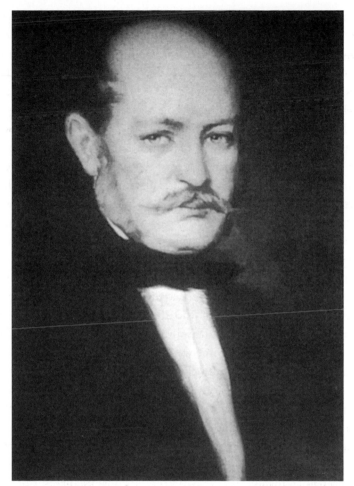

Figure 5.1 Ignaz Semmelweiss (1818–65). (Photograph of an oil painting by
M. Schachinger, courtesy of General Hospital Vienna.)

all other women in labour would be at risk of being infected by him until several
weeks had elapsed; that if three or more cases occurred in his practice, he himself
was the source of the contagion; and that it was his duty to prevent the disease from
being spread by nurses and assistants.[22] A few of Holmes's compatriots supported
his views, but most disagreed violently. Hugh Hodge, in 1852, went so far as to
publish a paper entitled 'On the non-contagiousness of puerperal fever'. He was
supported 2 years later by Charles Meigs, who preferred to attribute cases to 'accident or providence, of which I can form a conception, rather than to a contagion
of which I cannot form any clear idea'. There was little more that Holmes could do
against such injured vanity.[2,14]

 In Europe, it was a Hungarian, Ignaz Semmelweiss (1818–65; see Figure 5.1)
who first showed that puerperal fever was infectious.[23,24] He undertook his medical

training at the University of Vienna and obtained his first post in that city at the Obstetric Clinic of the Allgemeines Krankenhaus. It was there, in the early 1840s, that he began his independent observations. The clinic contained two divisions: in the first, the mothers were attended by professors and medical students; in the second, they were attended by midwives. Checking on the figures for deaths from puerperal fever, Semmelweiss found that between 1841 and 1846, there were almost 2000 fatal cases among 20 000 patients in Division 1, whereas in Division 2 there were only 700 deaths among slightly fewer patients; i.e. there were nearly three times the number of deaths in the doctors' division as in the midwives' division. Semmelweiss could find no explanation for this until, in 1847, a pathologist friend of his died from blood poisoning following a scalpel wound incurred during a postmortem. The autopsy on the pathologist revealed changes identical with those in a woman who had died of puerperal fever, and Semmelweiss immediately realized that the 'cadaveric poison' that had killed his friend was being carried to the mothers on the hands of doctors and medical students, providing an obvious explanation for the difference in death rates in the two divisions.

Despite the resistance of his staff who, like most other members of the medical profession, considered it a gross affront that they should be accused of being the killers of their own patients, Semmelweiss insisted that all students and assistants should wash their hands in chloride of lime before touching a woman. The result was dramatic, the death rate falling from 18% before the precautions were instituted to 1.2% afterwards. But still his colleagues and students refused to believe the evidence of their own eyes. The few of his friends who were convinced urged him to speak about or publish his results, but for some reason, possibly because of his difficulty with the German language, he failed to do so; his reforms were actively fought, and he eventually returned to Hungary. From his post as Director of Obstetrics at Pest in 1861, he published his only article on the subject, 'The etiology, concept and prophylaxis of childbed fever', but it was either denigrated or ignored. Semmelweiss was deeply wounded and wrote a number of scathing open letters to his tormentors, because of which he became branded as crazy; eventually, at the age of 47 and showing signs of real insanity, he was placed in a sanatorium in Vienna. There he died, ironically of blood poisoning, in 1865. The day after his death, Lister's first publication on antisepsis appeared, but in the actual use of antiseptics, Semmelweiss had forestalled him by 15 years.[25]

The high death rates in lying-in hospitals and wards in England were nothing compared with the terrifying situation in France, a matter that came to cause deep concern to a French surgeon, Leon Le Fort.[26] Le Fort visited London in 1858 to study English surgical methods and was amazed to find that survival rates following amputation were far better than those in France. The following year, he visited other European hospitals and discovered that they too failed to reach British standards. On further study, he found that every aspect of hospital planning and hygiene

Table 5.4. Maternal mortality in 12 Paris hospitals in 1861–3

Hospital	Puerperal fever deaths/1000		
	1861	1862	1863
Hôtel Dieu	43.5	35.8	26.7
Pitié	72.6	45.4	44.1
Charité	154.2	62.9	66.4
St Antoine	71.4	61.0	63.4
Necker	29.9	52.6	38.8
Cochin	142.9	41.6	73.5
Beaujon	43.5	38.9	19.2
Lariboisiére	69.1	34.3	31.0
St Louis	58.6	79.5	23.0
Lourcine	24.4	22.2	27.9
Cliniques	75.4	79.3	30.6
Maison d'Accouchements	99.8	63.5	130.1
Average	95.1	69.7	70.3

Source: Abstracted by Nightingale[8] from *Statistique Medicale des Hôpitaux* (1863).

in England was superior to that in France, and that the incidence of erysipelas and purulent infections was also lower. He attributed this success to the work of Florence Nightingale. In 1864, Le Fort gave an account of his findings to the Society of Surgery in the hope of influencing the design of the new Hôtel Dieu, which was about to be rebuilt on much the same lines as the old one that had proved so disastrous.

It was at this time that, realizing as Gordon had done many years earlier the resemblance of puerperal fever to erysipelas and hospital gangrene, Le Fort turned his attention to lying-in hospitals and lying-in wards in general hospitals. He submitted a report to the Director General of Hospital Administration in 1865, only to have it returned to him on the grounds that it was too polemical, theoretical and expensive. In France at the time, all hospitals were charities and were organized and managed by the same bodies as were charities for the poor. Consequently, doctors played no direct part in hospital planning or administration. Le Fort was strongly opposed to this system, considering the exclusion of the medical profession from any say in its own working conditions to be one of the main reasons for the tragically high death rate from hospital infections. Regretfully, therefore, he published the rejected study as a personal report, *Des Maternités*, in 1866.

The Hôtel Dieu in Paris was, as we have seen, a byword in the rest of Europe for its hideous record of hospital infections, but of the 12 Parisian hospitals taking in lying-in women, Le Fort's study showed that it was by no means the worst (see Table 5.4).

Table 5.5. Mortality from all causes among women delivered in French provincial hospitals in 1860–63

City	Number of deliveries	Deaths/1000
Bordeaux Maternité	714	42
Bordeaux St André	547	65
Colmar	396	65
Lille	683	35
Orleans	301	9
Rouen	1275	7
Strasbourg	556	140

Source: Abstracted from Le Fort.[26]

All but two of the hospitals showed an improvement in the 3 years over which they were observed, but even in the final year the death rate was much higher than that in London hospitals. The death rate in the only exclusively lying-in hospital, the Maison d'Accouchements, actually rose from an extraordinary 99.8/1000 to 130/1000 over the period.

Le Fort considered an important reason for these shocking figures to be the gross overcrowding characteristic of all French hospitals, which arose from their status as charities. This obliged them to admit all who knocked at their doors, rich or poor, married or single, and to treat them all equally to the best of their ability. As far as lying-in women were concerned, this was an easier obligation to act on in France than it would have been in England, because of the differences in the moral attitudes in the two countries. In France, unmarried mothers were regarded as 'unfortunates' or 'victims', and as such deserved treatment equal to that of married women. In England, they were stigmatized as 'sinners' and shunned by 'respectable' hospitals taking in married women; if they were taken in, they were segregated from the married women. Other differences between British and French arrangements for lying-in women that would account for the overcrowding of French hospitals were that the organization for home deliveries was far less advanced in France than in England, and that in England the indigent poor were often delivered in workhouse infirmaries rather than in hospitals.

As well as studying Parisian hospitals, Le Fort collected maternal mortality figures from French provincial hospitals (see Table 5.5) and from hospitals in other European cities (see Table 5.6). Although these figures are for total deaths rather than for deaths due to puerperal fever alone, they undoubtedly indicate a much higher death rate from puerperal fever in most European hospitals than was occurring in England at the time.

Table 5.6. Mortality from all causes among women delivered in hospitals in northern Europe in 1858–63

City	Years	Deliveries	Deaths/1000
Graz	1859–61	3089	31
Vienna, First Clinic	1860–63	17 447	29
Prague	1860–62	8378	39
Frankfurt-on-Main	1860–63	804	20
Bremen	1858–63	139	71
Freiburg-in-Bresgau	1860–62	281	35
Jena (Cinique)	1859–62	308	67
Moscow	1860–62	7874	29
Dresden	1860–63	2523	8
Stockholm (Maternité)	1861	650	56
Zurich (Maternité)	1860	200	100

Source: Abstracted from Le Fort.[26]

In light of Nightingale's results on surgical wards, Le Fort then went on to study how puerperal fever spread in lying-in wards, providing statistics and examples to show that cleanliness, the isolation of infected mothers, and precautions against contagion were all-important. In particular, he emphasized the dangers of multiple occupation of beds. He stated specifically that contagion was the only way in which an infection could be carried from a sick person to a healthy person, and in the case of puerperal fever he considered that this could occur in three ways: (1) directly from patient to patient, (2) indirectly via students and attendants, and (3) via contagious miasmas adhering to walls, beds, curtains, dressings, etc. (his use of the term 'miasma' here is original and does not appear to imply aerial spread). He gave numerous examples of each method, and pointed out that the low infection rate among home deliveries proved that in hospitals contagion was an important factor. Finally, he enunciated ten rules for preventing puerperal fever outbreaks in institutions, including instructions to staff to wash their hands and clean their nails.

Little bodies *en chainettes* in the blood of a woman dying of puerperal fever had been described as early as 1869. Ten years later, Pasteur reported the presence of microbes in a similar pattern in the lochia and blood of puerperal fever patients, and stated clearly that these (almost certainly streptococci) were the most frequent cause of infection in women in childbirth. When contradicted at a meeting of the Academy of Medicine, he leaped to his feet, drew the organisms on the blackboard, and convinced his fellows. Pasteur's discovery, and the germ theory that developed from it, forced even the obstetricians to accept their role as harbingers of death in their own wards.[22] Florence Nightingale (1820–1910) (see Chapter 6) never accepted the germ theory of disease, although she did believe in contagion as well as miasmas. She achieved her remarkable results in the Crimean War by fanatical attention to cleanliness, space and fresh air; when, in 1862, the Committee of the Nightingale Fund came to set up lying-in wards in a new part of King's College Hospital for the purpose of training midwives, it was on these ideas that their plans were based. High hopes were entertained that this new training school would be of great benefit to the poor, among whom the need for trained midwives was greatest. But despite the apparently ideal circumstances in which the women were housed, mortality from puerperal fever averaged 33.3/1000 over the first 5 years of the institution's existence, and it had to be closed. This disaster precipitated Nightingale into writing her *Notes on Lying-in Institutions* in 1871,[8] at a time when she was already sick and badly overworked. It must be emphasized that her primary consideration was the training of midwives, but she was not prepared to do this at the expense of mothers. If a safe lying-in institution could not be devised, then midwives must be trained on domicilary cases, for 'lying-in is neither a disease nor an accident, and any fatality attending it is not to be counted as so much per cent. of inevitable loss. On the contrary, a death in childbirth is almost a subject for an inquest.' After complaining bitterly about the lack of meaningful statistics from both Britain and Europe, she set about extracting the maximum possible information from those that did exist. Quoting extensively from Le Fort,[26] she confirmed his finding that large hospitals had, in general, a much higher mortality than small ones; she too showed that a badly managed small hospital could be just as lethal as a large one. That the lying-in wards of workhouses had, in general, a much better record than those of normal lying-in institutions was an unexpected finding. Nightingale gave Liverpool Workhouse as an extraordinary example of what could be achieved. Averaging 500 deliveries a year, there were only three cases of puerperal fever in the 13 years from 1858 to 1870, one each in 1859, 1860 and 1861, and this despite the fact that the wards were in a wing of the female general hospital next to the surgical wards. Nightingale attributed such results to the fact that the wards were never full and the women were transferred out of them as fast as possible, so preventing the build-up of miasmas. In Liverpool, there was also scrupulous cleanliness, and the attendants in the lying-in wards never entered the general hospital.

Although in her *Notes* Nightingale never mentioned Semmelweiss, when she came to discuss the admittance of medical students, she quoted Le Fort's figures from the two Vienna clinics studied by Semmelweiss, concluding that students should be allowed in lying-in wards only for limited periods, and then only when they were not working on any other wards or attending autopsies. That erysipelas and 'blood poisoning' could lead to puerperal fever she fully accepted, but the reason for this remained a mystery to her: 'the disease puerperal fever develops spontaneously under certain unknown circumstances. When it is about to become epidemic, it is sometimes preceded by the prevalence of erysipelas.' Based on her huge experience of hospital infections, and on her study of the statistics of puerperal fever in different types of lying-in institution, Nightingale described the layout of the ideal lying-in hospital. It should consist of alternate one- and two-floored pavilions, each floor containing a four-bed ward and scullery, and the pavilions being connected by a wide passage. There would be a delivery room on each floor.

Despite Nightingale's emphasis on hospital design, it was not until Lister's methods, slowly and against medical resistance, crept into the lying-in wards that a real onslaught on puerperal fever could begin. At first, it was assumed that chemicals that would kill microbes in vitro would also kill them in vivo, and a huge variety were pressed into service, including mercury salts, oxycyanide, Lysol (a cresol), iodine, permanganate of potash, hypochlorites and dyes (see Chapter 11). The York Road Lying-In Hospital in London had had a particularly bad record for puerperal fever, with a rate of 30.8/1000 births between 1833 and 1860. From 1880 to 1886, this had dropped to only 6/1000 due to the antiseptic policy, although it would have been helped by the fact that the hospital had been closed for 2 years.[22] At Queen Charlotte's, the rate dropped from 26.8/1000 in 1875–9 to 4.5/1000 in 1900–2, and at the General Lying-in, it fell from 30.8/1000 in 1838–60, to 6.2/1000 in 1880–87, to 0.5/1000 in 1893–1903.[16]

By the turn of the century, and into the 1920s and 1930s, the relative safety of hospital and home deliveries had been reversed, for general practitioners and midwives, largely because they were so poorly trained, ignored the antiseptic and aseptic practice that was urged on them by official reports and that had become routine in hospitals. Because of the obstructive attitude of the teaching hospitals and of their medical colleagues generally to increasing the time spent by students on obstetrics, obstetricians now believed that large lying-in hospitals should be built all over the country and that as many births as possible should take place in them, while home deliveries should be phased out.[17]

The nineteenth century before Lister: military hospitals and wound infection, civilian hospitals and 'hospitalism'

The eighteenth century had seen many improvements in the medical care of military and naval personnel, due mainly to the efforts of Pringle and Lind in Great Britain and others in Europe, especially in France. However, these principles seem often to have been forgotten in the horrendous wars of the nineteenth century. The large numbers of casualties in battles during this century were commonly associated with severe infections, especially gangrene following gunshot wounds. Other infections such as typhus, dysentery and cholera continued to be common in the unhygienic conditions of the warfare of the time.[1]

In the early part of the century, Dominique Jean Larrey made notable contributions to wound treatment. He was a surgeon to Napoleon and was responsible for many improvements in the medical services of the French army.[2,3] In 1810, Larrey was made a Commander of the Legion of Honour and was given the title of Baron. He introduced ambulances for the rapid removal of casualties, debridement (surgical cleaning of wounds), and immediate amputations in field hospitals, and reintroduced open wound management. Dressings or linen soaked in camphorated wine or salt water were commonly used by him as an 'antiseptic'. He was also one of the first to describe the therapeutic effects of maggots for removal of dead material from wounds. He believed that a soldier with a healing amputation wound on reaching a large base hospital stood a much better chance of surviving and was less susceptible to gangrene if operated on immediately on arrival; he was also obviously aware of the hazards of hospital infection.

Almost immediately after the Battle of Austerlitz, an epidemic of typhus broke out and hospital gangrene became rife.[4] The hospitals for troops of the line lost a quarter of their patients, whereas the Imperial Guard, who were treated in almshouses distant from the large hospitals, largely escaped. These almshouses were well lit, aired and kept perfectly clean. The absence of overcrowding and of contact spread was probably the main reason for the minimal spread of infection, although good ventilation and cleanliness no doubt played a role as well.

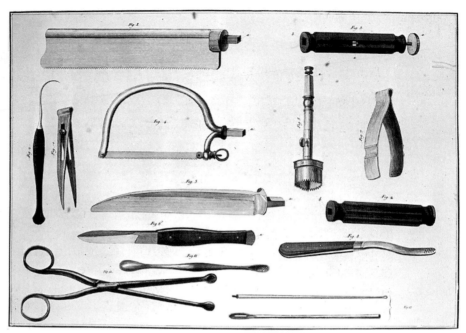

Figure 6.1   Portable amputating and trepanning instruments of the eighteenth century. (J.H. Sauvigny (1998). *Instruments Used in the Practice of Surgery*. London: T. Bentley. Wellcome Library, London.)

After the Battle of Waterloo (1815), every home in the neighbourhood, as well as stables and cowsheds, was used for British casualties. Gunshot wounds, unless superficial, almost certainly led to amputation, and it was estimated that 500 amputations were carried out after Waterloo and Quatre-Bras.[5] Amputations were carried out if possible within 24 hours, as recommended by Guthrie, a leading British army surgeon, following his excellent results in the Peninsular War. Guthrie had reported that 24 of 291 patients operated on in the field in the Peninsular War died, whereas of 551 secondary operations in hospital, 265 patients died.[6] The disastrous situation after the Battle of Waterloo was not always without humour. The future Lord Raglan was heard to call in his usual casual voice when his arm was amputated: 'Hello, don't carry away that arm until I have taken off the ring.' The hospitals in Brussels were overwhelmed, and many of the wounded had to be transferred to Antwerp, where there was a higher incidence of fevers, typhus and gangrene.[5]

The French army at the time of Waterloo had inadequate medical support compared with the excellent service provided in the early Napoleonic days, and their infection problems were greater.[1] Larrey was captured by the Prussians at Waterloo; he was going to be executed, until he was recognized and then released.

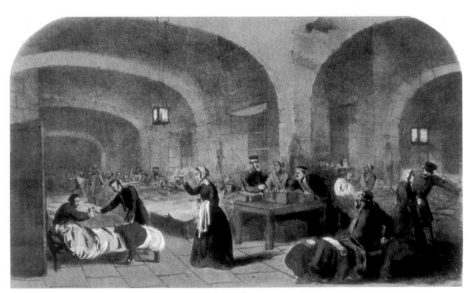

Figure 6.2   Florence Nightingale (1820–1910) in Scutari. (Wellcome Library, London.)

The deficiencies in the medical services of the British army during the Crimean War (1853–6) were exposed by Florence Nightingale (Figure 6.2), who was one of the first professional nurses to become involved in the care of battle casualties. She was born of wealthy parents in Florence in 1820 and showed an interest in nursing from an early age, but her parents objected to her becoming a nurse because of the poor hospital conditions at the time. Nevertheless, she was determined to become a nurse and to raise nursing standards. Despite the opposition of her parents and friends, she acquired experience of practical nursing in hospitals in England and on the Continent before going to the Crimea. On returning to England after the war, she continued to work for the improvement of hospital conditions and the training of nurses (Chapter 5).[7]

The conditions in the Crimean war were appalling. The general hospitals were little more than pest-holes. The largest hospital at Scutari was a hotbed of infection in which even those who began by being healthy could hardly survive. Men with hospital gangrene, typhus fever and cholera lay with vermin of all kinds crawling over them. Eighty cases of hospital gangrene were reported in 1 month.[7]

There were few beds, and patients lay on the floor with the same clothing or blankets they had brought with them from the front. There was a lack of linen to make bandages and a lack of other essential supplies.[8] There were no kitchens to prepare food on a regular basis, and the 2000 patients were expected to make do with only 20 bedpans.

These horrific conditions led Sir Sydney Herbert, Secretary of War in Britain, to send a contingent of nurses to the Crimea. He realized that there was only one woman who could do this job: he appointed Florence Nightingale as organizer and superintendant of a group of 38 nurses and arranged for them to travel to the barrack hospital in Scutari in 1854. Despite opposition from the military authorities, Nightingale and her nurses did much to improve the sanitary standards, and they reformed the entire hospital within 3 months.[9] She reorganized the provision of food and introduced simple hygienic procedures, such as providing clean bedding, changing sheets regularly, using hospital gowns, providing clean water, and washing the ward environment frequently, drastically reducing the rate of death from disease and infected wounds from over 40% to 2.2% in 6 months.[2]

Similar problems occurred with the Russians in the Crimean War.[10] A surgeon, Pirogov, stated that the wounds of all 120 patients, mostly amputations, in the splendid casino of Sebastopol were 'seized with a purulent edema, erysipelas and gangrene'. He considered these infections to be due to a miasma, but control procedures, such as evacuation of the rooms, whitewashing of walls, and improved ventilation, were all ineffective; the same wound complications were seen 3 weeks later. He thought the best way to tend the wounded was in hospital tents, and he attempted to avoid the use of large hospitals throughout the rest of the war.

The American Civil War (1861–5) was the last major conflict before germs were recognized as causes of infection. It was also probably the first to be dominated by the rifle, and more than 90% of wounds were caused by bullets. The number of casualties was huge and required a complex system of medical care, from first-aid stations to large general hospitals.[2,4,11]

Gangrene was the most feared of wound infections, occurring chiefly in hospitals and temporary shelters where sick and wounded were crowded together, usually with insufficient supplies of dressings and instruments. In one instance, a large number of wounded Federal prisoners were crowded into two churches, and hospital gangrene appeared a few days later; not a single soldier escaped.[4]

Asepsis was not recognized, and wounds were probed with unwashed hands and with instruments that were cleaned superficially but not sterilized. Sponges were used for washing wounds and conveyed infection from one wound to another. When these sponges were in short supply, clean linen or rags, which were washed or burnt between patients, were used, probably helping to reduce cross-infection. Erysipelas as well as gangrene was responsible for many deaths, and tetanus was common when stables were used as hospitals. Infected wounds were not the only problem: other diseases, such as pneumonia, were common, as were outbreaks of typhoid, dysentery and cholera due to contaminated water supplies and inadequately treated sewerage. Despite the availability of a vaccine, outbreaks of smallpox also occurred, and insect-borne diseases such as typhus, yellow fever, and malaria caused problems in certain areas. In a Southern prison, a third of 10 000 Federal prisoners died within 7 months of dysentery, scurvy and hospital gangrene.[4] It has been estimated that over half a million troops died of infections during the war. However, despite the terrible conditions in many of the field hospitals, the general hospitals in large urban areas were most excellent and had low mortality rates. They were usually of the pavilion type, with good ventilation and adequate bed-spacing.[12]

The American Civil War was responsible for considerable advances in traumatic surgery. For instance, infection was reduced by carrying out operations, especially amputations, during the first day after injury rather than delaying operation for several days when the patient was admitted to a general hospital.

In the Franco-Prussian war (1870–71), mortality after amputation was also extremely high at 80–90%,[13] despite Lister's studies of antisepsis, which were clearly unknown or not accepted at the time.

Hospital gangrene

Gangrene consists of a sloughing lesion of wounds due to loss of an adequate blood supply. It occurs in a number of forms as a complication of traumatic or surgical wounds, for instance gas gangrene. Descriptions in the literature indicate that all types occurred, particularly in military hospitals, and all could have devastating effects.

The date of the first appearance of hospital gangrene remains uncertain, but it is likely to have existed from ancient times;[14] a good description of an infection resembling hospital gangrene was given by Hippocrates:[4] 'The subject complained of severe pain in the toe with nausea and rigors on the first day. This was followed by swelling of the whole foot on the second day and the emergence of small bullae [vesicles], acute fever followed by death.' One of the first detailed descriptions of hospital gangrene as a distinct entity was given by Pouteau in the Hôtel Dieu in Lyons in 1781;[15] a good description was also given by Thomson, Regius Professor of Military Surgery in Edinburgh in 1813. Thomson believed that hospital gangrene was contagious and could be spread by sponges and dressings.[16] A detailed description was given by Blackadder in 1818.[17] He used the term 'phagedaena', or hospital sore, and described it as 'a foul and irritable sore which exhibits a constant disposition to spread and enlarge'. The symptoms were both local and general; Blackadder stated that local signs and symptoms were primary, while general symptoms were usually secondary, occurring a few days later. The infection was identified initially by the presence of one or more small vesicles about the size of a split garden pea. The vesicles contained a watery fluid, which could resemble 'bloody serum' or could be a less vivid, reddish-brown colour. In the course of 1 or 2 days, the appearance changed to a greyish-white, ash-coloured, or brownish-black slough. This extended to cover the whole surface of the original sore. A cavity with well-defined edges may then form which rapidly filled with 'thick glutinous matter'. Progress varied in different individuals, and often the discharge became more copious. The soft parts in the vicinity of the sore became more painful, and acute inflammation supervened. The spongy slough on the sore became more moist and of pulpy consistence. Over a few days, offensive matter is discharged at the edges and the slough begins to separate, preparing the way for extension of the disease by continued ulceration and recurrence of symptoms. During the progress of the disease, muscles and ligaments may be exposed and later destroyed, exposing bone. The disease may vary with the age and type of the original lesion and subsequent treatment; extending slough formation appears to be characteristic, but inflammatory symptoms may be variable.

Blackadder states that in no instance did he observe general symptoms preceding the local symptoms, unless an operation was performed on a stump following amputation for existing infection. Constitutional symptoms may emerge as early as the third or fourth day but sometimes as late as the twentieth day. Blackadder describes these as follows:

The countenance first begins to assume an anxious or feverish aspect, his appetite is impaired and his tongue is covered with a white mucus. His bowels are generally rather constipated and his pulse is rather what may be termed irritated than accelerated, but as formerly noticed with respect to local symptoms, the disease assumes more of an inflammatory, or typhoid character, as the particular causes producing these modifications have been predominant. About the end of the second week when acute inflammation of the sore becomes apparent, rigors with a rapid pulse may occur and if local symptoms progress the patient becomes more exhausted until death occurs. Diarrhoea is not constant, but infrequently occurs hastening the fatal termination.

In the American Civil War, descriptions of hospital gangrene were similar to that above, but the systemic symptoms tended to appear early in the disease; this may be an indication of greater severity rather than a difference in the disease itself.[11] Most descriptions of hospital gangrene include blue or grey spots and vesicles or bullae at the edge of the lesion before the emergence of a spreading greyish or greenish slough and typical appearances of gangrene.

It is likely that hospital gangrene was usually a haemolytic streptococcal infection in view of its resemblance to similar clinical infections described since bacteriological studies have become available and also because of its apparent transmissibility. For example, a more recent description in a 33-year-old woman consisted of a swollen arm and leg in which 'blue patches appeared in the centre of red areas of the skin of the thigh and also large blisters separate from the blue patches from which Lancefield group A haemolytic streptococci were isolated'. The organisms were isolated at postmortem from the bullae and blue necrotic patches, which were filled with dark brown fluid and fat necrosis.[18] If untreated, the blue-black areas slough and reveal subcutaneous tissue. Mortality before the introduction of sulphonamides was high, being 20%. A similar condition, necrotizing faciitis (Chapter 10), still occurs today, albeit rarely, and despite treatment with penicillin and good intensive care therapy, mortality is still high.[19]

Some other infections occurred more frequently than gangrene in hospitals. Erysipelas (red patches of inflamed skin) and cellulitis (a spreading inflammation of the skin or wound) are also caused by Lancefield group A haemolytic streptococci.[6,16] Pyaemia, which consists of a bloodstream infection with multiple abscesses, was the most important cause of hospital infection; this was probably caused mainly by *Staphylococcus aureus* or possibly occasionally a combined infection with haemolytic streptococci.

Civilian hospitals and infection

By the end of the eighteenth century, most provincial hospitals seem to have reached remarkably high standards, although overcrowding was becoming a problem, and many hospitals had to build new wings to accommodate growing populations. In general, hospitals were built on spacious sites, ventilation was good, and hygiene standards were reasonable. All this was achieved as a result of empirical observation and common sense, before there was any real understanding of why such measures should prevent the spread of hospital infections in hospitals.[20]

There has been some controversy over the part played by hospitals in the fall in the death rate during the latter part of the eighteenth century and the beginning of the nineteenth century. Some writers held that their mere existence and the steady rise in the number of beds available must have saved lives.[21] Others, basing their conclusions on the writings of Howard and other contemporaries, considered that infections were so serious a problem that hospitals did more harm than good.[22] Indeed, one author, quoting an earlier commentator, makes the unsupported statement: 'people who went to hospital in the eighteenth century, normally died there, generally of some other disease than that with which they were admitted'.[23] One reason for the bad name acquired by hospitals during this period is that conclusions drawn from the figures for a single hospital at an earlier period were sometimes applied to hospitals generally for a later period. Erichsen,[6] for instance, writing in 1874 about University College Hospital, reported a very high death rate and concluded that the rate must have been much worse in all hospitals in the previous century.

It is only by studying the returns for a number of hospitals for the actual period under review that some idea of the true situation can be obtained. For instance, between 1767 and 1820–21, Salisbury Infirmary treated 19 795 patients, of whom 11 695 (60%) were reported as cured and only 596 (3%) died. At Salop Infirmary, the death rate in 29 161 patients admitted between 1747 and 1846 was 12%. At the Gloucester Infirmary, 38 408 patients were admitted between 1747 and 1835, of whom 31 210 (80%) were cured or relieved.[24] Much more detailed, although inevitably still incomplete, evidence is available for York County Hospital. There, between 1740 and 1743, 90% of 18 717 patients were cured or relieved, as were 89.5% of 35 320 patients admitted between 1784 and 1842. When death rates were published again, in no year between 1825 and 1835 did they exceed 6.3%.[23] Alanson in Liverpool surprisingly reported no deaths in 35 amputations. In his book *On Amputations*, he gives instructions for cleaning and ventilating the wards, for isolating infected patients, and for disinfecting clothing and bedding by baking it in an oven.[25] However, John Bell from Edinburgh describing conditions at the end of the eighteenth century stated: 'our surgical patients are exposed to infection from the medical wards and especially to a disease, the hospital sore. This was likened to a plague, occurring twice a year and also infrequently affecting nurses'.[26] Other surgeons in Edinburgh operating at the same time described hospital gangrene as a minor problem and never in a contagious form. Munro, for instance, in 1832 reported a mortality rate of 8.3%. From the limited figures available, it is difficult to avoid the conclusion that the hospitals of the period, doubtless with some exceptions, especially in London and the larger cities, were astonishingly successful, although there were ominous signs of future problems of infection as the amount of surgery increased.

The arrival of the Industrial Revolution, however, bringing with it mass migration of the population to the cities, appalling living conditions, and gross overcrowding in the slums, led to a sudden massive surge in the demand for hospital beds with which the existing institutions were unable to cope. The number of reports of infection and high mortality increased throughout the nineteenth century. These were often associated with overcrowded hospitals and inadequate ventilation, water supplies and sewerage disposal. Outbreaks of pyaemia, cellulitis, erysipelas, sloughing of wounds and phagedaena were reported at some time in most hospitals. New wards often failed to cope with the problem, and later in the century many hospitals were pulled down and replaced.

In Bristol, for instance, new wards had been added to the infirmary in 1837, but when they were filled up the crisis was dealt with by packing in more beds. By 1863, the beds were 'nowhere more than one and a half feet apart' and two patients were often assigned to one bed. In July 1875, a subcommittee reported that 'septicaemia, erysipelas and every disease which could be caused or fostered by foul air and insanitary conditions were rampant, especially in the surgical wards'.[20] At Leeds General Infirmary, new extensions in 1821 had meant that one ward in rotation could always be kept empty for cleaning and whitewashing; by 1860, however, this was no longer possible and patients were sleeping two to a bed or on the floor, so that the recovery of all was retarded. Eventually, rebuilding on a new site was decided on, resulting in a dramatic improvement in the mortality rate.[24]

Table 6.1. Annual Registrar General's Report of mortality percentages in the principal hospitals of England in 1861

Number and site of hospitals	Number of special patients (8 April 1861)	Mortality (% of patients)
106	12 709	56.87
24 London	4214	90.84
12 Large towns	1870	83.16
25 County and large provincial	2248	39.41
30 Other	1136	40.23
13 Naval and military	3000	15.67
1 Royal Sea Bathing Hospital	133	12.78
1 Metro infirmary (Margate)	108	12.96

Source: Farr.[34,41]

Lawson Tait, a gynaecologist and statistician from Birmingham and a pupil of James Simpson, in his massive statistical survey of British Hospitals published in 1877, selected the new Leeds General Infirmary for special mention.[27] He pointed out that with the same staff and drawing on the same population, the mean length of stay had dropped from 32.6 days in the old hospital to 25.6 days in the new hospital, and that the death rate had fallen by 1.5%, the equivalent of 60 lives saved. He was in little doubt as to the reason for this improvement. The roofs of the old hospital had been low, the beds were crammed together, and the wards smelled. 'Ventilators had been provided, but they were found to be chiefly used by birds for building purposes.' In the new building, there was a margin of 30% of unused beds, and each bed was allocated an area of 106 square feet $(10 \, m^2)$ or 3000 cubic feet $(85 \, m^3)$. Tait also used the Leeds General Infirmary to cast doubt on the theory that the large proportion of accident cases received by the London hospitals, and the consequent high risk of wound infections, accounted for their often high rates of hospital infections when compared with the provincial hospitals. For instance, in a survey carried out in 1863, the mortality in 92 provincial hospitals averaged 7.5%, while that in 18 metropolitan hospitals was 9% (see Table 6.1). But Tait's figures showed that Leeds received more accident cases than many of the London hospitals. In this context, he pointed out that nine hospitals that were devoted entirely to accidents had an average death rate 2% lower than that of the London general hospitals.

At the Norfolk and Norwich Hospital we have, thanks to Dr Michael Beverley, a superb account of the situation in the third quarter of the nineteenth century.[28] Beverley had been appointed House Surgeon to the hospital in 1864 and was elected Assistant Surgeon in 1872. In the previous year, he had been ordered by the Weekly

Board to report to it all deaths in the hospital, together with their causes.[28] It was doubtless this duty that engaged his interest in the subject so deeply that, in 1874, he read a paper at a meeting of the Public Health Section of the British Medical Association entitled 'Hospital hygiene illustrated by references to the Norfolk and Norwich Hospital in the present, past and future'.[29] Up to the date of his appointment, the hospital had had an almost constant death rate of around 5.5% throughout its existence, less than half that of most of the London hospitals and well below many of the provincial ones. It had been famous all over England for the extraordinary success of its surgeons in the most severe operations and was especially well known for lithotomies (surgical removal of bladder stones). During this period, there had been two outbreaks of erysipelas. After the first, in 1829, it was recommended that an extra ward be built to allow the closing of beds for cleaning; however, although this was never done, the outbreak was contained. After further trouble in 1850, the solution was felt to be improvement of the drainage system and the provision of more effective WCs, but this could not be effected until a more adequate water supply could be obtained. In fact, the hospital had to make do with the old system for 16 years, until in 1866 Beverley himself, only 2 years after his appointment as House Surgeon, made representations on the matter to the board of management. Despite the lack of action on this matter at the time, the 1850 erysipelas outbreak was contained.

In the 10 years from 1864 to 1874, the overall proud record of the hospital had deteriorated and the average death rate had risen from 5.5% to 7.7%, still well below that of the London hospitals, but nevertheless worrying. Beverley put the blame for this squarely on the building programme, which had reached its peak at an earlier date. More wards, a board room, a chapel, a museum, a dead-house ('connected with and close to the wards and corridors'), and other facilities had been added in close proximity to the original buildings, cluttering up the site and preventing proper ventilation. 'Far better would have been the history of the latter days of the Hospital', said Beverley, 'had it retained in its hygienic simplicity its pristine form, that of the letter H, which could hardly be recognised in the sadly encumbered edifice of the present'. On top of the reduced standards of ventilation, the growth of the population and the mounting number of accidents had led both to the need for an increasing number of major operations and, although it was directly contraindicated, to overcrowding in the wards. After giving a detailed breakdown of the numbers of pyaemia/septicaemia cases occurring in various classes of operations and amputations, Beverley, becoming ever more impassioned, continued:

Now comes the question, what is to be done for the future? Are the surgeons of the Norfolk and Norwich Hospital to remain content to lose 66 per cent of their amputations for injury, and 10 per cent of their amputations for disease, from causes which are said to be preventable? Is pyaemia to be allowed still to reduce their lithotomy average to the present rate of one in 6.58?

Are there to be no means taken to prevent a recurrence during the next ten years of twenty-four deaths in ninety from pyaemia in the major operations, two in nine in the minor, and sixteen from accidental wounds? Is an annual death rate of four from pyaemia (liable to be increased in any year to seven or even twelve), not to be counteracted? the status quo cannot, must not, be allowed to continue.

He listed the attempts that had already been made to deal with the problem, including the closure and disinfection of wards, the adoption of the antiseptic system (Lister had first published on the subject in 1867), and the reduction in the number of beds. But to no avail. Surgeons were terrified and had almost ceased to operate in the hospital, most operations being carried out in an 'iron hospital' lent by the hospital corporation. Obviously, drastic steps had to be taken to provide premises safe for surgery.

There was much discussion at the time as to the relative merits, medically and financially, of small, single-storey, four- to six-bed wards, such as had been urged by Simpson of Edinburgh 6 years earlier, as against the usual large wards containing 20 or so beds and often two-storeyed. Beverley's drastic solution for the Norfolk and Norwich was to turn the existing building over entirely to chronic medical cases, after first eliminating the overcrowding, improving the ventilation, removing the outpatients department from the centre of the building, and moving the dead-house to a safe distance. Surgical cases, he said, should be housed in a series of single-storeyed wards dotted over the grounds, each holding no more than eight beds. These wards would be emptied, cleaned and disinfected in rotation. A brisk discussion followed Beverley's paper, a number of speakers disagreeing with his ideas, but almost all had encountered similar difficulties in their own hospitals and agreed that extreme hygienic precautions were essential. In the event, Beverley's recommendations were turned down. The Norfolk and Norwich was entirely rebuilt between 1879 and 1883 on an adjacent site and in an uncluttered H-shape. Only one wing of the old building was kept, and in it were housed the museum, the outpatients department and some staffrooms. The dead-house was relegated to a new range of outbuildings on the extreme perimeter of the site. Beverley remained at the hospital for the rest of his working life. In 1888, he was promoted to Full Surgeon, and on his resignation in 1897, after 25 years' service, he was given the rank of Consulting Surgeon.

The story of the Norfolk and Norwich Hospital is typical of that of many other hospitals in the nineteenth century, all of them affected severely by the rapid population increase and the consequent pressure on their wards and rise in the infection rate. Other examples are Manchester Royal Infirmary, Leeds General Infirmary and Lincoln County Hospital, which, like the Norfolk and Norwich, were completely rebuilt. The Bristol Royal Infirmary, Worcester Royal Infirmary and Leicester Royal Infirmary were extensively altered and extended.[20,24]

In 1832, the wards at the Manchester Royal Infirmary were reported to be unhealthy. Wounds became infected and poured pus, the mortality was high, and operations were an appalling risk. The situation had not improved in 1843, when the problems of surgical wards were described as a nightmare. No one knew the cause of infection, nor was it realized that skin inflammatory troubles such as erysipelas could be carried from patient to patient on apparently clean hands and dressings. The mortality was 25%. New wards were opened in 1848, but:

Infection continued and not a single patient after operation escaped erysipelas or some outward subsequent mischief. In consequence of the house surgeon's attention to numerous bad cases in the hospital and the want of dressers, he is confined to bed and quite unable to perform his duties.

Infections continued to be reported. In 1866, there were noted in the surgical wards 21 cases of pyaemia, of which 13 were fatal. In the same year, there were cases of sloughing and phagedaena in June, September and November, with several cases in each of the two latter months. Similar reports continued until 1876,[24] despite the opening of fever and convalescent hospitals following outbreaks in 1868.

Similar problems occurred elsewhere. The first county hospital in Lincoln was opened in 1769 in an existing building previously used for maltings, but a purpose-built hospital was opened in 1777.[30] Initially, problems were few. A surgeon wrote in 1779:

By the exclusion of air many compound fractures, of late years, have been cured in a short time, and with little trouble … It has been generally remarked that the cure of compound fractures does not succeed so well in London hospitals as in the country, where the air is more pure and conducive to health.[24]

However, the increasing numbers of patients caused problems in the following century. The hospital minutes in 1854 indicated a crowded state 'injurious to patients and that their recovery was retarded'. In 1860, the minutes stated: 'The very unsatisfactory condition of the hospital and the fatality after capital and other operations has of late been so great that your medical officers are anxious to avoid them, whilst patients operated in their own homes generally recover'. There was also evidence of defective ventilation and water closets, and a large cesspool in the garden, from which there was 'a continual supply of poisonous gas by regurgitation'. It was also stated that there was only one nurse to 12 patients, and that the night nurses were often old women worn out before their duties commenced. The disinfection of wards was implemented by a Mr Fox. He throughly heated wards, beds and bedding, as 'effectually to destroy disease germs they might be supposed to harbour'. He used three iron cases 4 feet (1.2 m) high and 2 feet (0.6 m) in diameter, and burnt a mixture of coke and coal for 3–4 days, maintaining a temperature of

82 °C or higher in every ward in the hospital. Despite this treatment, the hospital had to be closed.

T. Sympson states in his book that, due to the growth in the population by 1871, it was difficult to preserve purity in wards and prevent emanations from cesspools, and the water supply was polluted.[30] Hence, there arose outbreaks of pyaemia, erysipelas, sloughing of wounds and intractable diarrhoea not coincident with epidemics of similar infections outside of the walls. Bristowe and Holmes in 1863 stated that the hospital was inadequate and could not be brought up to modern requirements.[31] In the following year, the surgical staff described 'the present unhealthy conditions and high mortality among the patients'. A Mr Hewison advised rebuilding the hospital as the only means of getting rid of disease from his cases. A new hospital was opened in 1878, but no information is available on improvements in numbers of infections.

One of the oldest hospitals in England is St Mary's Hospital, Chichester. It reputedly came into existence in the second half of the twelfth century. Although built originally for the care of the sick as well as the poor, it mainly housed the poor; it still exists today as an almshouse. The first purpose-built hospital in Chichester, the Royal West Sussex, opened in 1826. Although only a small hospital (58 beds in 1864), it suffered the same problems as larger hospitals at this time, such as poor ventilation, imperfect drainage, and an inadequate water supply. Financial crises were common, such as the need to replace wooden floors that had rotted due to frequent scrubbing. The hospital was closed in 1864 due to an outbreak of smallpox. In 1879, cases of scarlet fever of a 'peculiarly modified type and deadly contagious and infectious' were identified. This led to a consideration of new accommodation for the treatment of infectious diseases.

In 1834, a report from Birmingham General Hospital stated: 'in consequence of the prevalence of erysipelas amongst patients during part of the past years, it has been thought desirable to cause the hospital to undergo a thorough purification. This is completed and the house is now quite free from infectious complaints'.[32] However, in 1857–8, the annual report stated that 'beds in almost all of the wards are still closely crowded and the operation theatre and "chapel" are too small and inconvenient for the increased number of patients'. In 1859, it is stated that 'the inevitable results of overcrowding lengthened the period occupied in the process of cure and from time to time the appearance of diseases of a low order'. In 1860, it was reported that there were 'no less than 10 burned children in a ward containing 4 beds'. The 1862–3 report stated 'in December last the Medical Board called the attention of the Weekly Board to the bad sanitary state of the hospital, as manifested by the unhealthy appearance of wounds, etc, and the slow recovery of patients suffering from them'. Phagedaena first appeared in the annual reports in 1861–2, in which 23 cases were recorded. This was followed by 20 cases in 1862–3 and two cases in

1864–5. There were reports of four further cases in outpatients in 1864–5 and five cases in 1865–6, but it was not mentioned again after 1866, although erysipelas appeared to be quite common from the 1850s to 1883, usually with about 20–30 cases per year. Cellulitis was not mentioned until 1855–6, when there were 25 cases in inpatients. Pyaemia was also mentioned infrequently, but 11 cases were reported in 1865–6 and subsequently only the occasional case in an outpatient. There was obviously a problem of all types of surgical infection between 1860 and 1866, but it is not known whether the disappearance of these was associated with the erection of a new wing that included a fever ward.

A lecturer at Leeds General Infirmary, T. Nunnelly, stated there was hardly a large hospital in which erysipelas had not been responsible for closing the whole or part of the ward.[33] He mentioned St Thomas's, St George's, Leeds General Infirmary, Birmingham General Hospital and Edinburgh Royal Infirmary. He attempted to distinguish this from hospital gangrene, which he considered to be infrequent, rarely severe or occurring as an epidemic in civilian practice.

Problems of gangrene and outbreaks of erysipelas occurred at York, where the hospital was closed for 2 months in 1859. In 1863–5, several cases of sloughing of wounds were reported at the beginning of an outbreak, and in 1886, 21 cases of pyaemia (13 fatal) and cases of phagedaena occurred. In 1867, hospital gangrene, erysipelas and pyaemia were still present in the surgical wards; in 1868, eight cases of hospital gangrene occurred, but no cases were reported after this year. In general, pyaemia was a greater problem than hospital gangrene; following amputations e.g. in 1859, pyaemia was responsible for deaths in 42% of all fatal cases following amputation.[24]

Outbreaks were therefore variable and could occur in hospitals with good air and ventilation; for example, the governors of St George's Hospital reported that phagedaena had been exceedingly prevalent during the 1860s.

Florence Nightingale continued her campaign on improving hygiene and design of hospitals on her return from the Crimea.[34] She used William Farr's figures to show that mortality was higher in the large London hospitals than in the smaller provincial hospitals (see Table 6.1). Although her interpretation of the figures was probably flawed, the conclusions were supported later by Sir James Simpson. She concluded that it was much safer to be treated at home. Despite her efforts to improve general hygiene, she still continued to believe in miasmas and never accepted, even in later years, the germ theory or the value of antiseptics.

Nightingale decried the use of the term 'contagion' because it implied the existence of certain germs and stated that there is 'no end to the absurdities connected to this doctrine. There is no proof that there is any such thing as contagion'. Nevertheless, she also stated that 'careful observers are convinced that the origin and spread of fever, appearance of hospital gangrene, erysipelas and pyaemia generally

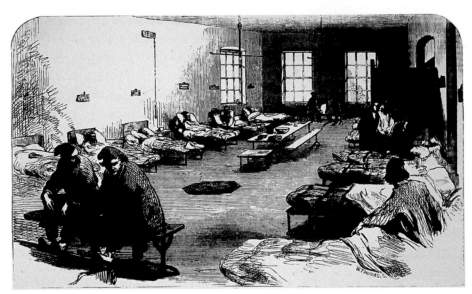

Figure 6.3   A ward in the military hospital, Portsea, in the nineteenth century. (*Illustrated London News.* Wellcome Library, London.)

are much better tests of the defective sanitary state of the hospital than mortality returns'.

Her belief in miasmas made her concentrate on hospital design and reducing the number of people under one roof. She described the Hôtel Dieu in Paris in 1788 as having 550 beds on a single floor with direct atmospheric communication between them. The whole hospital contained 1200 beds, and each bed contained two to four patients. One in four patients died, and the mortality after amputation was 60%. Wounds were washed daily with a sponge that went from patient to patient, and all were infected. She provided detailed instructions on optimal sizes of wards and numbers of beds, preferring pavilion-type wards. Fresh air, light and ample space were essential. Many plans of hospitals were included in her book. She also believed that good records should be kept of surgical operations, including registration of age, sex, occupation, date of accident or operation, constitution of the patient, and complications.

As an example, Nightingale described a hospital in which 800 operations were carried out, with 141 complications, 66 of which were referable to pyaemia, erysipelas, suppuration, gangrene or bedsores. Of 140 fatal operations, many deaths were due to infection. She appealed for a uniform system of publishing statistical records because, having applied everywhere for information, in scarcely an instance was she able to obtain hospital records fit for purposes of comparison. Nightingale identified the relevance of different infection risk factors in providing statistics, and her

Table 6.2. Mortality after limb amputations in Great Britain by size of hospital and degree of aggregation or isolation of patients

Size of hospital (number of beds)	Mortality
300–600	1 in 2½
100–300	1 in 4
25–100	1 in 5½
Fewer than 25	1 in 7
Cottage hospitals (isolated rooms in country practice)	1 in 9
Hôtel Dieu (Paris)	1 in 1½

Source: Simpson.[36–38]

statement on the problems of comparability of infection rates is still true today. The point on comparability of records in different hospitals was the subject of many arguments between surgeons during the latter half of the nineteenth century.

Sir James Simpson (1811–70), Professor of Midwifery at Edinburgh, was a pioneer in the study of hospital infection and one of the first men to highlight and attempt to explain the worsening situation in the country.[35] In his first publication on the subject of hospital fever in 1859, he stated that the probable route of spread of infection was by way of surgeons and nurses. He carried out a study on amputations in hospitals of various sizes and locations, and confirmed the results of Farr that mortality was related to the size of the hospital and degree of overcrowding. He stated that the risk was least in well-ventilated hospitals, and he believed that the fabric of the hospital was important.

He considered that amputation wounds provided a valid comparison as the operation was performed easily. He predicted that amputations carried out in rural hospitals were five times more likely to be successful than those carried out in a large city (see Table 6.2).[36–38] The overall results showed that the mortality of all amputations of upper and lower limbs in rural private practice was 10.8%, whereas that in the large hospitals of the metropolis and elsewhere was 41%. He believed a change was necessary to redress this balance. His study left him in no doubt about the dangers of large, crowded hospitals, and he put forward proposals for small cottage-hospital-type wards to ease the problem. He continued to work on hospital infection until his death, and it was he who, in 1869, coined the word 'hospitalism' to cover hospital-acquired septic infections.

Simpson's results and those of Nightingale and Farr were not accepted universally. A major critic was Holmes, a London surgeon, who commented that 'Sir James

Table 6.3. Infections admitted to and acquired in St George's Hospital 1865–8

Date	Infection	Cases acquired in hospital	Admitted to hospital
1865	Erysipelas	8	18
1868	Erysipelas	19	15
1865	Sloughing and phagedaena	29	22
1868	Sloughing and phagedaena	1	5
1865	Pyaemia	18	2
1868	Pyaemia	22	3

Source: Holmes.[39,40]

Simpson's name weighs far more than his arguments'.[39,40] He suggested that the rural figures consisted of small numbers of cases for disease that uniformly proved successful, and many of the amputations for injury were altogether different from those in London practice. As an example, four surgeons in a rural practice reported no deaths in 125 cases, a result that would be miraculous elsewhere. The length of stay in hospital was variable. In 1862, the hospital in Exeter with 233 beds showed a mortality of 28%, whereas Chichester, with 56 beds, showed a mortality of 50%, and a larger proportion of severe injuries were admitted to Guy's and St Bartholomew's hospitals than in rural hospitals. Infection was not only a hospital disease since the poor of London acquired most of their infections at home. Between 1865 and 1868, 80 cases of erysipelas were admitted from private homes and 43 acquired the infection in hospital; 60 cases of phagedaena were acquired in hospital and 55 were admitted with it; 81 cases of pyaemia were acquired in hospital and only nine were admitted with the infection. Erysipelas was mainly a community infection, whereas pyaemia was mainly hospital-acquired (see Table 6.3). It is surprising that so many cases of phagedaena were apparently acquired in the community. The exposure of the London hospitals to infection was obviously considerable, but infection was not the only cause of postoperative mortality.

The problems of 'hospitalism' were well reviewed by Erichsen, a surgeon at University College Hospital in a series of lectures in 1874.[6] He described 80 amputations of limbs between 1870 and 1873. Twenty-one died, of which nine deaths were from pyaemia. He defined 'hospitalism' as a 'septic influence occurring to a greater extent in hospital or any large building where large numbers of wounded or injured persons are aggregated under one roof'. Pyaemia and erysipelas were the most important infections, and he had not seen an outbreak of hospital gangrene in University College Hospital for 20 years. Pyaemia was considered to be a hospital disease and was due to septic permeation of a ward with organic atmospheric matter. He did not state that it was contagious, but nevertheless cases were isolated rapidly. Erysipelas was the most common septic disease, but it was not confined

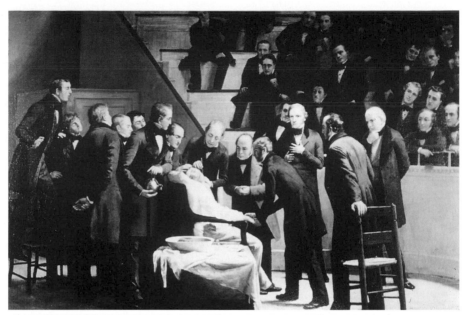

Figure 6.4   One of the first operations with the use of an anaesthetic, performed at the Massachusetts General Hospital, Boston, in 1846, showing the surgical team in everyday clothing and a large number of spectators in a gallery. (From a picture by Robert Hinckley in Boston Medical School. Wellcome Library, London.)

to hospital to the same extent as pyaemia. Erichsen accepted that erysipelas was contagious and was influenced by overcrowding and the weather and an 'epidemic influence'. It resembled puerperal fever in that it could be transferred by students from the dissecting room. He also talked about 'runs of luck' in a hospital when it remained healthy.

Despite his concern for miasmas, many of his recommendations suggest that contact spread was important, for instance isolation of all patients with septic disease, purification of bedding, removing patients' clothes, no personal communication between dissecting room and wards, and abundant carbonized water for washing.

The debate between Simpson and Holmes and their protagonists on hospitalism continued without agreement,[41] and a report in a leading article in the *Lancet* in 1869 concluded that 'it may well be the time for seriously considering the necessity for special arrangements in our hospitals for the treatment of all surgical cases with large wounds in single-bedded wards of cheap and temporary construction'. However, this argument was largely overtaken by the work of Lister, who achieved a considerable reduction in wound infection, often in rather doubtful environmental conditions (see Chapter 8).

The mortality from infected wounds was an even greater problem in many European hospitals.[42,43] The conditions in the Hôtel Dieu have already been described. Malgaigne (1806–65) published a mean mortality rate in amputation cases of 60%. Bilroth in Zurich reported that 'only 40%' of his amputation cases died. In Nussbaum's clinic in Munich it was stated by Lindpainter that '80% of wounds were affected by gangrene, and erysipelas was such an everyday occurrence that it could almost have been treated as a normal development. Eleven of 17 amputation cases died of pyaemia'.

Theories of infection: from miasmas to microbes

By the end of the seventeenth century, the idea that disease was a visitation from a punitive god that could only be cured by the intervention of that god after he had been suitably propitiated had been largely superseded by more materialistic and 'scientific' explanations. Other traditional ideas were, however, slower to disappear, one being the belief in the essential unity of all fevers. It was only as theories of the causation of fever came and went that it was slowly recognized that fever was a symptom of many diseases, not a disease in itself.[1] Ideas on the epidemiology of infectious fevers continued to evolve over the eighteenth century.

Throughout that century, the four main causes of epidemics were considered to be (1) the 'epidemic constitution' of the atmosphere, (2) local 'miasmatic' conditions brought about by climate, season, diseased bodies and putrefying organic matter, (3) contagion, and (4) variation in the vital resistance of individuals, the last being only a vague assumption used to explain extraordinary individual cases.[2]

The epidemic constitution of the atmosphere was used to explain the sudden onset of an epidemic in a previously healthy community; its qualities were considered to be undiscoverable and in any case beyond human control. For practical purposes, therefore, miasmas and contagion were the two theories on which preventive measures had to be based.

At the beginning of the eighteenth century, aerial transmission, whether over comparatively long or very short distances, was regarded by the medical profession to be of prime importance; contagion, either direct or indirect via fomites (inanimate objects), was only a secondary consideration. There were good reasons for the resistance of the medical profession to the contagion theory at a time when laymen, watching the plague spread from country to country and seaport to seaport, accepted it readily enough. The physicians knew that the theory as it then stood could not explain all the facts. Contagion, before the germ theory of disease, was thought to be due to the direct or indirect transfer of inanimate, poisonous particles from the diseased person to a healthy person, and doctors knew that there were many outbreaks for which this theory could not hold. For instance, epidemics could begin in new localities that had no known contact with any sick person, and could die out just as inexplicably without spreading further. Until it was accepted that living organisms were implicated in epidemic disease, and that transmission could occur by means of asymptomatic human and animal carriers, and through infected food and water, contagion could never be accepted by the medical profession as an adequate explanation for the transmission of infectious disease: hence, the emphasis throughout the century on thorough ventilation as the factor of overriding importance in the prevention of outbreaks of infectious disease in hospitals, jails, ships, army camps and other enclosed environments.[2]

It was Richard Mead who first put forward the idea that contagion was at least as important as aerial transmission, i.e. miasmas, in the spread of epidemics. Mead was a leading London physician when, in 1719, panic arose in England following an outbreak of plague in Marseilles. The Secretary of State asked Mead to report on whether the disease was a contagion that could be prevented from entering the country by quarantine measures, or a disease that was periodically generated in the atmosphere, as Sydenham had taught, and therefore beyond human control. Mead's studies were first published in 1720 (revised in 1744) and were a milestone in epidemiological thought.[3] Remarkably, although he had been asked specifically about the importance of the epidemic constitution of the atmosphere, he neither approved it nor combated it in his report; he simply barely mentioned it. His own theory he stated succinctly: 'Contagion [i.e. infection] is propagated by three causes, the air, diseased persons and goods transported from infected places'. If 'persons' and 'goods' are considered in the light of modern knowledge as a single cause, we are left with two causes: air and contagion. Mead enlarged upon this:

> Those who are strangers to the full power of [contagion], that is, those who do not understand how subtle it is, and how widely the distemper may be spread by infection, ascribe the rise of it wholly to the malignant quality of the air while others exclude all consideration of the air, but the contagion accompanying the disease, and the disposition of the air to promote that contagion, ought equally to be considered; both being necessary to give the distemper full force.[3]

As in earlier times, Mead had described miasmas as air corrupted by 'the stinks of stagnating water in hot weather, exhalations from the earth; and above all, the corruption of dead carcass's lying unburied'. But although miasmas could carry the poisons of plague over short distances, they could neither generate them nor carry them far without them being so diluted as to be rendered harmless. Mead quoted instances to illustrate his point. He concluded that quarantine was most important in preventing the onslaught of plague in England, and he so advised the Secretary of State.

Mead believed that plague, together with certain other infectious diseases, was endemic in southern and eastern parts of the world where the climate was especially suited to them, and that they were transmitted to colder climates either from person to person or through commerce:

For they have such force, that they may spread their pernicious seeds by emitting very subtle particles; which lighting on soft spongy substances, such as cotton, wool, raw silk, and clothing, penetrate into them, and there remain pent-up for a considerable time.[3]

Mead found no need to resort to the epidemic constitution of the atmosphere. Unlike his contemporaries, although he saw contagion as an essential prerequisite to the spread of plague, he was perfectly correct in agreeing with them that, on the evidence available, it could not account for all outbreaks. In the absence of modern knowledge of the part played by fleas and rats, some other explanation had to be found, and infection by means of miasmas as a secondary cause was entirely logical. But this concession was insufficient for some of his fellow workers. For instance, George Pye made a fierce attack on Mead's theory of contagion because it could not account for all the facts.[4]

Mead was much in advance of his time in another matter, namely his emphasis on the individual specificity of the plague and other infectious diseases. Fracastoro had hinted at this in the sixteenth century, but in the seventeenth century, Sydenham and many other workers still held the idea that most fevers were a single entity and could transmute from one form to another, depending on circumstances, a belief that continued to hold sway long after Mead's time.

John Pringle (see Chapters 3 and 4) was well acquainted with Mead's ideas, for in 1750 he addressed a monograph to him in which he referred to 'the authority of your own excellent writings on infectious diseases', and he proceeded to develop these ideas further. Pringle's military experiences are described elsewhere. Here, we must consider the theory of infection that grew out of his experiences not only with typhus but also with dysentery and scabies, which were brought into the hospitals from the camps. In the introduction to his account of his experiences, *Observations on the Diseases of the Army*,[5] Pringle made the following uncompromising statement: 'Among the chief causes of sickness and death in the army, the reader will little expect that I should rank, what is intended for its health and preservation, the hospitals themselves; and that on account of the bad air and other inconveniences attending them.'

Pringle went on to insist on free ventilation and the wide spacing of beds to eliminate the effects of 'bad air' and effluvia. The latter, he considered, could spread disease by contact, but not at a distance because, as Mead had postulated, they would be diluted until they could cause no harm. He strongly advocated cleanliness to control these effluvia, and made pertinent comments on the difficulty of persuading staff to keep up high standards of hygiene. However, it was on ventilation and the dispersal of patients that he laid the greatest emphasis.

Pringle, of course, adhered to the generally accepted theory that infection was spread by miasmas containing the poisonous particles from the putrid exhalations of the sick. But by 1764, his thoughts had taken a new turn. He had just read a dissertation by Linnaeus in which that author wrote favourably of Kircher's theory that living animalcules were the cause of disease. Pringle announced his intention to 'suspend all hypotheses, till that matter is further inquired into'. In the case of scabies, however, he came down unequivocally in support of Leeuwenhoek's 'certain small insects' as its cause, remarking that 'of all places the hospitals are most liable to the contagion, as receiving all sorts of patients'.

Pringle left the army in 1748 and settled down to private practice in London. It was at this time that Mead asked him to publish his experiences. That year, there was a disastrous outbreak of jail fever at the assizes, in which the judge himself was a casualty. Pringle considered that 'he could not comply more seasonably with your desire . . . than by communicating at present, that part of my observations, which related to this disease'. His advice was to wash the prisoners, and to destroy their own clothes and give them new ones before taking them to court, 'but if this method is not taken . . . the greatest security would arise from the use of ventilators', thus putting more emphasis on hygiene than ventilation, a slightly different approach from that in his writings on military hospitals.[6]

Like Mead, Pringle believed that climate affected the virulence of diseases, as did dispersal of the poisonous particles. For instance, he wrote that the true plague, 'with its subtle and diffusive virulence, can never be first produced in these climates'. In the case of 'malignant fevers', he took this idea a step further for he was convinced that when they passed from military hospitals to towns, 'it has always been with a lesser degree of violence, the contagious matter being weakened'.

Pringle's slightly younger contemporary, James Lind, did for the naval medical services what his senior had done for the army.[7] Lind was physician to the Haslar Naval Hospital near Portsmouth; his work on typhus is described more fully in Chapter 4, but here we can note how, compared with Pringle, he changed the emphasis on the relative importance of ventilation and hygiene in the control of infectious disease. On the basis of his own observations, Lind stated categorically in 1757 that typhus was not spread through the air and was not affected by ventilation; it could not even be contracted from the clean bodies of patients, but only from their filthy rags of clothes and bedding.

In 1771, William Alexander reported on some extensive laboratory experiments, which he carried out on the causes of 'putrid diseases'. He dedicated his study to John Pringle.[8] Alexander was well versed in the works of both Kircher and Mead, and his experiments were derived directly from those of Kircher. The underlying tenet of his investigations was the belief, commonly held at the time, that the mechanism of putrefaction was identical with that which caused 'putrid disease' of the living, and that both were forms of fermentation. But fermentation could also be beneficial, as in the digestion of food. Alexander held that if he could discover the mechanism of putrefaction, he would be well on the way to understanding the causes of putrid disease. With this in mind, he proceeded to investigate the effects of phenomena such as heat and moisture; putrid vegetable and mixed effluvia – whether they were septic or antiseptic; animalcules – whether they were the cause or effect of putrefaction; and the effect of various 'extraordinary' causes and particular states of the atmosphere. As a result of his temperature experiments on both live animals and meat, he came to the conclusion that heat alone did not necessarily bring on putrefaction or disease, but that the process probably started at 90–100 °F (33–38 °C). Moisture he decreed to be necessary for putrefaction in dead animals, but he could draw no inference for living ones. As to putrid (animal) effluvia, he agreed with Pringle that they could spread disease, but he could not make up his mind about mixed effluvia (from stagnating marshes), on which he proposed further work. Damaged and mouldy food he considered might weaken the patient but was unlikely to be a cause of disease. His experiments on animalcules were extensive, including the microscopic study of the liquids involved. He tended to disagree with the great botanist Linnaeus, who had been carrying out similar experiments, believing that the objects he saw in those liquids were probably the result of putrefaction rather than the cause; in this he was factually correct, for his microscope would not have been of high enough power to have disclosed bacteria. However, he made no dogmatic assertion to this end, and he obviously still had an open mind at the end of his experiments. Finally, he came to the conclusion that the 'states of the atmosphere' were probably not the 'proximate cause of any putrid distemper in this country'. But he held to the still prevalent view of the mutability of the fevers, rejecting Mead's pioneering suggestion that each was a separate and distinct disease; for he continued in explanation of his conclusion:

> ... as distempers of any kind are apt to change their nature, and to be transformed into others quite different from what they were originally; and as the atmosphere of this country has frequently been the cause of diseases of diverse kinds, when these have changed into putrid ones, the air has often been said to be the cause of them.[8]

Alexander finished his substantial book with a chapter headed 'An attempt to explain how putrefaction acts upon the living animal'. The core of his theory, as we have seen, was the importance of the fermentative, or putrefaction, process, not only in the corruption of dead organic matter, where it could be seen to take place, but in the putrid diseases as well, a theory not uncommon at the time. His starting point was the favourable effect of the fermentation of food in the stomach. It was only when this was overcome by the inhalation of putrid miasmas, which set up an unfavourable fermentation, that disease set in as the resultant poisons spread around the body.

Later in the century, a Frenchman, Guyton-Morveau,[9] writing as an old man in 1802 of his experiences 25 years earlier, was still concerned with miasmas and effluvia, apparently agreeing with Pringle that they were of equal importance with contagion in the spread of infectious diseases: 'Febrile contagions...may all be propagated by actual contact with infected persons, or things, or by breathing air charged with effluvia, whether proceeding from substances charged with contagious virus, or from patients labouring under pestilential disease'.

But Thomas Beddoes of Bristol, writing a year later on his conclusions on the transmission of fevers, made an important distinction between different fevers.[10] He fully accepted Lind's thesis that typhus could be spread only by contagion, stating specifically that the occasional case of apparent infection over a distance could always be traced to contact with infected clothing or sheets. He cited especially the 'miasmatist' opposition to a proposal to build a fever ward close to Newcastle Infirmary, pointing out that they could give no reason for their fears. However, he went on to state that 'intermittent and remittent fevers [malaria] in most cases spring from marsh exhalations, the concurrence of numerous observations compels us to believe [this]', thus accepting that different fevers could be transmitted in different ways and at least partially laying to rest the idea of the unity of all fevers.

It was during the nineteenth century that the contest between the miasmatists and the contagionists, and between those two groups and those who believed in the mutability of fevers and in spontaneous generation, reached its climax. One of the earliest physicians to oppose the miasmatists was Alexander Gordon of Aberdeen (see Chapter 5).[11] Most of his career was spent as a naval surgeon, but from 1786 to 1795 he practised and taught in his home city, taking a special interest in puerperal fever. After studying a series of 77 cases in cotton workers at a mill 2 miles from the city, he showed conclusively that all the cases were in those women who had been nursed by midwives drafted in from the city, where the disease was raging; women nursed by country midwives remained healthy. In 1795, he wrote: 'the cause of the puerperal fever...was a specific contagion, or infection, altogether unconnected with a noxious constitution of the atmosphere'.[12]

On the other side of the Atlantic, the field of battle was yellow fever (now known to be a virus infection spread by the bite of the mosquito *Aedes aegypti*). Devastating outbreaks of the disease had occurred sporadically in the USA all through the eighteenth century, and in 1793 a particularly severe one occurred in Philadelphia. Benjamin Rush, who was born near Philadelphia, went to Scotland, where he graduated in medicine at Edinburgh in 1768, then returned to his home town and set up in practice. Very soon, he was elected to two chairs at the College of Physicians and then became a physician at the city's hospital. He was involved in many aspects of the medical life of the city, but he is remembered chiefly for his contribution to the controversy over yellow fever.[2]

His first idea was that the outbreak originated in a damaged consignment of coffee putrefying on one of the city's wharves. The port physician disagreed, considering it to be of local origin attributable to 'morbid exhalations' from putrefying vegetable matter in local ponds and marshes. Rush then changed his mind and wrote to agree with the port official. Furthermore, he recognized two routes of infection: a primary miasmatic route involving exhalations, which could infect over a distance of 300–400 yards (300–400 m), and a secondary 'contagion', which could only travel across the width of a street.

The College of Physicians, however, believed (rightly, as we now know) that the disease had been imported by the ship bringing the coffee, pointing out, among other things, that some of the crew already had the disease when they arrived. Rush gave ten reasons for his belief in its indigenous origin, including the fact that in the West Indies (believed by the college to be the source of the infection) it occurred only where marsh exhalations were present, and that it was 'only a higher degree of a fever, which prevails every year in our city from vegetable putrefaction'. Here, Rush was accepting the still commonly held view of the unity of fevers, that the severe forms were merely a progression from the less severe. In the case of yellow fever, he considered that it was a more violent manifestation of 'bilious remitting fever', which in turn was a severe form of the common 'intermitting fever' produced by marsh miasmas. He even fought the idea of the specificity of fevers in print: 'Science has much to deplore from the multiplication of diseases. It is as repugnant to truth in medicine, as polytheism is to truth in religion.'[2]

Despite the fact that Rush changed his opinion on the source of the outbreak of yellow fever, his continued belief in contagion as a secondary form of infection (a dual view that would be common in the profession for many years) led him for a time to advocate the retention of quarantine procedures. But again he changed his mind. By 1799, he was laying such great stress on the epidemic constitution of the atmosphere as well as on putrefying organic matter that he was vehemently opposing maritime quarantine. In 1805, he made absolutely clear his final verdict on the epidemiology of the disease by publishing as essay entitled 'Facts intended to prove the Yellow Fever not to be contagious'.[2]

In Europe, a similar battle was raging, but here the struggle had economic and political, as well as medical, aspects. It was, of course, the belief in contagion that led to the imposition of quarantines both at seaports and inland, and this had resulted in a growing bureaucracy, limitations in trade, and financial loss.[13] Episodes such as the great French cholera epidemic of 1832, when quarantines and cordons completely failed to suppress its spread, provided all the evidence the anticontagionists needed for the futility of those precautions,[13] and quarantines gradually fell into disuse.

In England, the great sanitary reformer Edwin Chadwick was a thoroughgoing anticontagionist believing implicitly in the miasma theory. In his case, the belief resulted in an all-encompassing attack on London's filth and the disease-producing miasmas to which he considered it gave rise. His report, the *Sanitary Condition of the Labouring Population of Great Britain*, published for the Poor Law Commission in 1842, stated explicitly: 'Yet almost all [types of insanitary conditions] will be found to point to one particular, namely, atmospheric impurity . . . as the main cause of the ravages of epidemic, endemic and contagious diseases among the community'.[2]

The importance attributed in that period to filth and the miasmas to which it gave rise can probably be explained by the almost total lack of sanitation and the resultant stench that prevailed not only in the city slums but also in the better-off districts. At a time when the horse was the only means of transport, mountains of manure accumulated outside stables before eventually being carted away to the countryside. Street cleaning, if it took place at all, rarely kept place with the fouling. In the slums, cows were kept in basements and slaughterhouses were common. Until Chadwick took matters in hand, all sewers were open. While we now know that in these conditions disease was spread by direct contact and by flies, it is easy to see that to contemporaries, the time-honoured explanation of infective miasmas was perfectly satisfactory and was, indeed, reinforced when epidemic disease was reduced, even if not eliminated, following massive clean-up operations.[2] Measles and smallpox and, more recently, typhus (as a result of the work of James Lind) were the only diseases then recognized as contagious.

At about the same time that Chadwick was engaged in his drastic sanitary measures in England, F.G.J. Henle (1809–85) in Germany was also working on problems of epidemic disease. After taking his doctor's degree in Heidelberg and Bonn in 1832, Henle obtained the Chair of Anatomy at Zurich in 1840; in the same year, he published the results of his studies. It was he who realized at least that miasma and contagion theories were not mutually exclusive. He divided epidemic and endemic diseases into three groups: those that were solely miasmatic, of which malaria was the only known example; those that started as miasmatic but became contagious, such as smallpox, measles, typhus, cholera, plague and dysentery; and those that were solely contagious, such as syphilis and some skin diseases. He concluded that 'the matter of contagiousness is not only organic, but also indeed endowed with individual life and that contagion of infectious disease is a matter which may float in the air'.[14]

This ending of the conflict between miasmatists and contagionists allowed investigations to begin into the real nature of that ancient concept, the miasma.[2] Henle took another big step forwards when he proposed to combine the two aspects of the miasmatic-contagious diseases under the single term, 'infective material', stating unequivocally that this material was specific for each disease and that it could not arise spontaneously, thus undermining further the ideas of the mutability of the fevers and of spontaneous generation.

A few years later in England in 1849, John Snow, a Yorkshire-born but London-trained doctor, published a pamphlet entitled 'On the mode of communication of cholera,'[2] in which he came to the conclusion that, because the early symptoms are intestinal, the disease must be of alimentary rather than of atmospheric origin. A definitive edition of the essay followed in 1855, after he had studied further epidemics, in particular the infamous outbreak at Broad Street, Westminster, which he showed incontrovertibly to have been due to drinking contaminated water obtained from the street pump. As a result of his observations, Snow, like Henle, was left in no doubt that each disease had a specific cause, and that each cause had a specific mode of transmission. He went further in all but denying the spontaneous generation of diseases. He believed that in virtually every case, if the cause of the infection was known, then the origin of each outbreak could be traced. Only in the case of erysipelas did he allow that it might appear spontaneously around an open wound. Snow's great contemporary, William Budd of Bristol, came to similar conclusions about cholera as had Snow, and at about the same time, although he did not publish until 1859. It is for his work on typhoid fever, however, that he is justly famous, for it was he who first showed that the 'poison' is contagious and is carried in the diarrhoeal discharges.[2,14]

By the mid-1850s, the age-old concept of the miasma had almost been superseded by modern scientific ideas, as had the belief in the mutability of the fevers. The theory of spontaneous generation, although it took much longer to die, was slowly losing its adherents. For many years, acute observers had been coming up with the idea that living organisms that could reproduce themselves were, in fact, the cause of communicable disease. A Frenchman, Pierre Bretonneau, was one of the first.[14] He showed in 1821 that diphtheria was caused by a specific germ that produced that disease alone, and no other, although he was unable to see the organism. The next important step was taken by Agostini Bassi, an Italian civil servant, in 1835. He was working on the economically important muscardine disease of silkworms, which is infectious and fatal to the caterpillars. After many years of study, he was able to show that it was caused by a parasitic fungus, now known as *Beauvaria bassiana*. What is more, Bassi realized that he had made a discovery of fundamental importance to the whole concept of infectious disease, for he wrote:

This production of mine ought to interest not only the breeder of silkworms, but also all the cultivators of the natural sciences, it being capable, perhaps, of removing some of the many anomalies which the doctrine of contagions, such as variola [smallpox], petechia, pest, syphilis etc. are produced by vegetable or animal parasitic entities, but also that many, not to say all, of the cutaneous diseases are due to the same cause.[12,14]

Bassi was born in Mairago near Lodi and studied natural science in Padua. He held several posts under the French and Austrian governments before retiring due to ill health. He continued with the help of a legacy and wrote on a number of subjects in addition to silkworm disease and contagion, including cultivation of potatoes, wine, cheese and pellagra.

Four years after Bassi's discovery, J.L. Schoenlein (1793–1854), a German clinical pathologist, in a paper of only 20 lines became the first man to attribute a human disease to a specific micro-organism when he showed that the scalp infection, favus, was caused by the fungus now known as *Trichophyton schoeleini*.[14] That the first two diseases to have been proved to have been of parasitic origin were mycoses is no coincidence but is accounted for by their greater size compared with bacteria. Although the achromatic objective (a type of lens) had to a great extent already been perfected by Lister's father, Joseph Jackson Lister, in 1826, it would be a few years before the full results of those technical advances become apparent.

In the middle of the nineteenth century, medical opinion was still divided between those who believed that diseases were caused by micro-organisms entering the body from outside, and those who adhered to the old fermentation theories, in which zymes or ferments produced poisonous secretions, which were the ultimate cause of the symptoms. The theory of spontaneous generation still had a firm hold on the medical profession as late as 1864 according to no less an authority than the *British Medical Journal*. Indeed, Murchison, in his authoritative work of 1873, could account for the outbreak of a limited number of epidemics in no other way.[15]

Since most surgeons still believed in miasmas throughout much of the nineteenth century, it is not surprising that overcrowding and poor ventilation in hospital wards were considered to be the main factors in the spread of infection. However, it was recognized by some doctors that overcrowding was also likely to be associated with the spread of infection by contact. Spread by direct or indirect contact spread was suggested following the statement by Fracastoro in 1546, and since then many others had suggested the possible importance of cleanliness of hands and instruments in the spread of wound infection. In particular, the early military and naval practices of Pringle and Lind, as described previously, had a continuing influence, although not as great as might have been expected, on future practice.

Pouteau in 1772 in the Hôtel Dieu in Lyons pricked his finger whilst working on a cadaver. The finger became inflamed and gangrenous and he surmized that infection was contagious (see Chapter 8). He was also the first to demonstrate the erysipelatous nature of puerperal fever and gangrene, recognizing the similarity beween them. He observed that reused, inadequately washed dressings could be responsible for disease in a wound and, on the basis of these observations, insisted on clean hands for preparing dressings and carrying out operations.[16,17]

Rollo, a French surgeon, concluded following observations on military casualties that infection was spread by contact and that a 'sponge could spread sores'. Ollivier, a surgeon in Napoleon's army in Spain, in 1810 carried out experiments in which he inoculated himself with a lancet dipped in pus from a soldier dying from 'pourriture', a contagious emanation from wound discharge. He contracted a severe cellulitis (spreading inflammatory area on skin) extending to the axilla.[16,17]

Thomson stated that he believed hospital gangrene was contagious and could be spread on wound sponges, dressings and clothing, and that cases should be isolated in one ward.[18] Others, such as Blackadder, also recognized that spread by contact was a major route. Blackadder stated that most cases of wound infection were produced by 'a direct application of mortified matter to the wounds or sores through the medium of syringes, instruments, dressings, etc.'[19] He describes an experimental situation in which three patients with clean wounds were placed alternately in beds between three other patients severely affected by 'phegedaena'. The beds were not more than 2 feet (60 cm) apart, but all 'direct intercourse' was forbidden. None of the clean wounds became infected.[19] Erichsen suggested that erysipelas could be transferred by instruments, ward nurses and surgeons.[20] He would associate different mortalities not with hospital size but more with overcrowding and suppurating wounds. Although aware of the work of Semmelweiss and others on puerperal sepsis, surprisingly Erichsen did not recommend disinfection or washing of hands before surgery. Contact spread was not recognized by all surgeons until the end of the nineteenth century.

Franceso Redi in the seventeenth century had been one of the first to cast doubt on the theory of spontaneous generation, and Marcus Plenciz of Vienna in the 1760s maintained that infectious diseases were caused by micro-organisms and that nothing else but living organisms could cause disease. These views were obviously speculative,[21] but Spallanzani in 1765 was ahead of his time in his studies, disclaiming the existence of spontaneous generation.[14] He showed that heating prevented the emergence of animalcules in infusions and that they never appeared in the infusion unless new air entered the flasks and came into contact with the sterile infusion. Others in the nineteenth century, especially Theodor Swann in 1836, carried out experiments similar to Spallanzani's.[14] Other bacteria and fungi were observed and grown occasionally but were not isolated as individual organisms.[21] However, it was Louis Pasteur (1822–95) who finally elucidated the process of fermentation and so rendered untenable both the chemical theory of its mechanism and the theory of spontaneous generation.[14,22,23] Although not a physician, he was responsible for some of the greatest advances in medicine. In addition to being a unique laboratory worker, he was a deeply religious, humane and intensely serious man. He was born at Dôle in the Jura mountains, close to the Swiss border, the son of a tanner who had previously been in Napoleon's army. He was initially interested in art at school and possessed some talent, but he was converted to an interest in science by lectures given by Professor Dumas at the Sorbonne, graduating from the prestigious Ecole Normale Superiore in Paris in 1847. Here, he demonstrated his early scientific skills by defining the laevo- and dextro-polarizing crystals of tartaric acid. After several other appointments, he became Dean of Science at Lille University in 1854. He showed that fermentation was related to the living 'globules' that he could see in the fermenting liquors, and that it was not due to contact with some inanimate 'ferment'. A little later, he produced alcohol by inoculating a simple solution of sugar, ammonia and mineral salts with yeast cells, a result that he reported in 1860 – but the scientific world remained sceptical. Pasteur carried out a whole series of experiments to settle the matter. In addition to confirming the results of his predecessors, he showed that if a fragment of the cotton-wool plug that had kept a flask sterile was placed in the flask, then the culture medium became contaminated. He exposed sterile flasks in cellars and on the tops of mountains where the air was pure, and only a few became contaminated, whereas if he opened them in the street all were spoiled. This and much other work he published in 1862, and from then on any idea of the spontaneous generation of disease was seriously weakened. However, it was not entirely dispelled, as apart from the fungi in mycoses, no one yet had seen the germs that were supposed to cause disease. Pasteur eventually served as Professor of Chemistry at the Sorbonne (1867–89), but in 1868, at the age of 46, he suffered a minor stroke; however, his mind remained active and he soon returned to his work. Whilst investigating the souring of wine, he demonstrated that it was due to a parasitic organism, *Mycoderma aceti*, which could be eliminated by heating to 122–140 °F (50–60 °C). The term used for this low-temperature process was called 'pasteurization'; the method is still used for rendering milk safe from pathogens. He discovered with Joubert and Chamberland that *Clostridium septicum* was the cause of malignant oedema and thus it became the first anaerobic pathogenic organism. In 1879, he commenced work on cholera in chickens and on anthrax in sheep, developing vaccines for both, but his major effort in human (and veterinary) medicine was the development of a vaccine for rabies. The principles of his studies therefore provided the experimental foundation for future immunology and vaccine development. The Institut Pasteur was set up in 1888. He became Director, and in his last years he received honours from all over the world. Many famous workers joined him at the institute, including Metchnikoff, Yersin (the discoverer of the plague bacillus), Roux, Calmette and Chamberland. After his death, he was buried in the institute, and Joseph Meister, the first person to be treated successfully with his anti-rabies vaccine, became the first doorkeeper of the institute. The Institut Pasteur has since remained at the forefront of medical microbiological research, and many studies have been carried out on antibiotic resistance. The human immunodeficiency virus (HIV) was discovered there in the 1980s (see Chapter 16).

The *coup de grâce* to the miasma theory was dealt by Robert Koch (1843–1910), who was probably the greatest bacteriologist of all time.[14,22,23] He was a typical East Prussian, dignified, modest, fair-minded and highly intellectual. He was born in Clausthal, Hanover, and was the son of a mining engineer. He studied in the University of Göttingen and was influenced greatly by Wohler, Meissner and particularly Jacob Henle, whose theory of contagion may have started him on his life's work in bacteriology. Having graduated in medicine in 1866 and served as a surgeon in the Franco-Prussian war, in 1872 he was appointed to a post as a country physician in Wollstein. Working alone in a corner of his office, unsupported by professional colleagues, he elucidated the whole life history of the anthrax bacillus and succeeded in producing the disease in animals by inoculating them with a pure culture of the organism. He reported his results to Cohn, who published them in 1876. Pasteur, too, persisted with work on anthrax, and between 1877 and 1880 he succeeded in confirming Koch's work. By 1880, Koch's work was regarded so highly that he was given a laboratory in the Imperial Department of Health, where he founded the famous school of bacteriology. He pioneered the development of reliable and reproducible laboratory methods for culturing and staining bacteria, and the summit of his achievement was a paper on tuberculosis read before the Physiological Society of Berlin in 1882. This was one of the most important achievements in the history of infectious diseases. Until then, nothing was known of the aetiology of the disease, but Koch, using his new laboratory methods, showed unequivocally that the tubercle bacillus was present in tubercular lesions of a number of different kinds in both man and animals, and that the organisms could be grown in pure culture. Finally, he produced tuberculosis in guinea pigs by inoculating them with those cultures. He also propounded what are now known as Koch's postulates, which he considered necessary in proving that an organism was the cause of a disease:

1 The organism can be isolated from all cases of the disease.
2 The organism obtained from the disease can be produced in a pure culture.
3 The organism can reproduce the disease in experimental animals.
4 The organism can be recovered from the experimental animals in pure culture.

Koch also showed that bacteria were killed by aqueous solutions of mercuric chloride and other disinfectants, including chlorine, bromine and iodine, some of which were introduced later into surgical techniques. He also showed that bacterial spores were relatively resistant to heat but could be killed by exposure to steam at high pressure for 3 hours.

In 1883, Koch was sent to Egypt to study cholera, where, with his team, he identified the *Vibrio cholerae*. From 1896, he travelled extensively, investigating rinderpest in South Africa, sleeping sickness in Uganda, plague in Bombay, and protozoal diseases in the Far East. He became Professor of Hygiene and Bacteriology (and later Director) at the Institut f. Infektionskrankheiten in Berlin in 1885, remaining so until he retired in 1904. As Pasteur had done, he gathered around himself many of the leading bacteriologists of the day, such as Gaffky, Loeffler, Welch, Pfeiffer, and Kitasato. In 1890 at the International Medical Congress in Berlin, he described tuberculin as a remedy for tuberculosis; this was hailed all over the world as a major success in therapy. Unfortunately, it was a premature statement and his only mistake. Nevertheless, it did not tarnish his reputation to any extent and he received the Nobel Prize for Medicine in 1905. Soon after retiring, in 1906 he returned to Africa at the head of a commission on sleeping sickness, introducing atoxyl as a treatment for the disease. He died of cardiac failure in 1910 at the age of 67.

Even after the studies of Pasteur, Koch and their colleagues, the deeply entrenched theories of miasmas, spontaneous generation, and the mutability of fevers lingered on in a few minds for a few more years, but for all practical purposes observation at the laboratory bench had ushered in the era of the modern theory of infection.

As discussed already, the germ theory of infection was propounded by others over the years.[14,23] Of particular note was Frederick Cohn (1828–98), a prominent botanist and one of the important founders of bacteriology. He was one of the first (in 1875) to show that bacteria could be classified into genera and species, and he was a supporter of Pasteur's ideas on the absence of spontaneous generation. He recognized Koch's talents, and they became friends. Davaine, a French pathologist (1812–82), was also one of the early writers on infectious disease, publishing a classical work on anthrax and septicaemia.[14] He was the first to see anthrax bacilli in the blood of a rabbit, keeping his experimental animals in the garden of a friend!

Possible causes of hospital infection were described by several workers in the 1870s, including Pasteur and Koch. In 1878, Pasteur gave a talk at the French Academy of Medicine providing evidence that micro-organisms were responsible for disease and that particular organisms produced specific symptoms. Although not interested in taxonomy, he described 'staphylococci' in boils and 'streptococci' in puerperal sepsis. He also recognized the dangers of exposure to germs during surgery, stating that he would use only clean instruments and bandages and sponges that had been exposed to an appropriate heating process. Von Recklinghausen in 1871 found micrococci in the kidneys of patients with pyaemia. Klebs (1834–1913), a pioneer in all phases of bacteriology, described various structures that he regarded as different forms of one organism, *Microsporon septicum*, recognizing them as a probable cause of disease. He also recognized (in 1872) that traumatic septicaemia was of bacterial origin. Theodor Bilroth, a distinguished Viennese surgeon, presented his 'coccobacteria' as a type of alga that could change into cocci or bacteria, which he called bacilli, in 1894. Following Koch's recognition that specific organisms cause specific diseases, Bilroth abandoned his ideas on pleomorphism, but he did see 'streptococci' and 'staphylococci' and was probably the first person to describe streptococci. Koch applied his knowledge of anthrax to the study of wound infections in which six types of surgical infection, pathological processes and organisms are described in a short book, *The Aetiology of Traumatic Infective Diseases* (1878). He produced septicaemia in mice by injecting 'putrid fluids' into the skin of animals, which died 4–8 hours later.[24]

Salomonsen, a Danish bacteriologist, described the morphology of streptococci in pus from a patient with an inflamed knee joint in 1873, and he isolated the streptococci from the peritoneum of a rabbit that had been inoculated with the pus. He also noticed a motile rod in the pus following treatment. This pseudomonas-like organism may have been the first bacteriologically verified case of hospital-acquired infection in Denmark.[25] A pupil of Koch, Frederich Fehleisen, in 1882 also described morphological streptococci as a cause of erysipelas.

By then, it had become clear that surgeons using the same operating table and instruments without adequate cleaning between patients were contaminating the wounds with streptococci and causing infections.

Although Koch intended to determine whether infective diseases of wounds were of parasitic origin, he was unable to obtain suitable clinical material to complete the study, and it was left to Alexander Ogston, using Koch's methods, to confirm that 'micrococci' played a major role in the aetiology of acute purulent infections and that these could give rise to septicaemia and pyaemia.[26] Ogston graduated from the University of Aberdeen in 1864. He was good at languages, especially German, and as a student studied in Prague, Vienna and Berlin. Thus, he came into contact with many eminent European doctors, including Rokitansky, Virchov and Langenbeck. He became a junior surgeon at Aberdeen University in 1870 and immediately accepted Listerian principles. Having become a full surgeon in 1880, in the same year he gave a talk at the ninth Congress of the German Chirurgical Society in Berlin on abscesses. He described the presence of micrococci in almost 100% of acute abscesses, but not in chronic ones, and confirmed these results by studies on mice. In 1882, he became Regius Professor and in a paper suggested that micrococci were of two kinds: one in chains (streptococci (as identified by Bilroth)) and the other in bunches, which he named staphylococci (a bunch of grapes) (Figure 7.1).[27] However, following this appointment, he had little time for research.

Joseph Lister based his ideas of antisepsis on the work of Pasteur and repeated some of his experiments (see Chapter 8). By 1888, Watson-Cheyne, a surgeon and colleague of Lister, had already shown a good understanding of pyogenic (pus-forming) organisms and their mode of spread. He showed that the size of the bacterial dose and depressed vitality of tissues were important contributory factors in infections and that *Staphylococcus aureus* could be isolated from the air of surgical wards, from the surface of the body, including the hands of the surgeon, and from the healthy nasopharynx.[28]

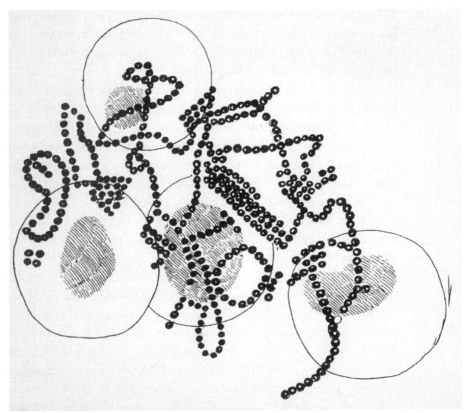

Figure 7.1   Drawings of streptococci by Alexander Ogston (1844–1929). (From A. Ogston (1880). Ueber abscesse. *Arch. Klin. Surg.*, **21**, 588–600.)

By the end of the nineteenth century and the early part of the twentieth century, most of the disease-producing bacteria had been isolated.[14,23,27,29] Many bacteriologists were involved in growing and staining newly described bacteria following the initial studies of Koch and Pasteur. Christian Gram, a Danish physician, requires a special comment as he described in 1884 the Gram stain that is still used as the initial basis for classification of bacteria today. Gram-positive organisms stain a purplish colour and Gram-negative stain red.

Many of the newly described organisms were aerobic Gram-negative bacilli, which were the normal flora of the intestinal tract and were later found to play a major role in hospital infection in addition to the staphylococci and streptococci already discussed. *Bacillus coli commune* (now *Escherichia coli*), the most numerous of these aerobic Gram-negative bacilli, was described in 1885 by Theodor Escherich, a young German paediatrician, who later became a professor in Graz and then in Vienna in 1902. He also described the green-pigment-producing organism of major importance in hospital infection, *Pseudomonas pyocyanea* (now *P. aeruginosa*).

Gustav Hauser provided the first account of *Proteus* spp. in 1895, and Carl Friedlander discovered *Bacillus pneumoniae* (later called *Klebsiella pneumoniae*) at about the same time.

Other Gram-negative bacilli were found to cause gastrointestinal infections and food poisoning (see Chapter 9). *Salmonella enteritidis* was one of the first described by Gärtner in 1888. He was a professor at Jena and isolated the organism from an outbreak of gastroenteritis in 58 people. The name 'salmonella' was derived from Dr Samuel Salmon, who worked in the USA in the Department of Agriculture. *Bacillus typhosus* (later *Salmonella typhi*), the causative organism of typhoid fever, was discovered by Carl Eberth in 1880 in Zurich and was first cultured by Gaffky, who later succeeded Koch in Berlin.

Dysentery is caused by shigella and was first described by Dr K. Shiga; many serotypes have since been identified of which *Shigella sonne* and *S. flexner* are the most common.

Plague was found to be caused by a Gram-negative coccobacillus that shows bipolar staining. The organism was discovered by Alexandre Yersin, a French bacteriologist, with coworker Shibasaburo Kitasato in 1884 when they were working on an epidemic in Hong Kong. It was initially called *Bacillus pestis*, later became *Pasteurella pestis*, and is now known as *Yersinia pestis* (see Chapter 9). Alexander Rennie in 1894 provided evidence that it was transmitted from the rat; Ogata, in 1887, implicated the flea as the vector.

Rickettsia are the causative organisms of typhus and related infections. They are small, intracellular coccobacilli, resembling viruses in that they cannot be grown in the absence of living cells. In 1909, Dr Howard Ricketts was able to transmit a rickettsial disease, Rocky Mountain fever, to guinea pigs and monkeys; Charles Nicolle, also in 1909, succeeded in transferring typhus fever to chimpanzees by means of infected blood, proving that transmission of human typhus was by the body louse. This provided the control strategy for typhus, and Nicolle was awarded a Nobel Prize. Five years later, Da Rocha-Lima and others isolated the causative organism and called it *Rickettsia prowazeki* after Ricketts and Prowazek, who was also involved in identifying the organism (see Chapter 9).

Antisepsis to asepsis

Although overcrowding, poor ventilation and inadequate facilities may be factors associated with surgical infection, and elimination of these necessitated new hospitals, the development of antiseptic and later aseptic techniques was of much greater importance since contact spread from patient to patient via the surgeon's hands, and clothing or instruments were the main routes of spread. The studies of Semmelweiss are often discussed, but his work seems to have had little immediate influence on surgery, and Lister was probably the major influence on the introduction of sterile techniques in modern surgery. Lister confirmed Pasteur's experiments, demonstrating that bacteria were responsible for putrefaction and that spontaneous generation did not exist.

Antiseptic surgery

Before Lister, phenols and other disinfectants had often been used for wound dressings.[1,2] Wood tar was used as a disinfectant by the Crowther brothers in Halifax in 1802 and as an antiseptic by Larrey in 1842. Of particular interest, the antiseptic treatment of wounds was used in England by Bennion of Oswestry before Lister. He successfully used tincture of benzoin for treating compound fractures. Phenol (carbolic acid) itself was first used as a dressing for wounds by Kuchenmeister in 1860 and in France by Lemaire at about the same time. Savory in England in 1867 reported that solutions of carbolic acid and chlorine compounds were effective in the treatment of pyaemia. Other antiseptics had also been used, e.g. Nélaton (1807–73) in Paris had successfully used alcoholic soaks on open wounds postoperatively, and continued to apply them until the wound looked healthy.[1] Nélaton's overall mortality for elective surgery rarely exceeded 4%, but unfortunately his method was not generally accepted, one of the reasons being that it prevented suppuration, i.e. the presence of 'laudable pus', which was still considered to assist wound healing.

Joseph Lister was born at Upton in Sussex in 1827 and grew up in a Quaker family.[3,4] His father was a wine merchant but was well known for his interests in

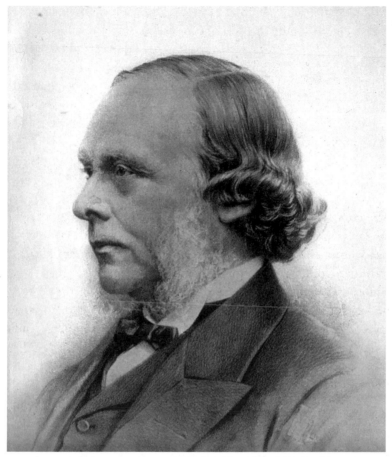

Figure 8.1   Joseph Lister (1827–1912). (R. Burgess (1973). *Portraits of Doctors and Scientists in the Wellcome Institute.* London: Wellcome Institute.)

microscopy. Lister qualified at University College London, and, in 1851, became a house surgeon to Erichsen, who was interested in surgical infection and probably influenced Lister at an early stage in his surgical career. Two years later, Lister obtained a house surgeon post with Syme in Edinburgh; he later married Syme's elder daughter. Lister was appointed Professor of Surgery in Glasgow in 1860 and then succeeded Syme in Edinburgh in 1866. His last move was to King's College London in 1877, and he remained there for 17 years, dying in Kent in 1912.[4] Lister was the first British surgeon to be given a peerage. He was a good practical teacher, but he was a shy man with few professional friends. He was apparently notoriously unpunctual but always very courteous. Although his early interests were in anatomy and physiology, he later developed an interest in inflammation and putrefaction, stimulated by his observations that two large wards in the Glasgow Royal Infirmary were most unhealthy and that hospital gangrene and pyaemia were common. In addition to his knowledge of Pasteur's work, he was also influenced by the effects of carbolic acid on sewerage, which reduced the odour of land irrigated with treated refuse material and destroyed the entozoa that commonly infected cattle feeding in these contaminated pastures. Antiseptics, including phenol, had previously been used for preventing infection (see above) but there was clearly little communication between Lister and these European (and English) workers, and he seemed to be unaware of other studies.

Initially, Lister instilled pure carbolic acid into wounds and soaked the dressings in it; later, he reduced the concentration and introduced a spray. Although he still considered airborne spread important, he also soaked his instruments, sutures and sponges in carbolic acid, but he did not realize the major importance of the hands and did not scrub with soap and water, although he did dip his hands in 1/20 carbolic acid and sublimate (a mercury-containing antiseptic). He also failed to wear protective clothing, apart from a towel pinned across his chest, when operating. Godlee, in discussing surgical techniques at the end of the century, stated: 'the modern refinements of surgery had not been worked out and that even Mr Lister was remiss by our standards. He did not boil his instruments or wear gloves'.[4] St Clair Thomson, who was Lister's house surgeon, said that Lister did not wear a mask, gown or gloves and usually rolled up his coat sleeves without removing his coat, yet his wounds healed as well as those subjected to the full aseptic practices.[5]

Lister showed that following the introduction of his carbolic acid technique, there were no large putrid exhalations, pyaemia or gangrene in his wards at the Glasgow Royal Infirmary, and although he did not carry out a controlled trial, the reduction in mortality was convincing. Of 35 patients operated on before he introduced his antiseptic treatment, 16 (45.7%) died, whereas only six out of 40 (15%) died after the introduction of the antiseptic method.[6,7] A similar result was obtained in Edinburgh. The wards were small and overcrowded, often with two to three children in one bed and with mattresses on the floor, but there was only one case of pyaemia and no cases of hospital gangrene reported over a period of 6 years following the introduction of the antiseptic system. Lister's methods were not followed by all surgeons, particularly in London, and when he arrived at King's College Hospital in 1877, conditions were similar to those in London when he had been there 20 years previously. Most wounds in King's College suppurated, but instruments were not boiled or disinfected, and a single probe was circulated, unwashed, from patient to patient. Lawson Tait, a Birmingham obstetrician, was one of Lister's major critics and did not believe the antiseptic system was effective, although he did use clean instruments and washed his hands before operating.[3] Sampson Gamgee, a Birmingham surgeon who had been a classmate of Lister, did not agree with his antiseptic methods. He believed in keeping wounds dry with

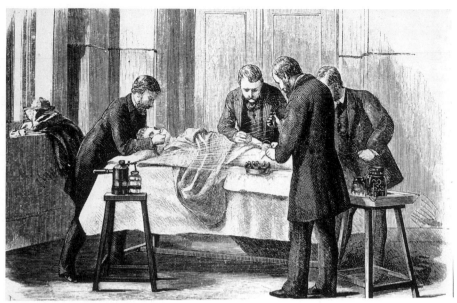

Figure 8.2   The use of a Listerian carbolic acid spray, showing surgeons in everyday clothing with no masks, hats or gloves. (Sir William Watson-Cheyne (1882). *Antiseptic Surgery*. London: Smith, Elder. Wellcome Library, London.)

an absorbent dressing and described in 1880 the well-known Gamgee dressing: a sandwich of absorbent cotton wool between two pieces of gauze. Gamgee was also a believer in absolute cleanliness and was said to be the first surgeon in Birmingham to wash his hands before operating.[8]

European surgeons were much more enthusiastic about Lister's methods.[9] Professor Saxtorph in Copenhagen reported that before the use of carbolic acid, pyaemia was frequent, even after small operations, but this and hospital gangrene disappeared after the introduction of antiseptic treatment. Reports from other distinguished surgeons in Munich, Berlin, Halle, Bonn and other towns in Europe and the USA described similar results. However, many American surgeons, especially the older ones such as Gross, were unconvinced at this time. Champonnière was also a Lister supporter and championed his cause in France. Bilroth in Vienna introduced carbolic acid in 1875 but because of tissue damage soon substituted thymol, mercuric chloride or iodoform. Von Bergman in Berlin also substituted bichloride of mercury for disinfecting his hands and instruments. Von Volkmann from Halle was also particularly enthusiastic about Lister's methods. Gustav Neuber in 1885 opened a private hospital in the middle of a wood and filtered air to remove germs. In this hospital, doctors and assistants washed their faces, arms and hands in mercuric chloride and sprayed walls, windows and floors. A separate operating theatre

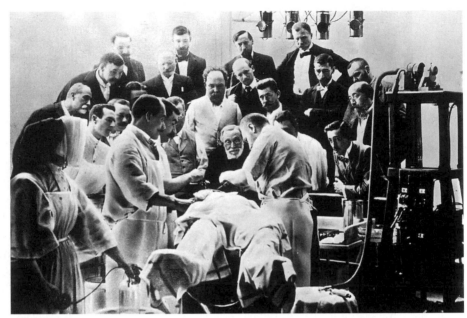

Figure 8.3   Rudolf Virchov (1821–1902) observing an operation on the skull in 1900 in a Paris clinic, showing surgeons in operating theatre clothing but no masks or gloves. (Berlin: Historischer Bilderdienst, 1900. Wellcome Library, London.)

was used for infected cases. Neuber also introduced plain-surfaced instruments that could be cleaned easily, as well as glass shelves and other cleanable surfaces. In 1892, Neuber introduced a cap and gown to exclude the surgeon's own clothing from the operating field; he also advocated the abandonment of surgical drains.[10]

Watson-Cheyne, a colleague and admirer of Lister at King's College Hospital London, wrote an excellent review of antiseptic surgery in 1882 (see also Chapter 7).[11] He stated:

Fermentation of wounds occurred as a result of the entrance of micro-organisms from without and if a wound is kept 'aseptic', infected diseases are avoided. On all objects in the external world septic dust is present on the skin of the patient, the hands of the surgeon, on all instruments, in the air, and when a wound is made the introduction of this dust must be carefully avoided and also afterwards by some sort of dressing. The term septic is derived from the Greek word for something that causes putrefaction.

He recommended that all these sites should be washed with diluted carbolic acid according to Lister's recommendation, but he considered the spray to be of less importance. He believed that dressings should be changed if there was a discharge from the wound, or at least every 8 days.

Most surgeons gradually accepted Lister's results, although there was a general move towards aseptic surgery at the end of the century.

Aseptic surgery

The change from antiseptic to aseptic surgery at the end of the nineteenth century was only partial. The use of antiseptics continued, and they are still used for disinfecting the skin of the operation site and the surgeon's hands; occasionally, they are also used to prevent infection in traumatic wounds and for cleaning dirty wounds. Nevertheless, the basis of aseptic surgery really started in Lister's time by Neuber and others, who were already using hats and gowns. Other aspects of aseptic surgery, including wearing sterile gloves, face masks and other protective clothing, and the sterilization of instruments, were developed from the end of the nineteenth century.

Although the hands of staff are now recognized to be one of the main routes of transmission of hospital infection, this was not commonly realized until bacteria could routinely be isolated and grown, but occasionally in the past hand-washing had been introduced before surgical or other aseptic procedures. For instance, as far back as Theodoric in the thirteenth century, it was considered advisable for surgeons to wash their hands. Alexander Gordon in 1773 recognized the contagiousness of puerperal fever and noted its resemblance to erysipelas many years before Simpson made a similar suggestion. He controlled the disease by washing his hands and putting on clean clothes before examining a pregnant patient (see Chapter 5). Pouteau, in 1775, also stressed the importance of clean hands for dressing wounds. The recommendations of Oliver Wendell Holmes (1843) and the subsequent work of Semmelweiss (see Chapter 5) indicated further the importance of clean hands in midwifery. Although this was not accepted uniformly, by the end of the nineteenth century some surgeons recognized the importance of presurgical hand disinfection.

Schimmelbusch, working in Von Bergman's clinic in Berlin in 1893, made recommendations for hand disinfection,[10] quoting Furbringer, who had previously described the use of alcohol for this purpose. Schimmelbusch also commented that 'surgeon's hands should be treated with suspicion' and that the skin of the surgeon's hands should be scrubbed with soap and water for 1 minute, dried and then wiped with sterile gauze in 80% alcohol. He also stated that 'one of the most deplorable relics of bygone times is the examination of wounds with fingers and probes' and, surprisingly, this practice was still being condemned at the end of the twentieth century. The relevance of the hands in the transmission of infection in surgery became increasingly clear when bacterial contamination was demonstrated by Meleney[12] and others in the 1930s using bacteriological methods, such as sampling the hands after dressing an infected wound.

The first major quantitative laboratory study on skin disinfection was carried out by Price in 1938.[13] He distinguished between the transient and resident flora. Transient organisms are those that do not normally colonize the skin and that are removed easily by washing or disinfection; resident organisms grow on normal skin and are removed with difficulty by the usual washing procedures and incompletely by most disinfection processes. Price showed that scrubbing with soap and water removed about half the residents in 6 minutes and two-thirds in about 10 minutes. 70% alcohol applied for 1 minute was as effective as prolonged scrubbing. The process of scrubbing for 10 minutes followed by immersion in 70% alcohol was used as a preoperative scrubbing procedure for many years. Since then, many similar laboratory studies have been carried out (Chapter 11), although none has been as conclusive as the clinical study of Semmelweiss.

Hand-washing with soap and water before carrying out hygienic procedures in wards was used in most countries, although this was replaced by antiseptics, including alcohol, later in the century.

Hand-washing or disinfection never completely removes micro-organisms, and the wearing of gloves was suggested in the eighteenth century. Walbaum described a 'glove' made of the caecum of a sheep for vaginal examinations, and in the early nineteenth century, Joseph Plenk, a dermatologist, described a glove to protect the midwife from venereal infections.[3] Thomas Watson of King's College Hospital, in 1842, suggested that a glove should be worn by accouchers to prevent the transmission of puerperal fever,[1,3] but the first sterile rubber glove used to protect the operator in surgery was probably produced by William Halsted at Johns Hopkins Hospital in 1889.[14] This was originally made for his 'scrub' nurse (who later became his wife), who was allergic to corrosive sublimate hand rinse. It is not certain when gloves were first worn routinely for surgery, but surgeons in the Johns Hopkins Hospital wore them in the 1890s. Robb, an associate of Halsted, wore gloves in 1894 and also scrubbed his hands and forearms with soap. This was followed by soaking in potassium permanganate and then in bichloride of mercury. Another surgeon in the hospital, Bloodgood, may have been the first to wear sterile gloves routinely for surgical operations. Halsted was also one of the pioneers of blood transfusion in surgery, although routine use was not possible until the immunological problems were sorted out by Karl Landsteiner in 1900.[3]

At a time when gloves were not commonly worn for surgery in Britain, Lynn Thomas (1905), a Cardiff surgeon, was one of the first to do so,[15] but they were not worn regularly for some years after. Lynn Thomas wore linen gloves for clean surgery, reporting a decrease in suture line infections, and rubber gloves for septic cases to protect himself. He introduced other important innovations. Instead of washing his hands in a nonsterile basin, Lynn Thomas recommended running water and the use of a nailbrush followed by brisk scrubbing in alcohol before putting on sterile gloves. He also recommended taps with elbow or knee levers or with a sterilized shield covering the tap. He recognized that hands were the 'high veldt' for sheltering undesirable organisms, and he suggested that gloves would remove

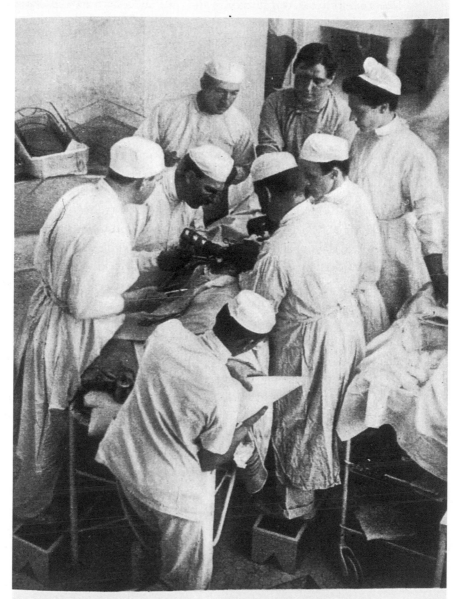

Dr. Halsted's First Operation in the New Surgical
Amphitheatre in 1904

Figure 8.4   William Halsted operating in 1904 in Johns Hopkins Hospital, showing surgeons wearing
operating clothing and gloves but not masks. (W.G. MacCallum (1930). *William Stewart
Halsted.* Baltimore: Johns Hopkins. Wellcome Library, London.)

the necessity for antiseptic treatment. He also wore a sterilized overall covering his forearms, a bib covering his mouth and nose, and a sterilized cap, stating that 'when a clean operated wound suppurates, the surgeon should put his house in order'. He visited Professor Axel Iverson in Copenhagen, who insisted that all entering the operating theatre should wear a sterile gown and rubber boots, and in addition suggested that operating rooms should have a good light, no ledges, and rounded corners to improve ease of washing, and that theatres should be washed down daily with boiled water. In recent years, gloves have also been worn to protect the surgeon from viruses in the blood of the patient (Chapter 16).

Sterilization of instruments by heat was also an important development in aseptic procedures,[16] and the difference between sterilization and disinfection was recognized early in the twentieth century. Sterilization is the killing of all micro-organisms, including spores, whereas disinfection reduces micro-organisms to a safe level but does not necessarily remove all organisms or spores. The term 'sterilization' has been, and sometimes still is, mistakenly used for a process that only disinfects, such as boiling. 'Decontamination' is a term sometimes used for the removal of organisms and can include sterilization, disinfection or cleaning alone.

Decontamination has taken place since biblical times. The process of flaming metal objects by passing them through fire to cleanse them was described in the book of Numbers in 1450 BC. Aristotle recommended that boiled water be used for drinking by Alexander the Great's army, and Hippocrates also recommended it to cleanse wounds, although he was not a supporter of the theory of contagion.[17] In 1681, Denis Papin described a closed vessel into which steam was introduced (a 'new digester') for softening bones and tissues but not for destroying 'contamination'.[18] However, most of the advances were made by Pasteur, Koch, Tyndall and others based on the need to obtain pure cultures of bacteria.[19]

Curt Schimmelbusch, an early exponent of asepsis (see above), wrote a classic book, *The Aseptic Treatment of Wounds*, in 1893.[10] He was probably the first to use a sterilizer for surgical dressings in 1885, although Louis Champonnière in 1887 claimed he had used steam for 'sterilizing' in the operating room before Schimmelbusch, who was in Von Bergman's unit. Paul Redard, a French orthopaedic surgeon, demonstrated in 1889 that steam at raised pressure was effective against spores. Hugo Davidsohn, in Koch's laboratory, suggested that boiling water was suitable for 'sterilizing' surgical instruments and this method remained in use in hospital wards for at least another 60 years, despite the inadequacy of the method in killing spores.[16] Surprisingly, there were few reports of spore-bearing infections due to deficiencies in sterilizing surgical instruments over this period.

A sterilizer using steam at high pressure is similar to a pressure cooker and is known as an autoclave. Steam was originally used by a physician, William Henry of

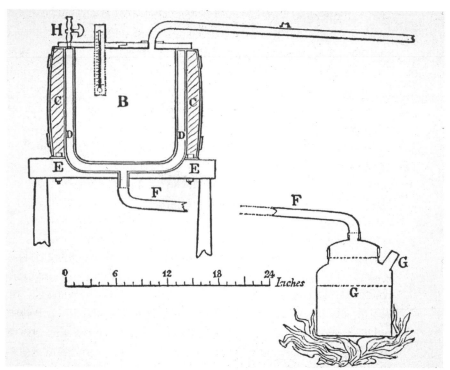

Figure 8.5   A hot air 'sterilizer' for the disinfection of clothes of scarlet fever patients. Steam from the boiler G passes to jacket D, heating the wall of the chamber. (W. Henry (1832). Experiment on the disinfecting powers of increased temperatures. *Philosoph. Mag.*, **II**, 22–3.)

Manchester, to decontaminate clothes of sufferers from typhus and scarlet fever. His method involved heating a jacket surrounding a closed container with steam produced in an adjacent vessel (Figure 8.5).[16,20] Autoclaves in use until the mid-twentieth century were of a downward displacement type, where steam is introduced, thus displacing the air, which is heavier than steam. By the end of the nineteenth century, most of the problems of autoclaving were recognized, mainly by German scientists.[16] These problems included the adverse effects of air mixed with steam, and the protection of bacteria by oil and grease; the advantage of using gravity for the removal of air was also realized. Improved sterilizers of varying designs were described by Magath in the USA.[21] Over the next 50 years, surgical techniques were the dominant interest and there was little further work on sterilization, presumably because there was no evidence of infection following the methods in use.

The relative roles of airborne and contact spread in wound infection and infectious diseases, and the need to wear face masks, have remained controversial,[22] but the potential risks to the open wound from droplets from the respiratory tracts of surgeons and their assistants were recognized as early as the sixteenth century by

Wurtz. Flugge and his colleagues in 1897 showed that numerous droplets are liberated into the air during talking, sneezing and coughing, and a colleague, Mickulicz, was the first to describe the use of a mask in surgery.[23,24] These workers showed that masks would reduce the number of bacteria expelled from the mouth by putting *Bacillus prodigiosus* in the mouth and showing a reduction in the number of colonies on culture plates on speaking or sneezing when wearing a mask. They believed that talking enhanced the chance of infection during an operation. Others, for example Hamilton in 1905, suggested the use of masks for the prevention of infectious diseases. A number of other studies involved the efficacy of masks,[25] but masks were rarely used for surgical operations in the early part of the century.

The belief in the role of airborne spread diminished in the early part of the twentieth century, due mainly to Charles V. Chapin, who wrote a comprehensive book, *The Sources and Modes of Infection*, in 1910, which considered the evidence for and against airborne spread.[26] Chapin was Superintendent of Health in Providence, USA; he received many honorary degrees, and he was also a president of the American Public Health Association. His thinking on the transmission of infection was far ahead of his time. He believed, correctly, that most infections were transmitted by contact, but he would not accept that some, such as chickenpox, were spread in the air. He suggested that the poor correlation between numbers of pus-forming organisms in the air and wound infection rates indicated that airborne infection was unlikely. This was supported by the fact that the low numbers of streptococci in small droplets also indicated that they were unlikely to cause infection. He also commented that 'a successful surgeon will operate with as little wound infection in a tenement as in the best operating room'. He quoted Parente that germs have low viability outside the body and that prompt transfer of germs from the infected patient or carrier is necessary for infection to occur. He also stated:

… contagiousness included the number of germs, their virulence and the volume of excretions or secretions and the surroundings; the virulence of organisms causing wound infection is reduced by drying and exposure to sunlight; sources of infection are people and not the inanimate environment and therefore fomites including walls and floors are not of great importance.

The controversy continued until the 1930s, when Wells and Wells re-established the role of airborne spread. They showed that droplets expelled from the respiratory tract often evaporated until they were dry (droplet nuclei), and their contents remained in the air for long periods.[27] Some of these dried droplets contained viable organisms and could travel for long distances: thus, airborne organisms were again considered to be a possible source of infection

Meleney in the 1930s, after finding that a nurse carrying haemolytic streptococci in her throat was responsible for a wound infection, introduced the wearing of masks during operations, and demonstrated a reduction in the infection rate if this was done.[12] The necessity of wearing masks was confirmed by others, although the evidence that this practice in surgery reduces infection has never been demonstrated clearly in controlled trials.[25]

Surgical-type masks usually contained an impermeable insert (deflector), but airborne organisms could still enter or leave the respiratory tract around the edges of the mask. A helmet completely covering the head and extending down to the neck, with a four-ply gauze mask, designed by Cone in Montreal, was worn by Meleney in the 1940s.[12] This was also fitted with an air-suction tube to improve comfort. Interestingly, a similar ventilated helmet was used as part of an ultraclean air system for prosthetic joint surgery by Charnley many years later (see Chapter 14). The studies of Wells and Wells, and the finding of haemolytic streptococci in the noses and throats of healthy subjects, convinced surgeons and obstetricians that masks should be worn during operations, when carrying out dressing techniques, and when delivering babies, and they continued to be worn for these purposes until the second half of the century.

The possibility of organisms entering the wound from the air of the operating room and causing infection was recognized by Lister, but later he considered this to be a minor route of spread and discontinued the use of his antiseptic spray. Others in the early part of the century still considered airborne organisms to be important, basing their judgement on the high numbers in the air of the operating theatre[28] and possibly on remaining beliefs in miasmas. The work of Wells and Wells and others in the 1930s led to the introduction of mechanically ventilated operating theatres.

The wearing of protective clothing, e.g. caps and gowns, when carrying out surgical operations was also in general use from the beginning of the twentieth century. These were made of cotton, and although they provided some protection against contact spread, they did not prevent the passage of organisms. New materials impermeable to bacteria were introduced later in the century.

Separate rooms for operating had first been used in the eighteenth century but not in all hospitals. Later, amphitheatres that could hold up to 700–800 spectators were built around the operating table for teaching and demonstration purposes.[1] The potential hazard of large numbers of people in the operating room was recognized in the early twentieth century, and new theatres with small viewing areas and with ventilation systems to reduce the numbers of airborne bacteria were designed. The effectiveness of these systems remained uncertain, but they were investigated extensively in the latter half of the century (see Chapters 12 and 14).

Quantitative information on surgical wound infection in the nineteenth century was based mainly on mortality, and little is available on infection rates, although annual reports suggest that streptococcal and staphylococcal infections were common. Following the introduction of antiseptic and aseptic techniques, mortality

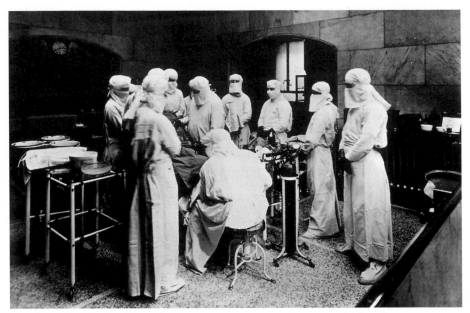

Figure 8.6   Surgical operation at the Middlesex Hospital, London, in 1927, showing surgeons wearing full operating clothing, including hats, masks and gloves. (Anon, 1927.) Wellcome Library, London.

fell considerably, and information on infection rates was of increasing interest. For instance, a reduction in infection rate of hernia wounds was reported in a small study by Bloodgood in 1899 following the wearing of gloves during operations, and there was a surprising reduction in hernia repair wound infection from 20% to 1.7% when face masks were worn.[14]

A few surgeons kept information on infection rates. For example, in one study, infections in 117 out of 6825 (1.7%) clean operative wounds were reported by Berkman. Brewer, in 1915, at the Roosevelt hospital in New York carried out an extensive study over a number of years.[29] He reported an infection rate in clean wounds of 39% in 1896, which was reduced to 9% in 1897 by the use of a modern operating room and an autoclave for sterilizing surgical instruments. The rate was reduced further to 3% in 1899 by the introduction of sterile gloves, by treating wounds and dressings with dilute solutions of formaldehyde, and by general improvements in asepsis. In 1912, a patient would be given a tub bath the night before operation, and the part of the body to be operated on was shaved. A soap poultice was applied to the operation site preoperatively, followed by a dressing impregnated with mercuric chloride. The dressing was removed in the operating theatre and the site was cleaned with ether/alcohol and 1/5000 mercuric chloride. The wound site was then surrounded with sterile towels. Sterile caps, gowns and gloves were worn, but masks were worn only for operations on knee joints and open fractures. The percentage of infected clean cases was 2.4%. Brewer then persuaded surgeons to watch each other's operative techniques, following this with a discussion of possible errors. The infection rate of 474 clean cases in 6 months was 1.8% in 1913 and 1.6% in 1914. If three cases of infection following the use of unsterile novocaine were excluded, only one infection occurred in the 1914 period, results that compare well with those obtained with modern surgical techniques for clean surgery, although the operations were less complex. This early introduction of a form of audit was of particular interest.

Meleney,[12,30] at the Presbyterian Hospital in New York, reported a clean infection rate in 1925 of 13.6% of 558 operations. This was reduced by 1940 to 2.1% of 1852 operations following improvements in aseptic techniques. However, Howe[31,32] reported an increase in wound infections from 1.2% of 401 operations in 1949 to 5.3% of 321 operations in 1955. He suggested that the increase was due to lapses in aseptic techniques following the introduction of antibiotics. In general, wound infection rates in the 1940s and 1950s were about 5%, but the staphylococcal epidemics in those years led to an increased interest in infection rates (see Chapter 12).

The twentieth century: hospitals and miscellaneous infections

Hospitals at the end of the nineteenth century continued to be of the pavilion type, with large, open wards containing 20–30 beds each, as suggested by Tenon in 1787 and later by Florence Nightingale.[1] The wards were oblong, with long side windows, high ceilings, and beds separated by curtains. A hospital block usually consisted of two to three floors, with wards on each side of a central corridor. Although Nightingale did not believe in the germ theory of disease, the wards in general hospitals were designed to provide good light and ventilation; single rooms for isolation of infection were uncommon.

The pavilion-type hospital continued in use, with modifications, through much of the twentieth century, particularly in the UK, where few new hospitals were built until after the Second World War. Hospitals in the USA and Europe tended to have wards subdivided into bays or with beds in separate, single rooms. In the USA, new hospitals were usually built with wards containing a maximum of four beds, and many had only one- or two-bedded rooms. European hospitals had rooms of six, four and two beds; they also had single rooms, which from about 1911 were provided mainly for privacy, although they were also useful for the isolation of infected patients.[2,3] Pavilion wards took up a large amount of space and were expensive, so tower blocks were built in the USA.

During the twentieth century, Nightingale wards were upgraded and hand-washing basins and electric 'sterilizers' were fitted, but overcrowding and infection remained a problem. By the mid-twentieth century, the idea of subdivided wards was generally accepted in the Western world, resulting in small wards or bays coming off long, single corridors, T-shaped wards, or wards with double corridors, often called racetrack wards.[4] Single rooms were included, but there was some discussion as to the numbers required, usually suggested as varying between 20 and 25%.[5] Centralized wound-dressing rooms in which patients from several wards were treated were also popular, increasing the risks of inter-ward cross-infection, although no evidence of this was obtained. Evidence for reduced staphylococcal infection in mechanically ventilated or non-ventilated racetrack

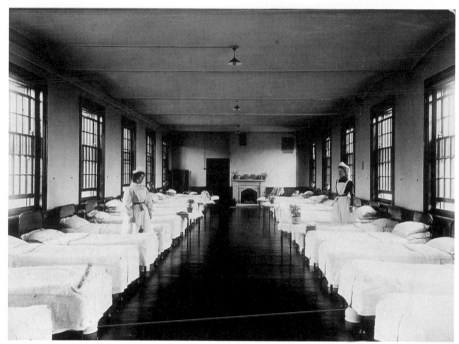

Figure 9.1   Interior of a large 'Nightingale' ward in 1900. (London and County Photographic Co., Bromley, Kent. Wellcome Library, London.)

wards was variable,[6] although small wards showed less cross-infection than the large Nightingale wards.[7]

Isolation wards for infectious diseases had been in use since the days of leper hospitals and of infirmaries in monasteries (Chapter 2).[8] These were followed by the setting aside of wards in general hospitals or by makeshift arrangements in other buildings until, at the end of the nineteenth century, specialized isolation hospitals were built. As infections such as typhus and cholera became less prevalent or disappeared altogether, the isolation hospitals in the mid-twentieth century were used mainly for diseases such as scarlet fever, erysipelas, measles, diphtheria, whooping cough, typhoid fever and poliomyelitis. Examples of new isolation hospitals included Bristol (Ham Green), built in 1894,[9] initially with 76 beds, and the Edinburgh City Hospital with 600 beds, opened in 1903.[10] Special hospitals were built for smallpox patients, and sanitoria were built for pulmonary tuberculosis patients.

At the beginning of the twentieth century, there was much discussion on the spread of infectious disease. Many physicians, such as Chapin, believed that spread was mainly by contact and that the air and fomites played a minor role, quoting results showing the absence of cross-infection in the Pasteur hospital (see Chapter 8).[11] Chapin was supported by others such as Rundle, who surprisingly found little spread of infection, even of varicella.[12] However, others disagreed:[7] Harries in 1935 found some spread of measles and varicella but also stated that cross-infection was the 'bane of staff in both children's wards and fever hospitals' (Chapter 10).[13]

Staff of fever hospitals sometimes became infected, and in 1905, 6% of 230 staff members at the new Edinburgh City Hospital acquired an infection (three cases of enteric fever, three of scarlet fever, three of diphtheria, one of measles and four of erysipelas).[10]

The wards in fever hospitals were commonly of the pavilion type, with two floors and often with cubicles opening on to corridors.[10] A study in the 1970s of different hospitals with non-mechanically ventilated, cubicled wards showed that cross-infection was low in the cases of varicella (1.68%) and measles (0.68%), but it advised that small wards and open corridors rather than central, closed corridors were associated with less cross-infection with these diseases.[14] This was confirmed by Tom Parker and colleagues in the case of staphylococcal infections.[15] Single cubicles with extractor fans were thought to be useful for preventing airborne infection with varicella and pulmonary tuberculosis, but the need for airlocks remains uncertain.[7] The role of isolation for staphylococcal infections is also considered in Chapters 12 and 14.

Miscellaneous infections

In the Western world, both the incidence of infection and the associated complications in most of the common communicable diseases decreased considerably during the twentieth century due to immunization, the introduction of antibiotics, and generally improved hygiene. However, food poisoning has remained a major problem throughout the world. Smallpox has been eradicated, but initial efforts to eliminate other infections such as poliomyelitis have not been successful so far. Some of the older infections, such as plague and cholera, remain a potential hazard, mainly in developing countries. Leprosy has almost been eradicated in developing countries, but many cases still remain in the tropical regions. Tuberculosis was also reduced considerably in the mid-twentieth century due to improved hygiene and antimicrobial agents, but it is now re-emerging because of its association with acquired immune deficiency syndrome (AIDS) and increasing antibiotic resistance. Some of these infections are discussed in this chapter, although few, except for occasional viral infections such as respiratory syncytial virus, Norwalk and rotavirus, are responsible for significant hospital infection. Tetanus and gas gangrene are also considered in this chapter, although cases of hospital-acquired tetanus and gas gangrene are now rare.

Viral diseases

Epidemic viral diseases, such as smallpox and measles, were recognized in antiquity but emerged as epidemics in Europe mainly in medieval times.[16] Most viral infections, however, were not characterized until the viruses were identified in the twentieth century. Viral communicable diseases are mainly community-acquired infections, but they have often required admission to hospitals for treatment and for single-cubicle isolation.

Viruses are small infective particles 20–200 nm in size (1000 nm = 1 μm) that contain either deoxyribonucleic acid (DNA) or ribonucleic acid (RNA); they grow only in living cells. The possibility of the existence of viruses was suggested by Ivanovski in 1892, when he discovered that tobacco mosaic organism could pass through a filter that retained the smallest bacteria. Then Beijerinck, in 1898, postulated that the agent must be incorporated into the living protoplasm of a cell to propagate itself and that it could not multiply outside the cell. In the same year, Loeffler and Frosch demonstrated that the agent causing foot and mouth disease in cattle could pass through a filter. Viruses capable of destroying bacteria (bacteriophage) were described by Twort (in 1915) and d'Herelle (in 1917). Subsequently, vaccinia viruses were grown in egg embryos, and other viruses were grown in tissue cultures in the 1930s. Viral structures were first observed in detail following the invention of the electron microscope by Ruska in 1930, and later observations were made by Burton and Kohl in 1942.[17,18] In more recent years, new viruses have been discovered and rapid diagnostic tests have been developed.[19]

Smallpox

Smallpox (variola) is a generalized febrile disease associated with vesicles and pustules on the skin. It spreads mainly by direct contact, but airborne spread can occur. In the early stages, there is a profuse growth of virus in the skin lesions and in the throat, which heavily contaminate bedding and dust. Small, stainable structures known as inclusion bodies were described within epithelial cells of smallpox lesions in 1892 by Guarnieri, and the virus was later grown in egg embryos, producing the characteristic pocks on the chorioallantoic membrane.[18] The disease was described in China in 1122 BC and was recognized in India before the Christian era, gradually spreading westwards.[19,20] Smallpox was often confused with measles, chickenpox and syphilis, the distinction between smallpox and measles being made by an Arabian physician, Rhazes, in AD 910. Nevertheless, smallpox appeared to be uncommon in England and probably the rest of northern Europe and America until the sixteenth century. It existed in epidemic form in Great Britain from the seventeenth century and had a high mortality, outbreaks of varying size continuing until the twentieth century (see Chapter 2).[21] Cases of smallpox were regularly admitted to hospitals, often to isolation wards or smallpox hospitals in the nineteenth century, the numbers varying from year to year; for instance, in Birmingham General Hospital, there were 94 cases in 1857–8 but only one case in 1861–2.[22] There is no indication of the number of cases that were due to cross-infection, but it was probably common in the absence of vaccination. Smallpox (variola major) was mainly replaced in 1919 by a milder disease, variola minor. The numbers of cases of variola minor were still high in 1927, when 14 467 cases were reported, with 47 deaths, in England and Wales.[21] The numbers dropped considerably from 1930, and in 1935 there was only one reported, nonfatal case, although small outbreaks continued. In 1946–61, seven of 53 smallpox fatalities in Britain were in unvaccinated hospital staff, and in the 1962 outbreaks, 64% of indigenous infections were hospital-acquired; these accounted for 84% of the 25 deaths.[5] The last few cases in Britain occurred in Birmingham in 1977. The index case was a university photographer. The infection was probably laboratory-acquired, but she apparently had no direct contact with the smallpox laboratory, which was on the floor below. The possibility of airborne transfer along a service duct was considered but never proven. Smallpox experts thought it was unlikely, and the route of spread was never found. The World Health Organization (WHO) declared smallpox to have been eradicated from the world in 1980.[20]

Inoculation of material into a healthy person from a smallpox patient for protective purposes was introduced by Lady Mary Wortley Montagu in the early eighteenth century, but although this procedure generally proved successful, it also caused fatal smallpox in some people. The procedure (variolation) was used by others, but Jenner is given the main credit for the use of cowpox material in 1798 and was mainly responsible for its widespread use.[20] Vaccination with cowpox was introduced in the first part of the nineteenth century and became available at public expense for all infants in England in 1840; its use became compulsory in 1853.[21]

Measles

Measles is also an ancient disease, characterized by upper-respiratory symptoms and a rash; it was often confused with smallpox (see above). The name 'mezils' was first used by John of Gaddesden (1280–1361), who applied it to measles and certain leprous lesions.[20] In the Middle Ages, the mortality was high, particularly in young children, but it fell considerably from the mid-nineteenth century. Measles was recognized as a separate disease in the early 1600s, and a death rate of 795 was reported in the London Bills in 1674.[21] Epidemics continued in children and susceptible populations into the twentieth century. Measles is a highly contagious disease transmitted by large respiratory droplets that can be airborne. Spread in hospitals was still common in the 1930s,[12] and cubiclization of wards reduced but did not eliminate the spread in the 1940s; death from measles-related pneumonia still occurred. Since immunization was introduced in the 1960s, the disease has almost been eliminated in developed countries, but failure by authorities to promote immunization has allowed outbreaks to continue in many countries.

Chickenpox

Chickenpox (varicella) is the most contagious of the communicable diseases of childhood, but it is relatively benign. It is characterized by a vesicular rash. It spreads by means of respiratory droplets and is commonly transmitted by the airborne route. It can also be transmitted by direct contact with the vesicles. The disease received little attention before the sixteenth century and was confused with measles and later with smallpox. It was the most common cause of cross-infection in children's wards in the early twentieth century. It is still particularly hazardous to immunosuppressed patients, and an outbreak in a children's ward is still a source of anxiety.[5] A live vaccine is available but not yet widely used. *Herpes zoster* infection (shingles) is caused by the same virus but affects mainly elderly people. This infection is due to reactivation of the virus in the nervous system. It is less transmissible than chickenpox, but a susceptible person can acquire chickenpox from the infection.

Influenza

Influenza is a disease of the respiratory tract. It has an acute onset, a very high attack rate, and usually a low mortality, although mortality can be high in some epidemics, particularly in elderly people. The virus was first described by Wilson Smith and colleagues[23] in 1933, and it was later grown in mice, in egg embryos, and more recently in tissue culture. Influenza is highly contagious and spreads mainly by heavy dispersal of large droplets. There are two main types, influenza A and influenza B, and a less common type, influenza C; type A is the usual pandemic strain.[16,21] The first identifiable epidemic in Britain was in 1510; epidemics recurred at intervals until the present time. Influenza has been confused with sweating sickness or English sweat, a severe disease associated with heavy sweating and rapid death, but with less prominent respiratory symptoms than influenza.[16]

A pandemic of influenza occurred in 1889–92, but the largest was in 1918–19. This was the greatest outbreak of pestilence that the world had ever known, and it is estimated as being responsible for 21 million deaths, including fit and healthy people as well as elderly people. Smaller outbreaks have occurred since then, and vaccines have been developed. However, influenza A has the ability to change, i.e. to undergo genetic drift, and careful surveillance is required so that new vaccines can be produced when necessary.[19,21]

Hospital cross-infection is not normally a major problem, presumably because patients are usually admitted with the disease in the later stages of the infection when spread is less likely,[5] but residential institutions for the elderly are often badly affected. Infections may be introduced into hospitals by nurses during community epidemics, when they infect other nurses and patients; for this reason, epidemics cause a strain on available hospital beds due to the sudden increase in numbers of admissions of patients with severe respiratory complications and due to a shortage of staff because of sickness. Death may be caused by influenzal pneumonia, but it is often due to a superinfection with staphylococci causing a staphylococcal pneumonia. Vaccination of hospital staff and elderly people is recommended.

Other viral infections

Many other viral infections can spread in hospital, particularly in paediatric wards, but these are mainly community-acquired diseases,[18,19] including adenovirus, para-influenza virus and rhinovirus infections, often with upper rather than lower respiratory symptoms.

Respiratory syncytial virus (RSV) is the most common cause of lower respiratory infections in young infants. The more severe cases are often admitted to hospital, and spread from them to other infants and staff is common. As well as droplet spread, these respiratory viruses may be spread on the hands of staff or on fomites, i.e. inanimate surfaces and toys.[19]

Rubella is a common childhood infection not often requiring hospital admission. The main hazard in hospital is the transfer of infection to susceptible women during pregnancy, with subsequent development of congenital abnormalities in the baby. Immunization is the optimal method of control and should include all hospital staff unless they are already immune.

Sporadic transmission of mumps to patients and staff may occur in hospital, but this is primarily a community disease. Immunization of children is usually recommended.

Human parvovirus B19 is another common childhood disease associated with a rash and fever. Transmission to hospital staff is the main hazard, when it can be associated with aplastic crises in people with sickle cell disease or in immunosuppressed patients; uncommonly, it is associated with death of the fetus in pregnant women.

Epidemic poliomyelitis was not recognized as a defined clinical entity until the late nineteenth and early twentieth centuries, although the disease was described in the eighteenth century.[20] Sporadic cases probably occurred in ancient Egypt[21] and have continued to appear since then, but epidemics were first reported in the developed world during the first half of the twentieth century. Many symptomless carriers are present in the community during an epidemic; others develop only a febrile disease; a minority develop paralysis, and a small number of these patients die. Spread is by droplets from the respiratory tract in the early stages but later occurs by the faecal-oral route, the virus being isolated from faeces for about 6 weeks. A probable causal virus was identified by Landsteiner and Popper in 1909, who transferred the infection to monkeys, producing a flaccid paralysis,[24] but it was not until 1936 that Sabin and Olitsky reported the propagation of the virus in human nervous tissue.[25] Enders and colleagues in the late 1940s first grew it in extra-neural embryonic tissues.[26] 'Killed' and 'live' oral vaccines were then developed. The disease rarely spreads in hospital, but patients in the early stages of infection require isolation and all healthcare staff are vaccinated routinely. The introduction of vaccines for all children and improved hygiene have almost eliminated the disease from developed countries, but the virus remains uncontrolled in many developing countries. Efforts are being made to eliminate the disease from the world, but the presence of numerous symptomless carriers makes this a more difficult task than the elimination of smallpox.

Miscellaneous gastrointestinal viruses

A number of other enteroviruses, e.g. Coxsackie and Echo, have been described, but these diseases are usually less severe than poliomyelititis.[9] These viruses may spread occasionally in children's wards.

Rotavirus is one of the most common gastrointestinal infections of children, and it is a major cause of mortality in developing countries. It was identified as a cause of hospital-acquired infection in the 1970s, and since then many outbreaks have been reported in children's wards as well as in geriatric establishments. The virus spreads by the faecal-oral route, probably mainly on the hands of staff, but there is a possibility that aerosol spread can also occur.[19] Another group of viruses, called the small round viruses, which includes the Norwalk virus following its isolation from an outbreak in Norwalk, Ohio, is responsible for outbreaks of gastrointestinal infection, mainly in the community. They are commonly transmitted in food, especially shellfish, and water. Person-to-person spread can occur in hospitals.

Gastrointestinal bacterial infections

Typhoid fever

Typhoid fever is caused by *Salmonella typhi*. It is a systemic rather than a diarrhoeal infection, although it is transmitted by faeces. It is likely that typhoid fever is an ancient disease and was known to Hippocrates. It was particularly devastating in armies in the nineteenth century, and large outbreaks have continued in developing countries in the twentieth century, e.g. in Mexico in 1972.[20] Typhoid fever was probably first recognized as a separate disease by Thomas Willis in 1684, when it was called 'putrid fever', but at that time it was still often confused with typhus. Its waterborne and food origin was identified by William Budd (Chapter 7), who thought, mistakenly, that it could be transferred in the air. Typhoid fever was a leading cause of death in hospitals up to the beginning of the twentieth century.[27] In Birmingham General Hospital, for instance, admissions for typhoid ranged from six to 57 a year between 1859 and 1878, but there are no records as to how many cases were due to cross-infection.[2] However, it was generally recognized as being not very contagious.

Typhoid fever is now a relatively rare disease in developed countries due to improved sanitation and a vaccine. Effective antibiotics, especially chloramphenicol, have been available since the 1950s, but the emergence of resistant strains is now a cause of anxiety. Typhoid now spreads rarely in hospitals, although transmission is still occasionally reported in maternity units or on medical equipment.

Other salmonella infections are common causes of food poisoning (see Chapter 13) and occasionally have caused large outbreaks in hospitals.

Dysentery

Dysentery is a diarrhoeal disease caused by *Shigella* (see Chapter 7). It is a major problem whenever sanitation is poor, and it is associated with overcrowding and malnutrition. Spread is normally from person to person, usually on the hands, but it can be transferred in food or on inanimate objects, such as toilet seats or bedpans.[27]

Dysentery is an ancient disease: severe diarrhoea, probably dysentery, apparently influenced the retreat of Xerxes' army in 480 BC.[16] Since then, it has commonly affected armies in the field, often influencing the outcome of wars. Dysentery was almost certainly responsible for a large outbreak in France in 580 AD and much later contributed to the defeat of the crusaders. It did not become epidemic in England until the seventeenth century, when it was described by Sydenham in 1670:

sometimes accompanied with feaver and sometimes without but always with great torment in the bowells upon going to stoole with frequent dejections and these for the most part not stercorous but mucous which are mixt with streaks of blood in the beginning, but in further progress of the disease bloud in larger quantitys and umixed often is evacuated to the great hazard of the patient's life.[28]

Although mainly a community disease, there were outbreaks in hospitals in the eighteenth century, and person-to-person spread was described by John Pringle in 1764. He stated that 'it was a most fatal distemper incident to every place illaired and kept dirty [i.e. jails and hospitals]. It spread by septic ferments with diarrhoea as a common symptom and showed a high degree of contagion'.[29,30] It was also described by Lind, who made suggestions for its prevention in the Royal Navy.[31] Dysentery often occurred at the same time as typhus and was sometimes confused with it. With improvements in hygiene, outbreaks became less frequent in developed countries. In Birmingham General Hospital in the 1850s, the number of cases reported annually remained low, at one to ten cases per year,[22] but epidemics continued in armies. In the American Civil War, 233 812 cases of acute dysentery were reported, with 4084 deaths.[20] Large outbreaks have continued to occur in developing countries in the twentieth century. In 1970, 200 000 cases, with 11 500 deaths, were reported in Mexico and Central America. It has been estimated that between 1966 and 1977, there were 164.7 million cases in the world, of which 163.7 million cases were in developing countries.[32] The strains causing outbreaks are showing increasing antibiotic resistance, but the extent of hospital spread in developing countries is unknown.[33]

Outbreaks of dysentery, caused mainly by *Shigella sonne* and *S. flexner*, have been reported in mental hospitals and occasionally in children's wards or infant nurseries in this century,[5] but hospital-acquired infections are now reported rarely in developed countries due to improvements in hygiene, despite the fact that the infecting dose is very low (about 100 organisms).

Cholera

Cholera has been described as the classic epidemic disease of the nineteenth century. Its symptoms are mainly profuse, non-inflammatory diarrhoea, and death is usually due to severe dehydration.[27] The causal organism is a curved Gram-negative bacterium known as a vibrio. *Vibrio cholerae* was identified by Koch, but the disease and evidence of its spread were known much earlier (see Chapter 7).[16] Exactly when it was recognized remains unconfirmed, but descriptions of probable cholera have appeared in Asia from about 500 AD and more certainly in the fourteenth and fifteenth centuries. The disease was endemic in India and the Far East in the nineteenth century and from there spread to most countries of the world, including Europe and the USA.[16,20] Epidemics continued into the twentieth century, the largest caused by a new strain known as El Tor lasting from 1961 to 1974. Cholera remains endemic in 80, mainly tropical countries, but particularly in the Ganges Delta region, and large outbreaks are still related to natural catastrophes and wars. Although many cases may be admitted to hospital, cross-infection is not usually a problem, but hospital spread is occasionally reported in developing countries.[33]

Other foodborne organisms

In addition to the organisms described above, a number of others can cause food or waterborne infections.[34] These mainly cause outbreaks in the community, but they may also involve hospitals, although person-to-person spread is uncommon. *Campylobacter jejuni* is the most common cause of food poisoning; it is usually acquired from meat or dairy products, but transfer from person to person is, uncommonly, a cause. A number of other bacteria, such as *Yersinia enterocolitica*, are rare causes of hospital infection.[34]

Outbreaks of food poisoning can also be caused by toxin (poison)-producing strains of bacteria. Contamination of food with toxigenic strains of *Staphylococcus aureus* from a carrier or infected member of the hospital catering staff is sometimes a source of infection. The organism grows in the food usually at room temperature and forms enterotoxins, which are responsible for the symptoms. Toxigenic strains of *Clostridium perfringens* (originally *C. welchii*) may cause outbreaks in hospitals, mainly in geriatric units. These are Gram-positive, anaerobic, sporing bacilli; they are commonly isolated from stews, gravies and meat pies stored at room temperature and reheated, as the spores allow the organisms to survive moderate heating. *Bacillus cereus* is an aerobic, sporing bacillus that is responsible for infections from inadequately heated food, especially rice and chicken.[34] It is a rare cause of other infections, including meningitis, possibly acquired from contaminated hospital linen.

Protozoa, such as cryptosporidia, can also cause cause foodborne infections (Chapter 16), but these are infrequent in hospitals in developed countries.

Tetanus and gas gangrene

Clostridium spp. have already been discussed as causes of food poisoning and diarrhoeal disease. However, they are also commonly associated with traumatic wounds, but they are rarely a cause of hospital infection as they do not spread from patient to patient and they require special conditions to grow in tissues.

C. tetani, the causative organism of tetanus, was first grown by Kitasato, a Japanese bacteriologist. The lethal action of the neurotoxin it produced was reported by Kitasato in 1889.[35] The organism forms spores and survives well in the environment. It is normally found in the faeces of man and animals, especially horses. Its spores are often present in the air and on the surfaces in operating theatres, but postoperative infections are rare. Neonatal tetanus occurs in some developing countries due to the application of faecally contaminated materials to the umbilical site. Tetanus has always been a problem of war injuries causing numerous deaths, although data on incidence were rarely available before the twentieth century. The use of horses in war used to cause considerable contamination of the battlefield. In the First World War, 2385 of over two million wounded British soldiers developed the disease. Following the introduction of immunization, tetanus almost disappeared as a consequence of war or of civilian traumatic wounds.[20] In England and Wales, only 388 deaths were reported between 1954 and 1962, and the incidence has continued to decrease. In hospitals, *C. tetani* have been reported in improperly sterilized catgut, cellulose wadding, cotton wool, plaster of Paris bandages, injections of drugs, and some other environmental sources; infection has been reported from some of these items, especially catgut and injections of drugs, but outbreaks have rarely been reported.[5] In the 1940s, postoperative tetanus was reported to probably have been acquired by two patients from dust that was admitted from grazing pastures through an open window in the operating theatre during an operation.[36]

At about the same time in another hospital in the UK, tetanus occurred in two patients following operations for open reduction of fractures in the lower limb. No organisms were isolated from the wounds or the theatre, but *C. tetani* were found in the plaster, hair and dust from walls in another theatre under repair, and it seemed likely that the final vehicle was talc in gloves used at the operations.[37] In neither of these outbreaks could environmental strains be related to infecting strains, as the organisms were not isolated from the wounds and typing methods were not available.

Gas gangrene is also caused by a clostridium, usually *C. welchii* (now *C. perfringens*), named after an American pathologist and bacteriologist, William Welch, althouth sometimes other species are involved. Infections usually occur in traumatic wounds, and until the twentieth century they were a common cause of death following war injuries.[20] Gas gangrene was a major problem in the trenches in the First World War, but few cases occurred in the Second World War. In civilian practice, it is commonly associated with a poor blood supply to tissues, e.g. following severe trauma, following injection of contaminated adrenaline, or postoperatively following amputation for an ischaemic limb.[5] However, the organisms are often present in wounds in the absence of clinical infection. Spores are normally present in the air and the environment and are part of the normal flora of the intestinal tract of man and animals. Spores are also commonly found in operating theatres, but hospital-acquired infection is now extremely rare. Surgical instruments were usually 'sterilized' by boiling in water from the end of the nineteenth century to the 1950s. The rarity of postoperative infections caused by spores was surprising. However, *C. perfringens* are apparently killed in 5 minutes by boiling water under laboratory conditions, but since that time instruments have been sterilized in an autoclave.[5] A possible outbreak of three cases over a period of 3 days was reported by Theodore Eikhoff in 1962.[38] Two operating theatres were involved, and airborne spread seemed to be unlikely. Surgical instruments were a possible common source, although the sterilization process appeared to be satisfactory. Endogenous infection also appeared to be unlikely, but typing methods were not available. This is one of the rare but unproven reports in recent years of possible infection due to inadequate sterilization of surgical instruments.

Hospital-acquired wound infection is mainly due to self-infection from the patient's own faeces, which often contaminate the surrounding skin, particularly in elderly and incontinent patients; typing of strains has confirmed the endogenous origin in several small outbreaks.[39] The spores of *C. perfringens* are resistant to antiseptics and are difficult to remove from the operation site for above-knee amputations in patients with ischaemic limbs. However, prophylaxis with penicillin is effective and is probably the main reason why postoperative gas gangrene has virtually disappeared in developed countries.

Pulmonary tuberculosis

Tuberculosis is an ancient disease and was well described in its various forms by Hippocrates. Fracastoro in the fifteenth century stated that it was contracted by people living in contact with someone with the disease, and later Benjamin Martin, in 1720, proposed that it was spread in the air by 'animalcules'.[20] A Dutchman, Franciscus Silvius, in the seventeenth century was the first to use the term 'tubercle' to describe the nodular lesions in the lung, and Johann Schoenlein coined the name 'tuberculosis' in the nineteenth century.[40] Villemin in 1868 was able to transmit tuberculosis using material from infected humans to infect guinea pigs and rabbits.[41] William Budd in 1857 proposed that 'germs' spread to susceptible individuals in tuberculous material and that this occurred in crowded conditions, but it was not until the work of Flugge and colleagues and later Riley in the twentieth century that it was shown to spread in airborne droplets.[42] The causal organism (*Mycobacterium tuberculosis*) was discovered by Koch in 1882. He recognized two types, the human and the bovine, the latter also causing disease in humans.[41] The bacterium is non-sporing; it stains poorly by Gram, and requires a special stain, the Ziehl–Neelsen. It grows slowly on culture and survives well in a dry state due to its fatty cell wall. Respiratory tuberculosis is now known to spread by the airborne route by means of droplet nuclei.

At the end of the eighteenth century, few hospitals were available for tuberculous patients; those that did exist were not popular because they were considered to be a sentence of death due to their unhygienic conditions. In the mid-nineteenth century, tuberculosis was responsible for about a quarter of the deaths in England and the USA, but the mortality soon started to fall due to improvements in hygiene.[16,23] Sanitoria were introduced in large numbers in the early twentieth century; for instance, in Bristol in 1950 there were 500 beds available for tuberculous patients.[9] The numbers of cases and mortality fell rapidly in the developed world, and by the late 1960s most of these sanitoria were closed. Nevertheless, in 1997 there were over seven million cases in the world, of which three million died.[40]

Leprosy

Leprosy is another ancient disease, probably existing in ancient Egypt and China. It was definitely known in Europe in the seventh and eighth centuries,[16,20] the problem being that it was confused with other skin diseases such as psoriasis and syphilis. It is caused by *Mycobacterium leprae*, discovered by Hansen in Norway in 1874, and it was one of the first bacterial causes of human disease to be recognized.[43] However, Neisser in 1879 was the first to give a clear account of the organism based on properly stained material.[44]

Leprosy is a chronic disease of the skin and mucous membranes, affecting the peripheral nervous tissue. It has a long incubation period of 2–10 years and is poorly transmissible. It is contracted following prolonged exposure to respiratory secretions, mainly in the acute stages of the disease. Lepers were ostracized from the earliest time because of their grotesque appearance, being isolated in leper houses (leprosaria) in the Middle Ages because of their appearance rather than because of any knowledge of contagiousness. The incidence rose to a peak in the eleventh to thirteenth centuries, but the disease gradually died out in Europe in the fourteenth and fifteenth centuries.[16] In France, there were 2000 leper houses in the eleventh century, and in Great Britain there were 362 in the fifteenth century; these were mainly in monastic institutions, which were destroyed in the Reformation of the sixteenth century (Chapter 2). However, there were still ten million cases in the world in 1965, but the numbers have since been reduced following the discovery of an effective treatment with dapsone and similar compounds.[27]

Plague

The first major pandemic appearing in Europe was in the fourteenth century, when plague was recognized as a contagious disease (see Chapter 2). The last pandemic spread from China to Hong Kong in 1893–4, then to India, and later to Europe.[20,27] In the UK, cases were few in the latter pandemic and usually confined to ports. Presumably hospital-acquired infection occurred during the pandemics, and a wide variety of isolation precautions were recommended. The cases reported in this century were mainly acquired directly from rodents and their fleas, and cross-infection in hospital has not been reported in the Western world. Patients with pneumonic plague are isolated under strict precautions. Cases of plague are still reported annually in Asia, Africa and the southern states of the USA.

Typhus

Typhus was a major disease of armies, prisons and hospitals in the eighteenth and nineteenth centuries (see Chapter 4). The discovery in 1909 that the body louse was the vector of typhus enabled Western European armies to organize defensive measures against the insect of such efficiency that the disease was kept at bay throughout the appalling conditions of trench warfare that characterized the Western Front in the 1914–18 war. The situation was different in the Eastern armies from countries where the disease was still endemic.[20] In 1915, typhus was rife in the Serbian army, until it was brought under control by British and French medical missions. At the end of the war, the Russian armies were badly affected, and a British mission was sent out to help. It began operations by separating typhus patients from others before evacuation from the front, insisting on keeping hospital beds well spaced, and it finally set up a special hospital for typhus patients only.

During the Second World War, there were outbreaks of typhus with a high mortality in North Africa and Iran. American troops were rarely affected due to the introduction of a vaccine and DDT (an insecticide). An outbreak in the ruins of Naples in 1943–4 among a louse-infested population of 500 000 was effectively controlled by DDT and vaccination, as were outbreaks in Germany and Japan at the end of the war. A final warning was given by Zinsser in his classic book, *Rats, Lice and History*.[45] He concluded: 'Typhus is not dead. It will live on for centuries, and it will continue to break into the open wherever human stupidity and brutality give it a chance, as most likely they occasionally will.'

Scabies

Scabies is caused by a mite, *Sarcoptes scabei*, that burrows into the skin and gives rise to lesions commonly involving the finger webs, and the flexures of the wrists, elbows, axillae, female breasts and male genital areas. It causes intense itching and spreads mainly by skin-to-skin contact. Scabies is associated with overcrowding, malnutrition and poor hygiene. The disease has been known since biblical times, but it has always been confused with other skin diseases, such as eczema and leprosy. Thomas Moffatt was probably the first to identify the location of mites on the skin in the sixteenth century.[46,47] One of the first major contributions to the understanding of the aetiology of scabies was made by Giovanni Bonomo (1663–96) in Florence, when he reported in a letter to Redi in 1687 his observations that mites burrowed into skin and deposited eggs. Bonomo also recognized the contagiousness of the disease.

Scabies remained a scourge of armies until the middle of the nineteenth century. For example, Schmucker, the Chief Surgeon of Frederick the Great's army during the Seven Years War (1756–63), stated that 'the number of cases of scabies increased tremendously in field hospitals because many of the patients were huddled together in small rooms, deprived of fresh air and were lacking in necessary cleanliness'. He believed that the dirtiness of the soldiers was in most cases responsible for the disease. Pringle, in his *Diseases of the Army*, made observations on 'the Itch', stating that 'it was communicated by contact, not "effluvia" as in dysentery or malignant fever. It seems to be caused by certain small insects (Leeuwenhoek) discovered in the pustules by the microscope' [a footnote also acknowledges the description of Dr Bonomo]. Infection occurs in ships, tents and barracks but of all places, the hospitals are the most liable to the contagion as receiving all sorts of patients'.[29,30] Wichmann, a physician from Hanover, in his publication *Aetiologie der Kratze* contended that 'field hospitals were permanently infected with scabies, mites being hatched and spread there continuously, due to the impossibility thoroughly to clean the mite infested woolen blankets used by the soldiers'.[47] Despite these descriptions of the mites and the disease, many physicians continued to believe that scabies was due to some disorder of the human body humours.

Outbreaks continued throughout the world in the twentieth century, particularly in overcrowded and unhygienic conditions, and especially in long-term care institutions. A condition termed 'Norwegian scabies' is especially likely to spread in hospitals and other residential institutions and to be transferred to healthcare staff, even under reasonably hygienic conditions, due to the very large number of parasites on the skin of infested patients.[48] These mites may also spread on clothing and bedding, although they tend to survive poorly in the environment. Scabies can be treated effectively by appropriate pesticides, and worldwide eradication should be possible in the twenty-first century.

The twentieth century: the emergence of antimicrobial chemotherapy and the demise of the haemolytic streptococcus

The discovery of bacteria at the end of the nineteenth century introduced a new search for possible antimicrobial agents that could be used for systemic treatment of infections. German workers were already interested in the effects of dyes on micro-organisms. In particular, Paul Ehrlich in Berlin described the use of aniline dyes for treating leishmaniasis and other protozoal infections; he also described a new arsenical, Salvarsan, for the treatment of syphilis.[1] Ehrlich is considered to be the father of modern chemotherapy and was awarded a Nobel Prize in 1908. He introduced the concept of selective toxicity in which organisms in the body could be killed without damage to the host tissues. He also discovered the phenomenon of acquired resistance of protozoa to chemicals. None of these advances influenced the treatment of hospital infections directly, but they led to the discovery of an important group of antibacterial agents, the sulphonamides, in the 1930s.

Franz Mietzsch and Josef Klarer, working for Bayer in Germany, synthesized a number of dyes. One of these, prontosil, was found by Domagk in 1935 to be effective against streptococcal infections in mice.[2] Domagk was awarded the Nobel Prize for his work, but he was prevented from collecting it by the Nazi regime. Colebrook and Kenny, in 1936, successfully treated puerperal fever patients with prontosil (p. 137).[3] French workers demonstrated that sulphonamide was the active principle in prontosil and was split off in the body by enzyme action. A series of other sulphonamides was developed, one of the most effective being a broad-spectrum compound, sulphapyridine, popularly known as M and B 693, since it was the six hundred and ninety-third substance to be tested by May and Baker.[1] Sulphonamides are particularly active against Gram-positive cocci, including haemolytic streptococci, and were often life-saving in severe infections caused by these organisms.

Streptococcal infections, such as erysipelas, cellulitis, scarlet fever and puerperal fever (but not hospital gangrene), continued into the twentieth century as important causes of hospital infection. The reason for the disappearance of hospital gangrene remains unclear, but techniques such as surgical debridement (cleaning and removal of damaged or dead tissues), drainage of wounds, and the introduction of antiseptic and aseptic techniques improved the prognosis and reduced the death rate. However, the mortality and morbidity from severe streptococcal infections remained considerable until the 1930s, when sulphonamides were introduced. Non-suppurative complications of streptococcal infections, i.e. acute rheumatic fever and kidney disease (glomerular nephritis), occurred in the first half of the twentieth century, but they have since almost disappeared in the developed world, possibly due to changes in the virulence of streptococci as well as to the use of penicillin for treatment and prophylaxis.

Bacteriological techniques improved in the early part of the twentieth century, and most common species of bacteria could be identified by staining and cultural techniques. Streptococci were recognized in pus as Gram-positive cocci occurring in chains (see Chapter 7). The destruction of red cells (haemolysis) by streptococci growing on blood agar allowed them to be classified into alpha-haemolytic, beta-haemolytic and non-haemolytic types. Alpha-haemolysis shows a greenish colouration, but those showing clear (beta) haemolysis caused most of the suppurative complications. However, this did not apply to all strains, and their epidemiology was elucidated further in the 1930s by the introduction of typing methods. Typing systems use specific markers to characterize individual strains and to differentiate them from other strains of the same species. Rebecca Lancefield[4] described a precipitin test in which a range of antisera is used to detect surface antigens (proteins specific to the group) of a particular species of streptococcus, which enabled beta-haemolytic streptococci to be subdivided into groups, of which A, B, C, D and G are of medical importance. Group A (*Streptococcus pyogenes*) was the predominant type causing severe infections, and a further subdivision of this group into 20 strains was made possible by use of another typing method described by Fred Griffith in 1934.[5]

Typing methods are particularly useful for recognizing cross-infection in hospitals and confirmed that outbreaks could be caused by transmission from healthy carriers. Cross-infection due to group A streptococci was demonstrated in burns wards, ear, nose and throat wards, and infectious diseases wards. As well as demonstrating the spread of different strains of group A streptococci in scarlet fever wards, typing showed that complications such as otitis and mastoiditis often followed the introduction of new strains.[6,7]

Major infections remained a problem. In Boston City Hospital, severe outbreaks of streptococcal infection occurred during an economic depression in the 1920s, and the disability and death from the disease were appalling. Wesley Spink stated that 'the strain on the overworked hospital staff was almost overwhelming and terribly frustrating at times'. Mortality from complications associated with bacteraemia (bloodstream infection) was about 75%, rising to 90% in patients with streptococcal pneumonia and empyaema (pus in the chest cavity). Cases of meningitis rarely recovered.[1]

Scarlet fever had been well described several centuries before in the 1700s by John Gregory, Professor of Medicine in Edinburgh,[8] and it was still treated as a very serious condition in the 1930s. Spink recalls:

> As a child I was incarcerated by the health department because I had been sent home from school with a sore throat and a rash. In addition my family was restricted in activity because of a large red placard nailed to the front of the house with the black letters 'scarlet fever' to be sure no one ventured near us. At the same time, those of my schoolmates without a rash and only a mild sore throat, probably harbouring the same strain, were allowed back to school after a day or two.[1]

In the 1930s, the sister of one of the authors (GA), also suffering from scarlet fever, was removed in a special fever ambulance to an isolation hospital, and a blanket soaked in disinfectant was hung over the stairs in the house.

Group A streptococci were responsible for about 50% of cases of puerperal fever in the 1920s, and it was still a problem in the 1930s, accounting for about 2000 maternal deaths a year in England and Wales. The number of deaths had not changed much in the previous 50 years.[9]

Leonard Colebrook (1883–1967) and colleagues was one of the major influences in the reduction of puerperal sepsis in the twentieth century.[9,10] He was a distinguished bacteriologist, but the alleviation of human suffering remained paramount in his career. He joined Almroth Wright's team at St Mary's Hospital, London, and worked on gunshot wounds during the First World War. Later, he studied streptococcal infections in obstetrics and burns patients and made significant advances in their treatment and prevention. Following the First World War, Colebrook commenced the study of puerperal sepsis. He soon realized that the doctrine of Semmelweiss was not being followed regularly, so he campaigned for the routine use of gloves and masks and hand-washing before attending a patient. Colebrook demonstrated that cursory washing of the hands with soap and water was not very effective and he sought a nontoxic disinfectant. Lysol and perchloride of mercury were much favoured at the time, but they were potentially toxic. He found that chloroxylenol (Dettol) was remarkably nontoxic and highly effective against streptococci, and it became used widely in midwifery for disinfecting the hands and the vagina. Griffith's typing of group A streptococci used by Colebrook and his younger sister, Dora, at Queen Charlotte's Hospital helped to demonstrate that the streptococci were more often transmitted from the staff than from the patient herself.[9] In the early 1930s, Dora reported that in 63 cases of puerperal fever, the infecting type occurred in the respiratory tract of two-thirds of contacts, and in one-third the organism was in the patient herself; in some instances it was present in both. This apparently confirmed the importance of preventing transmission

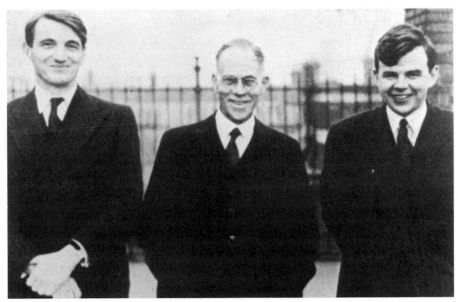

Figure 10.1   Ashley Miles, Leonard Colebrook and Robert Williams (left to right) at the Birmingham Accident Hospital in the early 1940s. (Peter London, FRCS; Birmingham.)

by wearing face masks and also the exclusion from duty of staff carriers (see Chapter 8).

Although there was a fall in deaths from puerperal sepsis over the period of 1930–35, it remains uncertain how much was due to hygienic measures and how much to loss of virulence in the organisms. A rather more impressive reduction was obtained by the use of sulphonamides. Colebrook and Kenny in 1936 found that in treated patients the mortality was 4%, while in untreated patients it was 20%; over 95% of infections were sensitive to the drug.[3] However, a controlled trial was not carried out, and the national mortality rate was already falling. Thereafter, the decline in deaths from puerperal fever was steep, possibly also due to the introduction of penicillin in the 1940s, a drug that is more effective than the sulphonamides.

In the Second World War, streptococcal cross-infection of wounds still occurred, and Sir Ashley Miles and his colleagues played a prominent role in elucidating the epidemiology and prevention of infection. Miles had a distinguished career in bacteriology.[11] He was appointed Professor of Bacteriology at University College Hospital in 1938 after posts at the London School of Hygiene and Hammersmith Hospital, London. He showed an early interest in hospital epidemiology, particularly in the use of quantitative methods and their statistical applications. In 1941, he became part-time Director of the Medical Research Council at the Birmingham Accident Hospital, studying war wounds (Figure 10.1). Miles and his colleagues, who included Robert Williams, showcd that only 8% of wounds acquired

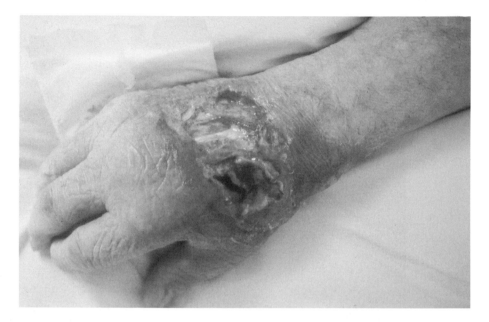

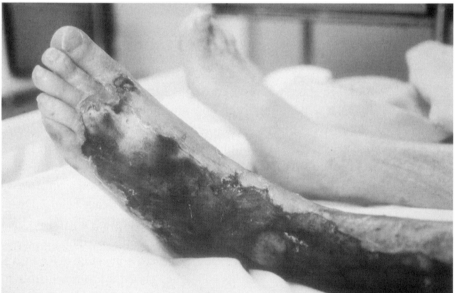

Figure 10.2 Streptococcal gangrene of hand and leg (necrotizing fasciitis). (Dr M. Barnham, Harrogate.)

streptococci in the first 3 days but that 30% were infected after 2–3 weeks, i.e. most infections were hospital-acquired.[12] Infection was mainly spread from wound to wound by contact and could be reduced by improved non-touch dressing techniques.[13] Infections were often associated with staphylococcal as well as streptococcal sepsis.

Streptococcal infection of burns remained a cause of severe sepsis and often death until the 1950s, and it continued to cause graft failure after that time. Cruikshank in 1935 believed that airborne spread was important, and he showed the presence of haemolytic streptococci in the air when infected wounds were being dressed.[14] Bourdillon and Colebrook, working in Birmingham after the Second World War, also showed that the acquisition of bacteria in burns could be reduced by using an air-conditioned dressing room, but they also realized the importance of contact spread (see also Chapter 12).[15] Bourdillon was responsible for developing the air sampler (slit-sampler), which, with slight modifications, has remained in use until the present day.

The group A streptococci are now usually only minor causes of throat or skin infection, and the presence of a generalized rash in combination with a throat or skin infection is uncommon in developed countries. They are some of the few organisms that have remained sensitive to benzylpenicillin after exposure to the drug for over 50 years, although they have occasionally acquired resistance to other antibiotics, such as erythromycin and tetracycline. Nevertheless, they still cannot be ignored, as severe systemic infections associated with virulent strains can occur, sometimes with septic shock, resulting in a high mortality. Occasional outbreaks of infection have been reported in postoperative wounds in recent years, and rarely, a severe gangrenous lesion of the skin (necrotizing fasciitis), described in the popular press as 'flesh-eating disease' and resembling hospital gangrene of the previous century, is reported (Figure 10.2). These cases require urgent surgery as well as high doses of penicillin[16]. Between 1955 and 1958, only 22 epidemics of more than four cases of puerperal sepsis were reported in England and Wales, and numbers have continued to decrease.[7]

Spread of infection

Bacteriological studies in the 1930s showed that group A streptococci could be isolated from 5–15% of the throats of healthy people, and sometimes from the nose.[7] The bacteria survive poorly on normal skin but have been isolated in large numbers from bedding and dust. Transmission on the hands, as shown by Semmelweiss, is probably the main mode of spread. The rapid spread of upper respiratory infections and the isolation of large numbers of streptococci from the air of military establishments during the Second World War suggested airborne spread, possibly by means of droplet nuclei, although evidence of particle sizes is not available. Hamburger and colleagues in the 1940s showed that nasal carriers were frequently heavy streptococcal dispersers[17] (i.e. they shed large numbers into the environment) and that they were often responsible for outbreaks. Although heavy nasal carriers were referred to as 'dangerous spreaders' at the time, these are now found rarely, and throat carriers or infected patients are the usual sources of infection. Dispersal is probably mainly on skin scales contaminated from an infected or colonized carriage site, similarly to *Staphylococcus aureus* (see Chapter 12), but again evidence is lacking. Either skin scales or large droplets from the respiratory tract, in addition to the hands, are probably responsible for most instances of transmission.

The role of the inanimate environment remains uncertain. Group A streptococci were frequently isolated from dust of wards containing clinical cases, and high air counts were found during bed making and floor sweeping. Oiling of bed clothes and floors reduced the air counts; in one study in a measles ward, oiling reduced cross-infection with group A streptococci,[18] but this was not confirmed in other studies. Most experiments that reduced the number of airborne organisms by oiling floors or bedding did not influence the spread of infection. There is also evidence from Rammelkamp and colleagues that dried group A streptococci have reduced virulence.[19] Military recruits issued with blankets contaminated with streptococci from infected patients did not acquire streptococcal infections, nor did volunteers become infected after infected dust was blown into their noses. Although the throat, especially of healthcare workers, is one of the main carriage site sources, other sources as well as the nose have been described, such as the umbilicus in neonates and, in recent years, the vagina and rectum. Less convincingly, environmental sources including dust, lavatory seats and showerheads have been suggested.[20]

The modes of spread are complex, and studies on transmission have decreased with the considerable reduction in outbreaks over the past 60 years. The number of cases of hospital-acquired group A streptococcal infection is now minimal compared with those caused by *Staph. aureus* and Gram-negative bacilli.

The twentieth century: sterilization, sterile services and disinfection

Decontamination of contagious materials by heat or cleaning has been used since biblical times, but most of the work on sterilization has occurred since the discovery of micro-organisms at the end of the nineteenth century.

After the initial studies by German workers (see Chapter 8), there was little interest in sterilizing processes in the twentieth century until the 1950s, when outbreaks of hospital infection led to a re-evaluation of aseptic techniques and it was realized that 'sterilized' items were not necessarily sterile. Faults in the installation, operation and maintenance of autoclaves were found, and poor packing of the contents was noted; in addition, many autoclaves were old and outdated, and autoclave operators were often trained inadequately. James Bowie in 1955 found that only five out of 64 autoclaves tested were satisfactory,[1] and similar results were obtained by James Howie and Morag Timbury.[2] One of the major influences on improving the reliability and efficiency of steam sterilizers was the Nuffield Provincial Hospitals Trust report, *Present Sterilizing Practices in Six Hospitals*, popularly known as the 'Yellow Peril'.[3] The Nuffield team was led by Brigadier Welch, the autoclaves were tested by V.G. Alder of Bristol, and other aspects of sterile supply provision were also investigated by two nurses, A.L. Amsden and D.F. Walker. In addition to the deficiencies of the autoclaves, the methods of use of metal dressing drums, ward boilers and forceps (cheatles type) for removing dressings from the drums were all criticized. The report led to recommendations on standards for autoclaves by a committee of the Medical Research Council (MRC) (1959–64).[4] Collaborative work between Alder and industry led to metal drums for dressings being replaced by cardboard boxes and disposable paper packaging replacing reusable cloth.

The Nuffield Report expedited the development of central sterile supply departments (CSSDs), which had been used in the USA by Perkins[5] for some time, Carl Walter having considered them to be essential by the late 1940s.[6] The idea of CSSDs was initially introduced in the UK by British military services following the Suez campaign in 1956, when the Americans demonstrated their techniques for transporting sterile equipment in packs. Until this time, nurses in the wards had

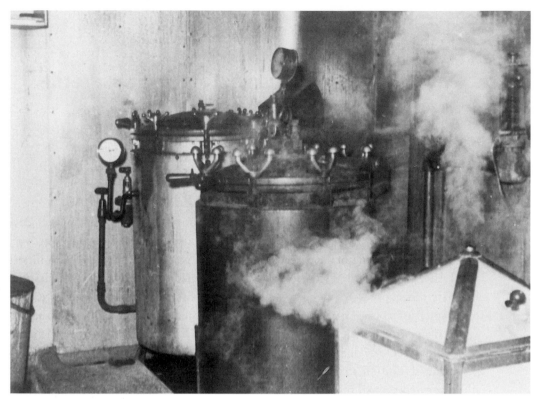

Figure 11.1   Laboratory autoclaves and a 'Koch' steamer, mid-twentieth century. (Hospital Infection Research Laboratory, Birmingham.)

prepared surgical dressings, packing them in drums that were subsequently sent to be autoclaved and were then returned to the same ward.[7] Centralization of sterile supplies enabled boilers and dressing preparation to be removed from wards and individual departments. Evidence was produced on the importance of removal of air and the use of vacuum pumps for high-vacuum autoclaves.[4,8,9] Tests of efficacy were introduced, in particular the Bowie–Dick test, which was a simple method of ensuring adequate steam penetration of autoclave loads.[10] Physical methods of testing autoclaves were preferred in the UK, although spore tests continued to be used in the USA and Europe. J.C. Kelsey and Ron Fallon were leading figures in the testing processes of sterilization and disinfection, and Kelsey became the first director of the Public Health Laboratory Service (PHLS) disinfection laboratory at Colindale.

A central syringe service was introduced in England during the Second World War by Stark Murray. This was continued and extended to other hospitals because of worries about hepatitis from inadequately cleaned and sterilized syringes and needles.[11] Then an infrared, dry-heat, movable-belt sterilizer for syringes was developed by E.M. Darmady and colleagues in 1957,[12] and the requirements for setting up a central service were described by the Nuffield Trust.[13] From the late 1960s, glass syringes were gradually replaced for most purposes by commercially produced disposable syringes and needles, and central syringe processes were gradually phased out.

The first purpose-built CSSD in the UK was at Musgrave Park in Belfast, and new accommodation was built at Addenbrooke's Hospital in Cambridge, soon to be followed by departments at Bristol Royal Infirmary and other major hospitals. These developed along the lines recommended by the Nuffield Hospitals Trust.[11,13]

Sterilizing processes continued to improve, but there were occasional setbacks, e.g. an outbreak of infection arose from contaminated commercially prepared intravenous preparations in 1972 due to a failure of the bottles in an autoclave to reach an appropriate temperature.[14] Improved standards for the design, engineering and testing of sterilizers were prepared by British Standards committees and the Department of Health of England and Wales, leading to the appointment of specialist engineers to monitor the routine performance of sterilizers and to advise on their use and management. Central processing of surgical instruments was standardized by the use of wrapped trays containing sets of instruments for each operation. This system was developed by James Bowie in Edinburgh and was known as the Edinburgh pre-set tray system. Sheila Scott, who later became a nursing officer in the Department of Health, was very much involved in persuading her colleagues to introduce the system in the operating theatres.[7] The system was gradually modified and introduced in all CSSDs, and it is still in use today. Wrapping techniques for dressings were also improved by various workers, especially R. Shooter and S. Allen at St Bartholomew's Hospital and V. G. Alder in Bristol.[11] Some of these departments became more specialized; those responsible for processing surgical instruments were attached to operating theatres and were known as theatre sterile supply units (TSSUs). Of interest is the recent return of metal or plastic containers, now fitted with bacteriological filters, for sterilizing dressings and instruments.

Central processing was often extended to include a hospital sterilization and disinfection unit (HSDU), as were many units in the USA. The HSDU was responsible for decontamination and processing medical equipment, such as respiratory and suction equipment and infant incubators. An early department was developed in Dudley Road Hospital in Birmingham by Ivor Ankrett, supported by the Hospital Infection Research Laboratory; the first purpose-built HSDU was established at Pinderfields Hospital, Wakefield, in the 1970s.[11]

Over the past 30 years, health and safety regulations and European directives and committees on standards have had an increasing influence on sterile supply practices. The range of single-use plastic items available has increased, and the role of commercial manufacturers making standard sterile commercial packs and

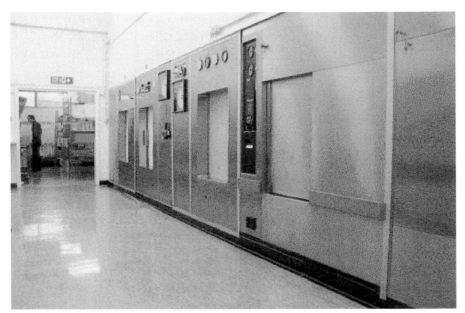

Figure 11.2 Bank of high-vacuum steam autoclaves in a modern central services department. (Sterile Service Department, City Hospital, Birmingham.)

supplementary dressing packs was outlined by a National Health steering committee under the chairmanship of Professor A.C. Cunliffe.[7] Implementation of these recommendations has enabled hospital-based departments to concentrate on their core function – to reprocess reusable medical devices.

New problems have arisen over the past 30 years in the sterilization or disinfection of heat-labile equipment. Ethylene oxide gas was initially used in industry before and after the Second World War, and was introduced for medical devices following studies by Phillips and Kaye.[15] It was used widely in hospitals in the USA and also in Europe, but it was used little in hospital CSSDs in the UK apart from in a few regional centres. Disinfection and sterilization with formaldehyde gas have been in use for many years,[16] and the sporicidal effect of adding formaldehyde to low-temperature steam at 70 °C was first demonstrated in 1902 by Esmarch in Germany. Alder in the 1960s developed a low-temperature steam formaldehyde (LTSF) autoclave that sterilizes items at 73 °C,[17] and a method for testing the efficacy was described by Line and Pickerill.[18] Later, George Gibson, Cameron Weymes and others were involved in further studies on the process and applications in hospitals.[11]

The considerable increase in the use of heat-labile fibre-optic endoscopes for diagnostic and surgical use created a decontamination problem that still exists today (see Chapter 17). Chemical disinfectants were required and sterilization processes were rarely possible. These fibre-optic endoscopes are often required quickly, but fast decontamination cannot be achieved by commonly available gaseous processes.

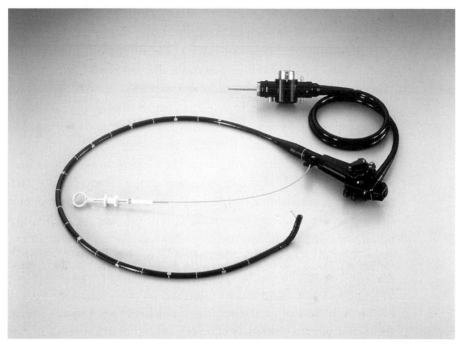

Figure 11.3 Fibre-optic endoscope (gastroscope). (Hospital Infection Research Laboratory, Birmingham.)

In addition, the narrow channels, especially of gastroscopes, are difficult to clean and disinfect (Figure 11.3). Early efforts at manual processing were often associated with inadequate cleaning and disinfection, followed by infection in the patients, especially with Gram-negative bacteria such as *Pseudomonas aeruginosa*,[19] until improved disinfection was obtained with glutaraldehyde. Many of the studies in this field were carried out at the Hospital Infection Research Laboratory, Birmingham, by John Babb and Christine Bradley. These problems were followed by the development of automated washer disinfectors, new disinfectants (see page 148), and gaseous sterilization methods such as gas plasma, using vapourized hydrogen peroxide. The production of autoclavable, rigid, operative endoscopes was encouraged, but flexible, operative endoscopes are still damaged by heat over 60 °C and require chemical treatment.[20]

The difficulties of reliably cleaning and disinfecting or sterilizing many of the heat-labile items, and the increasing costs of employing trained staff in developed countries, was associated with a considerable increase in the use of single-use items.[21] Although often cost-effective and improving the safety of patients and staff (e.g. disposable syringes and needles), some items, such as disposable anaesthetic circuits, are associated with a considerable increase in cost, which can reduce their use in developing countries. For example, the use of expensive, single-use cardiac catheters would reduce the number of patients treated. A major controversy is now developing about disposables. Most are made of nondegradable plastics and are responsible for increasing amounts of clinical (and other) waste. The disposal of waste creates problems either due to insufficient landfill sites or due to incineration producing toxic gases (unless very expensive incinerators are installed). The disposal of waste is a general problem of which clinical waste is only a part. Clinical waste disposal is particularly expensive, although apart from needles and other sharp instruments, the infection hazards are low.[21]

Another recent complicating factor is the emergence of prions (see Chapter 16), which are resistant to normal sterilization temperatures. The occurrence of bovine spongiform encephalopathy (BSE) in humans has increased the demand for single-use surgical instruments for certain operations. The possibility of prion disease going unrecognized in its early stages has increased the requirement for efficient cleaning of all reusable surgical instruments in a washer/disinfector, which can itself provide a reasonable degree of safety by removing protein and 10^2–10^3 organisms without a specific disinfection or sterilization process.

The early days of CSSDs and the problems of sterilization in the UK led to a meeting at Portsmouth in 1958 on the invitation of Darmady of a small number of interested people who initially were mainly hospital bacteriologists. This meeting led to the formation of the Central Sterilizing Club (CSC).[7,11] Since then, the club has expanded to include CSSD managers, hospital engineers, infection-control nurses, medical laboratory technicians, administrators and other interested parties. The multidisciplinary aspect has been particularly useful. However, the sterile supply administrators required a separate specialist organization to further develop training and standards, so the Association of Sterile Supply Administrators was formed in the 1960s. Training was initiated under the guidance of Eileen Holmes, and the first training manual was produced. In the 1980s, a need for more evidence of competence and training of CSSD managers led to the emergence of the Institute of Sterile Services Management (ISSM).[7] Max Cadmore and his team produced in 1989 the *Guide to Good Manufacturing Practice for National Health Sterile Service Departments*. This document was consolidated into the ISSM's *Quality Standards and Recommended Practices* in 2000.

In the last decade, international meetings on central services have been held, organized by Gillian Sills; European meetings have also become increasingly important in establishing European standards. The future of CSSDs (now called central services departments in the UK) remains uncertain, but recent emphasis on quality assurance of decontamination of medical devices has established more firmly a need for efficient hospital-based departments. However, the increasing number of European directives and standards, some of which are not met easily in small departments, are encouraging the use of commercial suppliers or larger hospital departments, but the campaign against general use of disposables could reverse this trend in the twenty-first century.

Disinfection

Although steam sterilization is used routinely for most surgical instruments, chemical disinfection has continued to be used for decontamination of the inanimate environment, of some heat-labile equipment, of dirty wounds, and of staff hands.[22,23]

Phenol (carbolic acid) was found to be too toxic for application to wounds, but a wide range of phenolic products have been developed since Lister's time, including 'white' and 'black' fluids, Lysol and clear soluble phenolics, for environmental use. Some phenol derivatives, such as chloroxylenols and hexachlorophene, have also been used for skin disinfection, but although they fulfilled a useful role for a time, they have mainly been replaced by newer compounds.[22]

Chlorine compounds continue to play an important role, mainly in environmental disinfection. Chlorine was discovered in 1774 by a Swedish chemist, Scheele, and Bertholet, a French chemist, discovered hypochlorites in 1789.[24,25] Hypochlorites were originally used to counteract noxious odours thought to be causing infectious diseases. Labarque in 1825 used calcium hypochlorite for washing mortuaries, hospital wards, and other potentially contaminated sites. He also reported that hypochlorites were used successfully in Paris on infected wounds in burns, and in England for the purification of drinking water. Alcock in 1827 used bleaching powder as a disinfectant. Nevertheless, the British Board of Health in 1832 stated that chlorine gas was ineffectual in preventing the spread of infectious fevers in hospital wards. Chlorine compounds were used successfully in obstetrics by Robert Collins, Semmelweiss and others in the nineteenth century (see Chapter 5), and their use continued in the twentieth century, particularly for the treatment of water and sewage. A chlorine solution (Dakin's) was used widely in the First World War for disinfecting wounds, and another chlorine-containing solution, Eusol, was used until recently as a wound-desloughing agent. However, Eusol is now used infrequently owing to its toxic effect on normal cells. A resurgence in the use of chlorine agents occurred in the 1980s as the emergence of bloodborne pathogens, such as hepatitis B and HIV, became apparent. A variety of preparations with different activities is now available; in addition to hypochlorites, these include sodium dichloroisocyanurate, chlorine dioxide and superoxidized water. Chlorine compounds have the advantage of being actively viricidal and cheap, but they are corrosive to surgical instruments unless effective anticorrosive agents are added.[25,26]

Mercury compounds have also been used since ancient times, and were employed in the fifteenth century and onwards to the twentieth century for the treatment of syphilis. Mercuric bichloride was used by Koch as a disinfectant. It was less corrosive than phenol, and surgeons tended to use it, or alternatives such as mercury oxycyanide,[25,27] for disinfecting the hands and instruments. Less toxic but more active organic mercurials were developed as antiseptics in the twentieth century. However, their use for purposes other than as a preservative gradually disappeared due to the development of other, more active and less toxic agents.[26]

Other disinfectants include hydrogen peroxide and peroxygens. Hydrogen peroxide was used to neutralize foul odours in 1858 by Richardson and was employed widely for the treatment of dirty wounds in the twentieth century. It is still used today for the disinfection of contact lenses and sometimes for instruments. Peracetic acid, another peroxide compound, is corrosive when concentrated, but in dilute solutions it is relatively noncorrosive and highly active against bacterial spores. Glutaraldehyde was introduced in the 1960s as a possible alternative to formaldehyde, which was often used with other agents for the storage of sterile instruments. Alkaline solutions of glutaraldehyde are noncorrosive and are still the standard disinfectants for decontaminating flexible endoscopes. Glutaraldehyde is toxic and allergenic, and environmental precautions are required when it is used. It is slowly sporicidal and mycobactericidal, and other more active agents, e.g. peracetic acid, chlorine dioxide and superoxidized water, have been proposed for the decontamination of flexible fibre-optic endoscopes.[22,23,25]

Despite the fact that Chapin indicated as far back as 1812 that fumigation was ineffective (see Chapter 4), the practice has continued; however, formaldehyde gas replaced sulphur dioxide and continued to be used throughout the twentieth century, particularly for fumigation of rooms occupied by patients with severe virus infections such as Lassa fever.[28] Formaldehyde was also used for the decontamination of woollen blankets in the 1950s,[29] and it is still used for the decontamination of protective cabinets in microbiological laboratories. 'Fogging' of rooms with formaldehyde or phenolics was introduced again in the mid-twentieth century for terminal disinfection of rooms previously occupied by patients with pathogenic *Escherichia coli* or virulent staphylococcal infections. This fell into disrepute when it was realized that prior cleaning with a detergent/disinfectant was necessary because aerosols or gases would not be effective on surfaces contaminated with organic matter unless they were precleaned.[22]

Disinfection of skin and wounds

Wine, vinegar and honey are among the oldest of antiseptics. Alcohol was recommended by Galen in 200 AD for treating wounds, and it has remained one of the most effective antiseptics.[25] In 1363, Guy de Chauliac used hot wine to treat wounds, while later surgeons used hot oils. Alcohol was used in French hospitals in the eighteenth century (see Chapter 8) and by a Portuguese surgeon, Barbosa, in 1855.[25] Harrington and Walker in 1903 showed that 60–70% ethanol and isopropanol were more effective than higher concentrations of alcohol. Alcohol is still the most effective agent for preoperative disinfection of the skin and disinfection of hands of staff.

Quaternary ammonium compounds (QACs) were described by Domagk in 1935[30] and were used widely in the Second World War. Although effective against Gram-positive organisms, QACs are less effective against Gram-negative organisms and inactive against spores. Their activity is mainly bacteristatic, which has reduced their value as a skin disinfectant. Their main advantage is their lack of toxicity. QACs often have detergent properties and are used for cleaning dirty wounds. Alcoholic solutions are still used for skin disinfection, although aqueous solutions are sometimes used as environmental cleaning agents, especially in food preparation areas.[22]

Iodine was discovered in the early nineteenth century and was used for treating wounds in 1839 by Davies.[24] Since then, it has been used as an antiseptic for application to traumatic wounds and as a tincture for the preoperative disinfection of skin. Iodine is an irritant and causes allergy, but in the 1960s complexes (iodophors) were developed that are non-irritants; these have mainly replaced iodine for disinfection of the hands and the operation site.[26]

Chlorhexidine is a substance with good activity against Gram-positive organisms and lesser activity against Gram-negative organisms. Developed by the Imperial Chemical Industries in the 1950s, it is a nontoxic, bactericidal agent that remains persistent on the skin.[31,32] It is commonly used as a detergent preparation for the disinfection of hands and in an alcoholic preparation for preoperative skin disinfection.[33,34]

Other agents used as antiseptics include aniline and acridine dyes, but these are not employed commonly. Silver nitrate was used to prevent eye infection in neonates until recently, and silver sulfadiazine is still in use today to prevent infection in burns. Hexachlorophene was introduced for surgical disinfection of the hands in the 1950s and was also used for bathing neonates (see Chapter 14). Its main activity is against Gram-positive organisms and it has a good persistent effect. However, neurotoxicity of hexachlorophene was demonstrated after repeated use in neonates. It has now been replaced mainly by chlorhexidine, povidone-iodine or triclosan, except for a powder that is still sometimes used to prevent staphylococcal infection in neonates and to treat staphylococcal carriers. Triclosan is another relatively nontoxic agent with a good residual effect on the skin. It is sometimes used as an alternative to chlorhexidine for skin disinfection.[34]

Disinfectant policies

The importance of cleaning the environment and surgical instruments was recognized by Schimmelbusch and others at the end of the nineteenth century. Disinfectants have been used widely for decontaminating the hospital environment throughout most of the twentieth century, despite the limited evidence of their efficacy in preventing infection. The general public mistakenly feels that a disinfectant smell in a hospital indicates that infection has been dealt with adequately. However, Gram-negative infections caused by contaminated disinfectant solutions, especially QACs, were reported in the 1960s and 1970s.[34] A wide variety of disinfectants was available and a PHLS survey in 1965 indicated that they were used inappropriately and indiscriminately.[35] Hospital policies were then recommended by Kelsey and Maurer in 1965 and later by Ayliffe and colleagues in 1993 in PHLS publications.[22] These policies recommended avoiding the use of liquid disinfectants when cleaning methods are adequate or when heating methods for disinfection or sterilization can be used, but although most hospitals have a policy, implementation is not always satisfactory. However, audits of ward procedures by infection-control teams are now improving implementation.

Cleaning the environmental surfaces with a detergent is considered to be adequate in many countries and has often replaced routine disinfection. However, disinfectants are still used for potentially hazardous situations, e.g. spillage of body fluids, and indications for disinfection and recommended agents vary from country to country. Chlorine compounds, phenolics, aldehydes and QACs for environmental disinfection have all been used in recent years, but some are potentially toxic unless controlled well.

Manufacturers are encouraged to produce heat-tolerant medical devices whenever possible, but they have tended to prefer single-use devices, which relieves them of any responsibility for recommending a method for cleaning and sterilization.

Disinfection of hands of staff

It became increasingly clear from many studies in the twentieth century that the hands of hospital staff were the main route of spread of hospital infection, although evidence from controlled clinical studies remained limited. Elaine Larson in the USA reviewed much of this evidence in 1988.[36]

As described in Chapter 8, the process of scrubbing for 10 minutes followed by immersion in 70% alcohol was used as a preoperative scrub for many years. Later studies by Lowbury, Lilly and other colleagues in the 1960s and 1970s[32,33] showed that a shorter disinfectant wash with hexachlorophene, povidone-iodine or chlorhexidine reduced the application time to 5 minutes or less. For surgical hand-washing/disinfection in the UK, the application time of the disinfectant has been reduced to 2 minutes, or possibly less if using an alcohol preparation. Brushing of the hands is carried out only before the first operation of the day to reduce damage to the skin.

Disinfection with alcohol has been used more widely in many European countries, and methods were published in Germany as standard tests by the Deutsche

Gesellschaft für Hygiene und Mikrobiologie (DGHM).[37] In the 1970s, a committee to investigate the standardization of disinfectants in Europe, chaired by Professor Schmidt from Berlin, was formed.[38] Tests on hand disinfection were studied by Reber in Switzerland, Rotter, Koller and colleagues in Vienna, Werner and colleagues in Mainz, and Ayliffe and colleagues in Birmingham. These studies eventually formed the basis of European standard tests (European Committee for Standardization (CEN)) in the 1990s.

Alcohol is being used increasingly throughout the world for preoperative skin disinfection and for disinfection of the hands of staff in hospital wards (i.e. hygienic hand disinfection for killing transient organisms). However, hand-washing with soap and water is still used commonly for routine procedures in hospital wards in many countries, although laboratory tests indicate that alcoholic disinfection is more effective.[39,40] Times of application of agents remain controversial owing to the lack of clinical evidence of effectiveness.

The importance of covering all surfaces of the hands with the agent during washing or disinfecting was recognized in Birmingham in the 1960s, when high postdisinfection bacterial counts were obtained on one subject in laboratory tests. This subject was found to have long thumbs, which were missed during the disinfection process. Lynda Taylor and a group of West Midlands infection-control nurses subsequently demonstrated, using a dye test, that certain areas of the hands were regularly missed during routine disinfection, and a new technique was developed by the Hospital Infection Research Laboratory to avoid this error.[41]

The main problem at the present time is not the agent used but the failure of staff, particularly doctors, to wash or disinfect their hands after contact with patients or after handling contaminated items. Persuading staff to implement hand-washing at the correct time seems to be as difficult in the early twenty-first century as in the time of Semmelweiss (see Chapter 17).

Disinfectant testing in the laboratory

Early testing of the activity of disinfectants before micro-organisms were recognized have been described, e.g. by Pringle (see Chapter 4). Davaine, who demonstrated that iodine was effective against anthrax bacilli, was one of the first, in 1873, to test disinfectant activity against a known organism.[42] Koch in 1881 compared the action of a number of disinfectants against a range of bacteria. He used pure cultures dried on silk threads, immersed them in a disinfectant solution, and demonstrated the concentrations of disinfectant that would prevent growth (bacteristatic activity) and those that would kill the organisms (bactericidal activity). He tested over 70 substances and found perchloride of mercury to be the most effective; however, Geppert in 1889 showed that if perchloride of mercury was neutralized, some spores could survive, i.e. it was highly bacteristatic. Nevertheless, despite this, and despite their toxicity, mercury compounds continued to be used for disinfecting the hands and equipment for some years. Kronig and Paul in 1887 were the earliest to describe disinfectant testing in detail, and their work formed the basis of modern methods.[43,44] They laid down requirements for testing, e.g. standard inocula, defined contact times, constant temperatures, optimal recovery media, and counts of survivors.

Other standardized testing methods were developed in the early twentieth century.[45] The phenol coefficient test (Rideal–Walker test) was introduced in 1903 and continued to be used by industry for most of the century.[46] A modification of this was the Chick–Martin test, which incorporated organic matter into the test medium and increased its practical value. A quantitative supension test for assessing QACs was published by the British Standards Institute in 1960 and formed the basis of such tests.[39] Most countries developed their own test systems, but none gave results comparable with each other, and all had problems with interpretation in terms of practical use. The most complete system of tests was developed in Germany by the DGHM and included suspension and surface tests, and tests on instruments, linen and hands.[37] However, the main problem with these practical tests was a lack of reproduciblity. The USA developed a surface test with penicylinders, which was approved by the Association of Official Analytical Chemists (AOAC); a system of testing was approved in France by the Association Française de Normalisation (AFNOR); a quantitative suspension test, 5-5-5, was developed by Mossel and colleagues in Holland; and the UK used the Kelsey–Sykes capacity test, modified by Kelsey and Maurer in 1974. International standardization of test methods and uses became an urgent need.[39] The first attempts at standardization of, and definition of requirements for, disinfection were made by a committee of the International Colloquium on the Evaluation of Disinfectants in Europe, funded by Schulke and Mayr.[38] Although progress was slow, due mainly to differences between countries in the philosophy of control of infection and lack of agreement on definitions in different countries, Reybrouk from Belgium and Werner from Germany produced a quantitative suspension test modified from the 5-5-5 and DGHM tests. This test formed the basis of the Council of Europe suspension test in 1987, and then later for the CEN test.[39] At the time of writing, the CEN disinfectant committees are developing carrier and suspension tests on mycobacteria and viruses, but international standardization is still some way off.

The mid-twentieth century: the emergence of antibiotic-resistant *Staphylococcus aureus*

Staphylococci were recognized as a cause of wound infection at the end of the nineteenth century and continued to be an important cause of hospital sepsis in the twentieth century, although early reports usually indicated less severe infections than with haemolytic streptococci. Studies in the 1930s and 1940s suggested that *Staphylococcus aureus (pyogenes)* was still the most common cause of clean surgical wound infection,[1] and this has continued up to the present time, irrespective of antibiotic therapy. *Staph. aureus* has also continued as a cause of abscesses in the skin, such as carbuncles and furuncles (boils), pyaemia, septicaemia (bloodstream infection) and osteomyelitis (bone infection).

Although the pigmented staphylococci (orange or yellow colonies on culture) were originally considered to be the most virulent, it was found later that pigment was not necessarily an indicator of virulence. A better indicator was the coagulase test. Coagulase is an enzyme that coagulates plasma. It was originally described by Loeb in 1903, although he did not recognize the significance of the finding.[2] The description of the role of coagulase in determining potential pathogenicity was made by Daranyi in the late 1920s, and the development of a simple test for coagulase in the late 1930s and early 1940s was a major advance. Coagulase-positive staphylococci were found to be potentially more virulent than coagulase-negative staphylococci and were named *Staph. pyogenes*. However, much discussion took place over the nomenclature and *Staph. aureus* is now used rather than *Staph. pyogenes*, irrespective of the colour of the staphylococcal colony on culture media. Coagulase-positive strains produce a range of other toxins. Stephen Elek wrote a large monograph on staphylococci and their properties in 1959, giving over 4000 references;[3] these include all the major references on coagulase, toxins and other properties of staphylococci up to that time. Nevertheless, there is still no laboratory test to identify a virulent or epidemic strain, although typing can be helpful.

The problems of staphylococcal cross-infection in the 1940s and 1950s followed the introduction of penicillin. Although penicillin G (benzylpenicillin) was discovered by Fleming in 1929,[4] it was not developed for clinical use until the time of the

Table 12.1. Bacteriophage typing of *Staph. aureus*

Group	Phages
Group 1	29, 52, 52A, 79, 80, (81)
Group 2	3A, 3C, 55, 71
Group 3	6, 42E, 47, 51, 54, 75, 77, 83A, 84, 85
Miscellaneous	94, 95, 96, 88
Supplementary*	CRF 616, 617, 618, 622, 623, 625, 626, 629, 630
Experimental*	88A, 90, 83C, 932

*There are many experimental phages in use throughout the world. Those listed are in use in the UK.

Second World War by Chain and colleagues in Oxford.[5] It was the first clinically useful antibiotic to be produced by a soil fungus, *Penicillium notatum*, and it was highly effective against group A streptococci and initially against *Staph. aureus*.

Natural resistance to penicillin in *Escherichia coli* was originally described by Fleming, but outbreaks of infection with penicillin-resistant *Staph. aureus* were soon described in patients in the 1940s by Mary Barber in London,[6] Kirby, Maxwell Finland and others in the USA, and Phyllis Rountree in Australia.[7,8] Resistance was naturally occurring and was due to the production of beta-lactamase, an enzyme that inactivated penicillin.

It became apparent in the 1940s that *Staph. aureus* was spreading in hospitals in all countries and was replacing haemolytic streptococci as the main infecting organism. This spread was demonstrated by phage typing. Phages are virus particles that are able to lyse (i.e. destroy) some strains of bacteria but not others. The discovery of phages in *Staph. aureus* by Fisk[9] became the basis of a typing system developed further by Wilson and Atkinson[10] and later by Blair and Williams.[11] The system has remained, with some additions, the basis for elucidation of staphylococcal epidemiology until the present day, although it is now being replaced by molecular methods. The patterns of lysis characterize certain strains, which initially occur in groups (1, 2, 3 see Table 12.1).

A new virulent strain, known as phage type 80/81, was reported from Sydney by Phyllis Rountree and colleagues in 1955.[12] This was responsible for very severe infections, especially in neonates. It soon appeared in many places, including Eastern Europe, the Netherlands, Uganda, the USA and Canada. An outbreak in Southampton gradually spread west and north and was responsible for 30% of outbreaks in the UK in 1957.[13] Type 80/81 *Staph. aureus* had become a real problem by then, but other, less virulent strains of *Staph. aureus* were causing outbreaks of surgical wound infection. Although it was not always possible to correlate a phage type with virulence, type 80/81 appeared to be particularly virulent and transmissible. In addition to neonatal sepsis and breast abscesses in mothers, it also caused characteristically severe furunculosis and septic fingers in hospital staff.

In surgical wards, epidemics were commonly caused by phage group 3 strains, for example 7/47/53/75/77, 53+,75/77. These mainly infected wounds, did not usually cause furunculosis, and rarely caused neonatal sepsis. Not all of these strains caused outbreaks. Shooter and colleagues in 1958 found over 180 strains in a surgical ward over a period of 8 months, but only 13 strains were responsible for clinical sepsis and only three types were responsible for sepsis in more than one patient.[14] Other evidence that some strains were more virulent was available from nasal carriers. A third of patients carrying these 'more virulent' strains developed sepsis whereas only 2.5% of patients carrying other strains in their noses developed sepsis. Gillespie and colleagues in 1959 found that most of the surgical ward infections were caused by tetracycline-resistant group 3 strains, but theatre-acquired infections were commonly due to group 1 strains resistant only to penicillin and tended to be more severe.[15] Nurses infrequently carried wound-infecting group 3 strains in their noses, and this led to the discontinuation of the use of masks when dressing wounds.

In the 1960s, the virulent type 80/81 strains tended to disappear, and although type 80/81 and related strains continued to be isolated, particularly from noses, they rarely caused severe infections. The reason for the disappearance of the virulent type 80/81 strains remains a mystery. Since then, predominant phage types have changed continually; in some instances, this may be a result of the emergence of resistance to new antibiotics, but usually the reason for changes in epidemic strains remains uncertain.

After the introduction of penicillin in the 1940s, a number of other antibiotics were discovered. A screening programme of soil fungi and actinomycetes was set up by Waksman's group at Ruttger's University in New Jersey; streptomycin was isolated and came into clinical practice in 1944.[8] Resistance emerged rapidly, but streptomycin continued to be used in combination with other agents for the treatment of surgical infections and tuberculosis.

The first of several tetracyclines, chlortetracycline obtained from fungi, was introduced in 1948 and was soon followed by a series of other antibiotics (chloramphenicol, erythromycin, novobiocin, lincomycin). Resistance emerged to all of these agents, often soon after their introduction but sometimes after a delay of several years.[7] Many of the studies on resistance were carried out by L.P. Garrod, Mary Barber and Edward Lowbury in the UK, Maxwell Finland, Wesley Spink and others in the USA, and Chabbert in France.[7,8,16] Several other antistaphylococcal antibiotics became available, but vancomycin was the main agent used for treating severe infections in 1960 and has remained in use until the present day. However, vancomycin is toxic, requires continual monitoring, and is not an ideal therapeutic agent.[16]

The 1950s were a period of disenchantment in hospitals; some bacteria, especially *Staph. aureus*, had demonstrated a remarkable ability to spread and to develop resistance, and it seemed possible that antibiotics might lose their usefulness only 20 years after their introduction.[7,17] However, in the early 1960s the problem of increasing resistance seemed to be solved for *Staph. aureus* by the introduction of new semisynthetic beta-lactamase-resistant penicillins, such as methicillin and cloxacillin. These and other penicillins were developed by Rolinson and colleagues from Beecham's Research Laboratory in England.[18,19] Ernst Chain was again involved in the project, and the early work was done in his laboratories in Rome. Cephalosporins were also developed, based on work by E.P. Abraham and colleagues at Oxford. These cephalosporins were also stable to staphylococcal beta-lactamases, but they showed some cross-resistance with methicillin (i.e methicillin-resistant strains were also resistant to cephalosporins).[7,16]

Methicillin and related agents were relatively nontoxic and very effective against staphylococcal infections, but Patricia Jevons at the Central Public Health Laboratory at Colindale found a naturally resistant strain in 1961.[20] Despite warnings by Mary Barber and others that methicillin should be used with care, the advice was generally unheeded,[21] as many, including Chain, felt that resistance would not be a problem. Methicillin was even sprayed into the air of infant nurseries. Nevertheless, resistant strains were reported in Poland, Turkey and India before methicillin was used clinically.[22]

During the 1960s, methicillin-resistant *Staph. aureus* (MRSA) was being reported increasingly in European countries such as Switzerland, Denmark, France and the UK, as well as in Australia and some other countries, but few outbreaks were reported at this time in the USA.[22] This was the beginning of the worldwide epidemic of MRSA. Current national patterns of nosocomial isolates of staphylococci were discussed in the first international conference held in Atlanta in 1970, but the epidemic strains were causing greater anxiety in Europe than in the USA.[23] Although there was an initial decline of MRSA in the 1970s (see page 215), it remains the main hospital epidemic 'bug' of today.

Epidemiology

The epidemiology of *Staph. aureus* was studied extensively between the 1950s and the 1970s, particularly by Sir Robert Williams and colleagues. Williams was Professor of Bacteriology at St Mary's Hospital, London, and he was one of the world's leading research workers on the spread of *Staph. aureus* and its prevention. He later became Director of the Public Health Laboratory Service in the UK and President of the Royal College of Pathologists. Workers in other countries, such as C. Solberg in Norway, G. Laurell and Anna Hambraeus in Sweden, and Kirsten

Rosendal in Denmark, contributed to the extensive literature on the spread of staphylococci.

Although considerable advances were made, general conclusions on controlling outbreaks have often been difficult to draw since the behaviour of the staphylococcal strains can vary in virulence and transmissibility, and with the environment. The results of studies on one bacterial population in one environment do not necessarily have a universal application. Obtaining significant data on control was also difficult due to the multifactorial aspects of infection, and the same problems remain today with MRSA.

Studies have shown that *Staph. aureus* is carried in the nose of 20–40% of healthy individuals, and about 3% of non-nasal carriers are perineal carriers.[13] Other areas of healthy skin, such as that on the wrists and hands, are not usually true carriage sites but may be contaminated from carriage sites such as the nose. As with streptococci, transmission of *Staph. aureus* is mainly on the hands of staff contaminated from infections or colonized sites in patients or from their own carriage sites. Duguid and Wallace[24] in 1948 and Hare and Thomas[25] in 1956 showed that staphylococci may be dispersed into the air by nasal carriers in small numbers during normal breathing and talking, and that the numbers may be increased with more vigorous respiratory activities, such as snorting, but that many more are disseminated from clothing and bedding. Contaminated nasal secretions may contaminate the hands, face and hair, and the secretions may then be shed into the environment on skin scales, as described by Davies and Noble in 1962.[26] A heavy disperser (shedder) is likely to be a major source of infection.[27] Robert Blowers and others showed that male carriers tend to shed more than females, but the reason for this remains unknown. Perineal carriers, especially males, are likely to be particularly heavy shedders.[28,29] Shedding is also increased after showering, probably due to the breaking up of clumps of skin scales. Carriers vary greatly in the numbers of staphylococci shed, but the extent of dispersal is related to the number present in the carriage site and the area of contaminated skin.[29,30] Antibiotic-resistant strains also tend to be present in greater numbers than sensitive strains in the carriage site, and to be present in larger numbers in the environment.[31] Dissemination of staphylococci from lesions and evidence of cross-infection has been described on many occasions, but spread can still occur from carriage sites not associated with heavy dispersal. Hare and Cooke in 1961 sampled the noses, hair, faces, chests, abdomens, fingers, nightwear, pillows and blankets of infected patients, and the adjacent floor.[32] They found that certain patients contaminated the environment more than others, particularly if the lesion could not be covered with an impermeable dressing. Widespread dermatological lesions, pneumonia and enterocolitis were usually responsible for considerable environmental contamination, whereas postoperative wounds, bedsores and varicose ulcers, if covered adequately, showed much less contamination. Nevertheless, soaked dressings from wounds or burns, bedsores and ulcers have frequently been associated with cross-infection. Heavy contamination of the environment of dermatological wards due to many heavy dispersers was shown by Sydney Selwyn and others.[31,33]

Nasal carriers probably have an increased risk of postoperative sepsis; for instance, in one study the wound sepsis rate was 2% in 342 patients who were never nasal carriers and 7.1% in patients who were carriers at some time. In half the cases with sepsis, this was caused by the same strain as that isolated from the nose. It seems likely that nasal carriers are more susceptible to infection, irrespective of whether they are infected with the strain present in their nose at the time or another strain. However, in another, larger study, the sepsis rate was similar, irrespective of whether the patient was a nasal carrier.[13] More recent studies confirm that nasal carriers are associated with higher wound infection rates.

Dispersal is apparently not always associated with shedding of skin scales; for instance, in burns, staphylococci may be shed on small particles (4μm in diameter). Staphylococcal-carrying particles have been disseminated in large numbers from the respiratory tracts of babies with respiratory infections;[34] these were known as 'cloud babies'. No recent reports of similar cases have been described. The spread of staphylococci in a nursery was also studied by Mortimer and colleagues in the 1960s.[35,36] Naturally colonized babies (index babies) were placed in two nurseries of seven or eight cots containing babies admitted directly from the delivery room. With no special precautions, most of the other babies were colonized from the index case, usually within 4 days. Staff washing their hands with hexachlorophene before handling a noncolonized baby reduced the colonization to about one-third. The use of different nurses for handling colonized and noncolonized babies reduced the acquisition rate to about 10%. This residual infection rate was due presumably to airborne spread, but transmission on the hands of the nurses was the main route of spread.

The role of the inanimate environment in the spread of staphylococci

The role of airborne spread in the dissemination of infection in general was discussed in Chapter 8. Although staphylococci can be readily isolated from the air of hospitals, it has been difficult to determine the role of the air in the spread of infection.[31,37] The air in a ward is contaminated mainly from clothing, bedding and infected dressings, and many workers found that large numbers of airborne staphylococci were present when sepsis rates were high in surgical wards.[12] It seems likely that airborne spread of staphylococci can occur in wards, especially in cases when a number of nasal carriers are suddenly identified in various sites in a ward in which there is a single heavy disperser of an epidemic strain, but it is likely that contact spread from the lesions and bedding is of greater importance. The evidence that reducing the number of staphylococci in the air of a surgical ward reduces sepsis is not convincing. However, infection and carriage are influenced by many factors, including the age of the patient and their length of stay, antibiotic use, types of wounds and lesions,[38] epidemicity of strains, and overcrowding.

The introduction by Colebrook in the 1940s of a burns dressing room with a positive-pressure ventilation (plenum) system providing filtered air at 20 air changes per hour considerably reduced the number of airborne bacteria.[39] A controlled trial of the same dressing room by Lowbury in 1954 showed a reduction in the incidence of infection with _Staph. aureus_ and also with Gram-negative bacilli, including _Pseudomonas aeruginosa_ and _Streptococcus pyogenes_.[40] Rooms used for the dressing of burns are subject to the release of much larger numbers of organisms into the environment than are other areas of hospitals, and results obtained from burns units cannot necessarily be applied to other wards. The use of an open-top plastic isolator did not reduce the acquisition of _Staph. aureus_ in patients with burns, although a reduction was obtained with _P. aeruginosa_. This further suggested that airborne spread can occur in burns units, although the introduction of window ventilators into the cubicles of a burns unit reduced air counts but not infection. Similar results were obtained in a busy surgical ward.[41]

Division of a ward into cubicles opening on to a partially enclosed corridor, as in a fever hospital, reduced acquisition of antibiotic-resistant nasal strains.[42] A mechanically ventilated hospital with cubicles has also been associated with a lower infection rate than an old hospital, but more recent studies on moving from an old to a new hospital or operating room have not confirmed this.[43,44] Isolation of infected patients or carriers in single rooms has been reported as effective in controlling outbreaks, but measures have usually been multifactorial.[13] However, in a study by Robert Williams and colleagues, the isolation of carriers or infected patients in ventilated cubicles attached to a 25-bedded ward reduced the spread of resistant strains from these patients and reduced the acquisition of infection in the larger ward probably by about half.[45] The evidence that airborne dispersal of staphylococci in wards, apart from burns units, is an important mode of spread is therefore limited and is usually related to specific conditions involving a heavy disperser.[31,46]

Surgical wounds are mainly infected during the operation, and one of the main efforts to reduce infection since the Second World War has been to introduce ventilation systems and to design theatres appropriately (Chapter 14). However, it has since been realized that most of the theatre-acquired infections are due to the patient's own bacterial flora. Nevertheless, surgical wounds are inevitably exposed to the air for varying times and _Staph. aureus_ can always be isolated from the air, although usually in small numbers. The number of organisms in the air depends on the number of people in the operation room, their activity, and whether they are male or female; the type of clothing worn; the air flows; the number of door openings; and whether any patient or staff member is a heavy staphylococcal disperser.[13] The susceptibility of the patient and the surgical technique are usually of greater importance as infection risk factors than the number of staphylococci in the air, but it is still recommended that the minimum number of staff should be in the theatre during an operation, that activity should be minimal, and that the doors should not be continually opened and closed. The source of staphylococci in wound infections at the time of the operation is still difficult to determine.[47] Burke in 1963 studied 50 postoperative wounds and recovered *Staph. aureus* from 46, with many wounds yielding more than one strain. Possible sources were the air (68%), a carrier site on the patient (50%), and the noses and hands of the surgical team (20%). Only two of the wounds developed a clinical infection.[48] Another study, by Bengtsson and colleagues, showed that 45% of infected wounds were associated with *Staph. aureus* and that about 60% were due to self-infection.[49] Outbreaks of staphylococcal wound infection in the 1950s frequently seemed to be due to acquisition from air in the operating theatre. Blowers and colleagues in 1955 obtained a reduction in the incidence of postoperative sepsis in a thoracic unit by changing an exhaust ventilation system for a positive-pressure system in association with a number of other improvements in asepsis and hygiene. Similar results were obtained by Shooter and colleagues, who also thought that an extraction system drew in contaminated air from the wards.[13] Theatres were then designed to reduce airborne infection, and the general design is similar today (see Chapter 14). Other workers did not necessarily report a reduction in wound sepsis by using a plenum system with filtered air, although airborne counts were usually reduced. In a study in a hospital in the Birmingham region in the 1960s, patients whose operations were performed in a plenum-ventilated theatre were not found to have a lower incidence of sepsis than those whose operations were performed in the same operating theatre with natural window ventilation during the previous year.[50] However, the comparison was not entirely valid as the type of operation differed in the 2 years of study. Air counts during the period of plenum ventilation were halved when compared with those during the period of window ventilation. Occasional outbreaks of theatre-acquired infection due to airborne spread have been reported to have been caused by unscrubbed staff.[13,31] These staff members have usually been heavy dispersers from desquamating skin lesions.

The limited evidence available in recent years suggests that most staphylococcal wound infections of clean wounds are self-infections, although the strains may have been acquired in a carriage site during the preoperative hospital stay and could be hospital staphylococci. Airborne spread clearly does occur in prosthetic surgery (see Chapter 14).

The increase in minimal invasive surgery in the past 10 years further reduces the importance of airborne spread in operating theatres since the size of wounds is much reduced and possible changes of design of operating rooms require consideration.[51]

In the 1940s, high bacterial counts in the air were often found during bed-making, and large numbers of staphylococci were isolated from blankets. Rountree and Beard in 1968 found that large numbers of staphylococci in the air were associated with heavy blanket contamination and increased sepsis.[52] Before the 1960s, most blankets were woollen and were rarely disinfected. These were gradually replaced with cotton blankets, which could be washed at higher temperatures. However, the role of blankets in the transmission of infection remained uncertain because oiling of blankets and floors reduced the dispersal of organisms from these sources but did not reduce the infection rate, and no reduction in air contamination was found by using cotton instead of woollen blankets whether disinfected or not.[13] Gillespie and colleagues in 1959 disinfected blankets with formaldehyde after use by each patient; they found that this alone did not influence cross-infection, but it did when combined with other measures.[15] In another study, only ten of 872 blankets in a surgical ward were contaminated heavily with *Staph. aureus*, and nine of these were with epidemic, multiresistant strains. The heaviest contamination was on the blankets of a disperser, and all except two were on blankets of infected patients, one of whom subsequently developed an infection with the same strain (G. Ayliffe, personal communication). Nevertheless, the number of heavily contaminated blankets was so small that it is unlikely that they play a major role in cross-infection, although they may be of importance on the bed of a disperser. Changing the bedding of a disperser has only a limited effect since recontamination occurs in about 1 day.

Curtains adjacent to the beds of heavy dispersers may show heavy contamination, but most show only a few staphylococcal colonies.[53] Changing curtains has only a temporary effect if the disperser is still present in the ward. Although staphylococci remain viable in the environment for long periods, the numbers fall on surfaces over a few days. The type of material of the curtain does not appear to influence staphylococcal survival.

Clothing of patients who are dispersers can be heavily contaminated, and large numbers of organisms are shed into the air on exercising; however, as with blankets, clean clothing is recontaminated rapidly. Anna Hambraeus and colleagues showed that the clothing of staff can also transfer staphylococci from an infected patient to a non-infected one in another room in a burns unit.[54]

Skin scales carrying staphylococci become attached to floors and other surfaces and are difficult to remove, so resuspension in the air of staphylococci is minimal under normal conditions and presents very little hazard of airborne transmission.[53] Cleaning or disinfecting a floor has a short-lived effect in a busy unit as rapid recontamination occurs, often in about an hour. After disinfection, bacterial counts on a floor increase to reach previous levels, and a state of equilibrium then exists in which the rate of deposition is equal to the rate of removal by death or other natural means. Sweeping with a broom disperses organisms from a floor, but dispersal is much less if a vacuum cleaner with a filter is used or the floor is wet-cleaned. Careful use of a dust-attracting mop is also fairly satisfactory, but less so than using a vacuum cleaner. Bacterial air counts are often less in carpeted wards than in those with conventional flooring, although counts from the actual carpet are often higher; there was no evidence at that time that carpets increase the infection risk.[55]

Walls are rarely contaminated heavily and tend to reach a low equilibrium as do floors, counts remaining unchanged over many months.[53,56]

Other environmental items have been suggested as possible agents of spread. There is some evidence that patients with open postoperative wounds acquired *Staph. aureus* from contaminated baths. Large numbers of organisms, including *Staph. aureus*, can be isolated from bath water and spread over the surface of a bath; they also contaminate face flannels, towels and the adjacent floor. However, disinfection of bath water alone was not shown to reduce cross-infection in a surgical ward, but formed part of a series of measures that together showed an effect.

Although staphylococci can be found readily in the inanimate environment, they do not grow and they gradually die. Finding airborne organisms does not necessarily mean that there is, or will be, clinical infection. Most of the evidence obtained in the 1950s to 1980s suggested that the inanimate environment has a minor role in transmission of *Staph. aureus* and that people are the main sources, hands being the main route of transmission. However, more recent studies suggest that the environment may have a greater role than thought previously, but this is probably not a major role (see Chapter 16).

The mid-twentieth century: Gram-negative bacilli

At the same time as outbreaks of *Staphylococcus aureus* were occurring in the 1950s and 1960s, increasing numbers of infections caused by Gram-negative bacilli were being reported, particularly in the USA. It seemed that they might replace *Staph. aureus* as the main causes of outbreaks of hospital infection, since methicillin and the new penicillinase-resistant penicillins and cephalosporins appeared to be controlling staphylococcal infections.

Finland and colleagues at the Boston City Hospital in 1959 reported an increase in Gram-negative bacteraemias, from 40 in 1935 to 180 in 1957,[1] the Gram-negative bacilli replacing *Streptococcus pneumoniae*, *Strep. pyogenes* and antibiotic-sensitive *Staph. aureus* as the predominant pathogens. McCabe and Jackson in 1962 investigated bacteraemias over 8 years and found a similar increase in Gram-negative infections, considering this to be due mainly to more instrumentation and to the changes in underlying diseases.[2] Others found similar changes in causes of bacteraemias, suggesting that increased ageing of the population and prior antibiotic therapy were also important predisposing factors.[3]

Escherichia coli are the most numerous of the aerobic Gram-negative bacilli in the normal intestinal flora. They cause, usually with *Bacteroides* spp., most of the intra-abdominal infections, including appendicitis, peritonitis, pelvic abscesses, septicaemia, and gallbladder and wound infections associated with abdominal surgery. *E. coli* was, and still is, the most common cause of acute urinary tract infection. Most of these infections are endogenous in origin (self-infections acquired from the patient's own natural bacterial flora). Other Gram-negative bacilli, including *Proteus* spp., *Klebsiella* spp., *Enterobacter* spp. and *Pseudomonas* spp., may also be part of the normal intestinal flora and can cause similar infections to *E. coli*, but they are more likely to acquire resistance to antibiotics and to cause cross-infection.[4] Most of these are opportunist organisms, are of low pathogenicity, and infect mainly patients with reduced immunity to infection, such as leukaemics, or susceptible sites such as the eye or meninges after operation.

Despite the number of new penicillins, cephalosporins and quinolones, some Gram-negative bacillary infections were almost untreatable by the end of the twentieth century, with little prospect of a continuing supply of effective new agents.

Antibiotic resistance

Resistance to streptomycin was shown in the 1940s to be due to selection of existing resistant mutants by continued use of an antibiotic on a mixed population of susceptible and resistant organisms. This was considered to be the main genetic mode of origin of resistance to other antibiotics such as tetracycline and ampicillin, but a more important mode of origin, transferable resistance, was discovered later. Transferable resistance is the transfer from one organism to another of a so-called R factor, consisting of extrachromosomal DNA (later termed a plasmid), which controls resistance to one or more antibiotics.

The existence of transferable resistance created major problems both in therapy and in controlling cross-infection. Watanabe and colleagues in Japan in 1963 reported the isolation of strains of *Shigella* resistant to streptomycin, tetracycline, chloramphenicol and sulphonamides in patients who had not been treated with these agents, and *E. coli* were also isolated with similar resistance patterns in the same patients.[5,6] They then showed that resistance to all these agents could be transferred together on an R factor by conjugation; that is, the transfer of DNA through a tube or pilus from one species of organism to another. Thus, the use of one antibiotic for treatment could select resistance to all agents carried by an R factor. Naomi Datta, in London in 1962, also found R factors in *Salmonella* and demonstrated transfer of resistance from them to *E. coli*, and vice versa.[7] Many other plasmids were detected, including one described by Lowbury and colleagues in 1969 controlling carbenicillin resistance in *Pseudomonas aeruginosa* in patients with burns.[8] Carbenicillin was the first nontoxic antibiotic to be effective against *Pseudomonas*, and resistance was a major setback at the time to the treatment of severe burns infections.

Plasmids have since been shown to be distributed widely in different species of bacteria, including *Staph. aureus*. They vary in transmissibility and may be transferred by other mechanisms, for example by bacteriophages. Smaller genetic elements that can move from chromosome to plasmid, or between plasmids, or between chromosomes, and that can transfer resistance have been described more recently and are termed transposons or 'jumping genes'.[9]

Mechanisms of the mode of action and resistance to antibiotics have been studied since their discovery in the 1940s, and antibiotic-inactivating enzymes were found to have a prominent role as resistance mechanisms. In addition to the inactivation of penicillins by beta-lactamases, other important inactivating enzymes were responsible for aminoglycoside resistance, for instance gentamicin acetylase. The enzymes are usually controlled by plasmids that are transferable between different species of Gram-negative bacilli.[9]

Opportunist Gram-negative bacilli

The opportunist Gram-negative bacilli are commonly found in the moist inanimate environment, but they can also colonize the gastrointestinal tract, particularly if selected by antibiotic therapy. They are commonly isolated from moist equipment and instruments, for example washing bowls, thermometers, endoscopes, enteric feeding tubing, and respiratory equipment, and from nonsterile fluids. They sometimes spread in aerosols but not usually in dried droplet nuclei, as they die rapidly on drying.[4,10] An exception is acinetobacter, which can survive drying, although airborne spread of infection is reported rarely. The main route of spread of all these organisms is on the hands of staff from infected or colonized lesions on patients or via equipment, but sometimes they spread directly, for instance from contaminated intravenous fluids.

P. aeruginosa (originally known as *Bacillus pyocyanea*) is of special significance. It was recognized in greenish pus by Gerard in 1882, and infections were reported rather infrequently until the 1940s. It is naturally resistant to several antibiotics and disinfectants, and it can grow in fluids with minimal nutrients.[10] It causes infections in immunocompromised patients and was (and still is, in many countries) particularly hazardous in patients with large burns, causing graft failure, septicaemia and often death. Treatment was difficult before the newer penicillins and cephalosporins were developed. *P. aeruginosa* replaced *Strep. pyogenes* as the primary burn wound pathogen after the emergence of penicillin therapy.

Small epidemics of *Pseudomonas* septicaemia were reported in patients treated with antileukaemic agents in the 1950s, and Gould in Edinburgh described 152 cases of wound, respiratory and urinary tract infections in a group of general hospitals during 1961 and 1963.[11] Many other outbreaks were reported, tending to occur in debilitated patients at the extremes of life. Some of the outbreaks originating from a single environmental source that occurred at this time were due to failures in cleaning and disinfection or sterilization of equipment or instruments.

Reports of Gram-negative infections from contaminated disinfectants began to appear in the 1960s.[12] These were due to weak solutions in which the organisms could survive or to 'topping up' existing solutions instead of replacing them and cleaning the container. Pseudomonads have a special ability to survive in solutions of certain disinfectants, such as quaternary ammonium compounds (QACs), and infections have been associated with cotton-wool pledgets soaked in these agents and used for cleaning the skin. Contaminated cork stoppers in bottles of disinfectant have also been associated with infection, and epidemics of meningitis caused by opportunist organisms have resulted from rinsing lumbar-puncture needles in water that has been sterilized inadequately. Washing bowls are often stacked so that a small amount of residual fluid allows a growth of *Pseudomonas* to occur overnight. Food processors have also been suggested as a possible source in an intensive care unit.[13] Floor mops and floor-washing machines are often contaminated heavily with Gram-negative bacilli, although these are probably rare sources since organisms on floors are unlikely to reach a susceptible site on a patient. A shaving brush used in neurosurgery before removing hair from the scalp preoperatively was responsible for a number of cases of postoperative meningitis in the 1960s.[10] The source was not detected for some time, as the brush was kept in the pocket of the ward orderly who shaved the patients; the brush was not decontaminated between patients. Also in the 1960s, failure to sterilize fluids used for washing the eyes during operations was responsible for severe postoperative eye infections; some patients lost an eye.[10] This was probably due to a failure to sterilize a whole batch of small bottles of saline, and it demonstrated the importance of good management in the prevention of infection. There were several major outbreaks of septicaemia from inadequately sterilized commercially produced intravenous fluids in the UK and the USA. In 1971 in a factory in the UK, bottles of dextrose for intravenous use were loaded into an autoclave in which the air was inadequately removed. A small number of surviving bacteria grew to large numbers and were responsible for four deaths; 54 bottles were found to contain large numbers of opportunist organisms (see Chapter 14). The largest outbreak in the USA in the mid-1970s associated with a manufacturing deficiency involved almost 400 cases of infusion-related septicaemia reported from 25 hospitals.[14] The actual numbers were almost certainly much higher. More than 20 microbial species were identified in the bottles, many of them unusual Gram-negative bacilli, such as *Erwinia* spp.

Bacteriologists in the 1960s and 1970s were isolating Gram-negative bacilli from all parts of the 'wet' hospital environment, and it became clear that the mere presence of bacteria was not a hazard unless there was a route to a susceptible site on the patient. Typical examples of this were contaminated sinks, which were rarely sources of infection; flower vases containing heavy growths of *Pseudomonas* were also causes of anxiety, but there was no route of spread to the patient unless nurses failed to wash their hands after handling the flowers. A study of 198 samples of flower-vase water in six hospitals showed the presence of *P. aeruginosa* in 25% of them, but none of eight *Pseudomonas* infections present in these hospitals showed the same strain as in the flower water.[15] Since the opportunist bacteria that were isolated were normally present in the moist environment of the same hospital, typing methods were vital in determining whether they were responsible for infection or for common-source outbreaks. In the 1960s and 1970s, appropriate typing methods for Gram-negative bacilli were developed (see also Chapter 12), such as phage, serological and bacteriocin typing. Bacteriocins are antibiotic-like substances produced naturally by bacteria, and a range of them can form a pattern for a specific organism in a similar way to phages.[10] Bacteriocin and phage typing methods were often used in combination, but they did not always give satisfactory results; more recently, molecular methods have been developed for typing these organisms. It is also of interest that *Pseudomonas* were isolated much less frequently in the home environment than in the hospital.

Medical equipment developed rapidly after the Second World War and became increasingly complex. Many items of dialysis, respiratory and endoscopy equipment were associated with a moist environment and, not surprisingly, Gram-negative infections were soon reported. Unfortunately, the designers of equipment rarely considered that equipment must be cleaned and possibly sterilized, and collaboration with bacteriologists and sterile services staff was rare until the problem arose, but this was often too late for a suitable decontamination process to be developed.

Many of the hospital-acquired infections in the twentieth century were associated with catheterization of the urinary tract, the vascular system and the respiratory tract. Instrumentation of the urinary tract was done from early times, and infection was presumably inevitable since instruments were not then sterilized. In the twentieth century, catheterization was used increasingly, and bacteriological advances enabled a more accurate assessment of infection to be made. Indwelling catheters were introduced by Foley in the 1920s to reduce bleeding after prostatectomy, and these catheters are still in common use. Cuthbert Dukes at St Mark's Hospital, London, in 1929 showed that indwelling catheters were major risk factors for infection, and almost all patients acquired a urinary tract infection following excision of the rectum for carcinoma. Kass in the 1950s reported an infection rate of 2–4% following single catheterization, and 98 of 100 patients were infected if indwelling catheters remained in situ for more than 96 hours.[16] Brumfitt in 1961 found infection in 9.1% of healthy women following single catheterization and in 22.8% of abnormal obstetric patients. These observations were repeated continually, and methods of prevention of infection were investigated by a number of workers (see Chapter 14).

The bacteria causing urinary tract infection are mainly Gram-negative bacilli, and *E. coli* are the still the most common isolates. Self-infection from the bowel is the usual route of spread of these organisms. However, the use of typing methods and more detailed identification techniques have demonstrated the importance of cross-infection, particularly in urological units, epidemic strains usually being highly antibiotic-resistant organisms such as *Klebsiella* or *P. aeruginosa*. Spread could occur from contaminated urine bottles or bedpans, often on the hands of staff, to the junction of the catheter and the urethra, and then proceed between the surfaces of the urethra and the catheter, or along the inside of the catheter, possibly in air bubbles. Macleod in 1958 isolated *P. aeruginosa* from 33 out of 44 urine bottles in a urological ward and suggested that these were major sources.[17] Although closed urinary drainage (urine drained into a sealed bag or bottle through a catheter) was used to reduce urinary tract infection from the 1960s (see Chapter 14), patients with indwelling catheters still became infected within a week due to colonization of the urethra. Cytoscopes were used for examination of the bladder early in the century but were often responsible for cross-infection due to inadequate sterilization or disinfection.

Endoscopes are used for viewing internal cavities such as the gastrointestinal tract, the bronchi, the bladder and the uterus and, more recently, for intra-abdominal or other surgery using minimally invasive techniques. Bozzini from Germany in 1806 described a system using a candle, mirror and tube for examining the bladder, rectum and vagina. This was improved when an incandescent lightbulb became available in 1880, when lenses of telescopes were then improved, and again in the 1950s when fibre-optics were introduced.

Flexible fibre-optic gastroscopes and colonoscopes were a major advance, but there were problems. They were long and the channels were difficult to clean and disinfect, and the endoscopes were damaged by heat at 60 °C and above. The earliest reported infections in these instruments were caused by opportunist Gram-negative bacilli, which grew overnight in the moist conditions within the endoscope and its accessories, such as the water bottle.[18] *P. aeruginosa* was commonly isolated, particularly when inappropriate disinfectants such as hexachlorophene or QACs were used. Surprisingly, despite the frequent isolation of large numbers of Gram-negative bacilli, clinical infections were few and were usually in patients with reduced immunity or following endoscopic operations for removal of gallbladder stones (endoscopic retrograde cholangiopancreatography, ERCP). A few outbreaks of *Salmonella* infection were reported also due to inadequate disinfection. Improvements in cleaning and disinfection methods almost eliminated infections[19] (see also Chapter 14).

Machines (haemodialysis) for removing waste products from the blood of patients in acute renal failure were introduced into routine clinical practice in the 1960s. The dialysis fluids could support the growth of large numbers of Gram-negative bacilli and although separated from the patient's blood by a membrane impermeable to bacteria, bacterial toxins could cross the membrane and enter the patient's bloodstream, causing severe reactions.[20] It is also possible for the bacteria to cross the membrane if it is slightly damaged, when they may cause septicaemia, particularly if large numbers are present in the dialysate.

Potential infection risks from respiratory and anaesthetic equipment have been recognized since the early days of anaesthesia. Skinner in 1873 stated:

If there be one evil, more crying, more disgusting than another, in the practice of inducing anaesthesia, it is the use of inhalers ... There is not one inhaler, my own excepted, where every patient is not made to breathe through the same mouthpiece, tube and chamber ... sweet seventeen is made to follow a devotee of Bacchus, saturated with the exhalation of cognac.[21]

Much later, in the early part of the twentieth century, Magath in the USA devised a water trap for filtering out bacteria.[22]

The warm, moist atmosphere present in respiratory ventilators (machines used for providing air mechanically) and in anaesthetic machines assists in the survival and growth of Gram-negative bacilli, particularly *Pseudomonas*, and infections arising from respiratory equipment were being reported by the mid-twentieth century. The acquisition of *Pseudomonas* infections from contaminated ventilators was reported by Phillips and Spencer in London in the 1960s,[23] and *Pseudomonas* pneumonia was also reported from aerosols from contaminated nebulizers by Reinarz and colleagues in Texas.[24] However, it was shown later in the 1960s by Johanson and colleagues that colonization of the mouth and throat with antibiotic-resistant Gram-negative bacilli often occurred in severely ill patients and was a more frequent source of respiratory infection.[25] Cross-infection on the hands of staff was (and still is) a common route of spread, particularly in intensive care units.

Outbreaks of Gram-negative infections, in addition to problems of staphylococcal cross-infection, led to a review of methods of decontamination of equipment, including the use of low-temperature sterilization methods, and to improved control of sterilization processes (see Chapters 11 and 14).

Gastrointestinal infections

Gram-negative bacilli are the most common cause of gastrointestinal infections. They are mainly community-acquired, but they continue to cause occasional outbreaks in hospitals and remain an important cause of morbidity and mortality, particularly in young children and the elderly (see Chapter 9).

E. coli infections

Enteropathogenic strains were the main causes of outbreaks of diarrhoea in children's wards in the 1930s to 1960s, specific types being identified by serological methods.[26] Outbreaks occurred most often in infants under 1 year. The diseases were mainly propagated in the community and introduced into hospitals by children with diarrhoea and vomiting, person-to-person spread occurring mainly from the hands or clothing of staff or via equipment. Environmental contamination was often very heavy, and possible airborne spread was proposed by Keith Rogers in Birmingham Children's Hospital in the 1950s and 1960s.[27] Spread also occurred on articles such as weighing scales, nappies (diapers) and feeding bottles. In recent years, the enteropathogenic and enterotoxigenic strains have largely disappeared from infant wards in the developed world, and airborne organisms have been detected rarely. The reason for their decline is uncertain, although it may be due to changes in the virulence of organisms as well as to improvements in hygiene.

Infections with these strains are still common in the developing world, and presumably hospital-acquired infections are still frequent in these countries, but little published evidence is available. A new highly toxic strain, 0157:H7, which is associated with haemorrhagic colitis and kidney failure, emerged in the community in the 1980s in many countries, but outbreaks in hospitals have so far been rare.[10]

Salmonella infections

These are the most common of the gastrointestinal organisms causing outbreaks in hospitals. In adult patients, they are usually due to food poisoning. Hospital outbreaks have continued since the 1950s. A large outbreak of *Salmonella* food poisoning in a psychogeriatric unit in the UK in 1985 was responsible for major changes in the administration of control of infection and a new interest in hospital infection by the government.[28]

Salmonella food poisoning usually comes from a common source, for example poultry, eggs or dairy produce, and large numbers of serotypes of the organism have been described in man and other animals.[29] The increase in the number of outbreaks has been associated with battery farming and feeding animals with antibiotics as food additives. Symptoms are mainly diarrhoea and occasional vomiting, and recovery is usually rapid with no specific treatment. Apart from geriatric units, hospital outbreaks are commonly in maternity and children's wards, but these have decreased in recent years. Spread in these wards is usually person-to-person rather than being due to food poisoning. The infection is often introduced into a maternity ward by a mother who may be a carrier or who has recently had a bout of diarrhoea, and who initially infects her own baby. This is then spread to other babies in the unit mainly on the hands or clothing of staff. Other less common modes of spread include rectal thermometers, infant feeds and feeding equipment, enteric feeding tubes, and suction equipment.[30] Infection is usually spread during the acute diarrhoeal stage, when most organisms are disseminated into the environment, particularly from infants or incontinent elderly patients. Nappies and bedding are likely to be contaminated heavily and to contaminate the hands of staff. Although the organisms do not survive well on drying, some may survive if large numbers are dispersed into the dry inanimate environment, and possible airborne spread has been proposed as suggested in an outbreak of *Salmonella typhimurium* in an adult ward in which person-to-person spread occurred.[31] Dust in a vacuum-cleaner bag was suggested as a possible source of another outbreak in a children's hospital.[32] Spread of *Salmonella* has also been reported from contaminated endoscopes. They have been isolated from mice and cockroaches, but there is little evidence that these have been sources of major hospital outbreaks.

The control of staphylococcal and Gram-negative infections

For infection to spread, microbes must reach a susceptible site on a patient in sufficient numbers and be of sufficient virulence to establish an infection. The main sources of infection are infected patients, including carriers.

To prevent infection, (1) sources or potential sources of infection, or more usually the disease-producing microbes from potential sources, must be removed, or (2) routes of transfer (airborne, direct and indirect contact) must be blocked, or (3) the patient's resistance must be enhanced.

The important measures for control of staphylococcal infection in the 1940–50 outbreaks were described in a report from a standing advisory committee of the National Health Service in 1959 in the UK and at a conference at about the same time in the USA.[1,2] The recommendations are still generally applicable; they include isolation of infected and immunosuppressed patients, effective aseptic and hygienic techniques, sterilization and disinfection procedures, the development of surveillance methods, and the setting up of infection-control organizations.

The discovery of bacteria at the end of the nineteenth century improved considerably the understanding of cross-infection and its prevention. The bacteriological studies on haemolytic streptococci, particularly the development of typing methods, provided the basis for control methods in the twentieth century. However, the control methods were rather less successful with the *Staphylococcus aureus* outbreaks, since carriage in healthy people was much higher than with haemolytic streptococci, and the numbers of carriers of epidemic strains continually posed problems of providing sufficient isolation facilities. In addition, routes of spread of staphylococci are multiple, and individual measures often fail.

Detection of carriers was, and still is, a problem in that the nose, throat, axilla, groin and perineum can all be staphylococcal carriage sites and sampling can involve a considerable amount of laboratory work if all suspect patients are screened. There are other problems, such as the facts that the treatment of staphylococcal carriers is often incomplete and that small numbers of organisms surviving treatment may re-emerge in large numbers in the same site days or weeks later.

The importance of the 'personal factor' had also become apparent, and it was believed that one of the failures in controlling staphylococcal outbreaks was a failure in asepsis. Sir George Godber in 1963 stated that when he was having tea in a general hospital, he was told by a surgeon who was having problems with infections that 'he would have to go back to asepsis'.[3] Failure in hand-washing by staff at appropriate times has remained a problem to the present day.

Postoperative wound infections

In the 1940s and 1950s, the number of wound infections appeared to increase with the emergence of epidemic *Staph. aureus* around the world. It was recognized that quantitative information on infections was required to assess the extent of the problem and to measure the response to preventive measures.

A few surgeons, such as Meleney and Howe (see Chapter 8), had already collected accurate data. A large study by Barnes and colleagues at the Massachusetts General Hospital showed a slight but significant rise in infections in clean operations from 3.6% to 5.6% between 1937 and 1957. There was no evidence of an increase in numbers of staphylococcal infections or of influence by prophylactic antibiotics.[4] A further study of 3000 gastrectomies from the same hospital showed incidences of 16% between 1932 and 1940, of 4.1% between 1941 and 1953, and of 9.4% between 1954 and 1958.[5] The initial reduction was thought to be due to the increased availability of blood transfusions and the subsequent changes in the population rather than to an increase in antibiotic-resistant organisms. A number of reports of wound-infection rates were published between 1955 and 1965, varying from 1% of 52 000 wounds in a report by Dineen and Pearce[6] to 26% in a study by Jeffrey and Sclaroff.[7] A careful study by Suzanne Clark in Bristol reported a rate of 13.6% in 1957.[8] It seemed that mean infection rates were of doubtful value in comparing infections in different hospitals with any accuracy as there were considerable variations between the different types of operation as well as in other contributing factors, such as host susceptibility and the age of the patient.[9] However, higher infection rates were often found during staphylococcal outbreaks, and recording could provide information on improvements in individual units or hospitals.

Although the fulminating wound infections of the past century had largely disappeared, there was no doubt that hospital-acquired infection was still rife during the post-Second World War period despite antibiotic therapy. New hazards had appeared with a wider range of operations and immunosuppressive drugs that lowered natural resistance.

Infections in surgical wards in the 1950s, such as empyema, abscesses following perforated gastric ulcers and inflamed appendices, and mastoid abscesses, have shown considerable reductions since then. Complicated fractures (fractures

Table 14.1. Infection rates in different types of surgical wounds in England and Wales in 1960[9,11]

Operation	Number	Incidence of infections (%)
Gallbladder	247	20.6
Breast	188	15.4
Stomach	240	8.7
Hernia	437	7.3
Thyroid	550	6.7
Appendix abscess	58	43.1

associated with a break in the skin) often healed slowly and were commonly infected initially with *Staph. aureus* and later with *Pseudomonas aeruginosa*; occasionally, if involving the lower limb, an amputation was required. Postoperative sepsis after abdominal surgery was often associated with sinuses and fistulae that took a long time to heal, and death from severe sepsis was not uncommon. The cause of these abdominal infections was probably mainly anaerobes, *Bacteroides* spp., although they were not usually identified at the time, but in colorectal surgery the introduction of metronidazole for prophylaxis considerably reduced the number of severe infections (see page 184). Aerobic Gram-negative bacilli, such as *Escherichia coli* were often the only organisms grown in the laboratory from these infected wounds but were often not the main pathogen.

In addition, wards were often overcrowded, with beds along the centre of the ward, and staff were commonly overworked, a situation that has always occurred when populations in an area increase or, as in present times, improved survival leads to increased lengths of stay in hospital by elderly patients. In 1946, a house surgeon at Dudley Road Hospital, Birmingham, greeted the consultant on the latter's arrival at the ward with 'Welcome to Scutari'; large numbers of patients were crammed in the wards like sardines,[10] and overcrowding continued throughout the 1950s. This information was not usually reflected in records of infection rates, and effective control of infection methods was rarely practised by nurses and doctors.

A large Public Health Laboratory Service (PHLS) study published in 1960 showed the differences in infection rates in different operations (see Table 14.1).[11] This study also indicated that the mortality attributed directly to wound sepsis was low but that the mean stay in hospital was 7.3 days longer than expected. Other studies showed variable results depending on the operation, but often the length of stay was longer than in the PHLS study.

Several large studies subdivided wound categories into clean, clean-contaminated and dirty.[12] These categories depended on the amount of bacterial contamination during surgery; for example, clean wounds were those in which the gastrointestinal

Table 14.2. Surgical wound infections in three large studies in the USA and Canada

Investigators	No. of operations	Infection rates (%)		
		Clean wounds	Clean-contaminated wounds	Contaminated wounds
National Research Council[12]	15 613	5.1	10.8	16.3
Cruse and Foord[15]	62 939	1.5	7.7	15.2
National Nosocomial Infections Study (1975–6)	84 691	2.1	3.3	6.4

tract or other potentially contaminated areas were not opened, clean-contaminated wounds were those that transected organs where contamination could occur but was not usually abundant, for instance the stomach, and contaminated wounds included operations on the lower intestine, which is colonized with large numbers of organisms. Although the extent of wound contamination during the operation was probably the most important factor, many other factors influenced the risks of infection, especially surgical technique.[13]

Owen Lidwell in the early 1960s used the PHLS study to carry out multiple-regression analysis on the factors influencing wound infections. He produced a table showing the number of observations required to demonstrate a significant difference between differences in the incidence of infection following the introduction of an infection-control procedure.[14] To show a significant reduction, the numbers of patients required in a study were usually large, particularly if infection rates were low. Unfortunately, this important publication was continually ignored over the next 30 years, and many subsequent studies were invalid due to an inadequate number of observations.

One of the largest and most influential studies was carried out by Cruse and Foord in Canada from 1967 to 1977 (see Table 14.2). They studied infections in 62 939 postoperative wounds and identified many risk factors for infection, for example age of patient, length of preoperative stay, technique of the surgeon, size of incision, duration of operation, type of operation, and wound drainage. Infections were fewer if surveillance (see Chapter 15) was carried out and the results fed back to the surgeon, if patients showered preoperatively with hexachlorophene, or if preoperative shaving was discontinued.[15] These results have mainly been confirmed by others, in particular following the development of mathematical models by Bibby and colleagues in Birmingham[16] and Simchen and colleagues in Israel,[17] and later in the USA by Culver and colleagues.[18]

On the basis of these and similar studies, some modifications to practice could be made, such as admitting patients as close to the operation time as possible, providing feedback of results on infections to surgeons, avoiding drainage of wounds when possible (or at least using closed drainage), and not shaving the operation site. Few surgeons could be convinced of the advantages of avoiding shaving altogether, but they could usually be persuaded to remove hair with clippers or an electric razor on the day of operation; later studies suggested that showering with an antiseptic probably did not influence the infection rate.

The site of acquisition of infection and the importance of airborne spread remained controversial, as we have already discussed in previous chapters, but it seemed likely that most wound infections were acquired in the operating theatre and might be influenced by design and facilities.

The period up to the end of the nineteenth century showed few advances in the design of operating theatres. Theatre tables were usually made of wood and were surrounded by tiers of wooden benches for onlookers. The word 'theatre' was used to describe the performance of surgeons before an audience. With the emergence of asepsis, antiseptics and more complex surgery, more thought was given to theatre design. Separate rooms for anaesthesia, instruments and scrubbing-up were built adjacent to the operating room. Smaller numbers of observers were allowed to watch the operations, and they wore theatre clothing. Later, extractor fans were introduced to remove steam and hot air from sterilizers.

The Medical Research Council (MRC) Subcommittee on Operating Theatre Hygiene in the UK in 1962 introduced an improved zoning system, depending on the degree of cleanliness required, which was generally accepted.[19] This included an outer protective zone separating the theatre suite from the rest of the hospital, a clean zone that included anaesthetic and scrub rooms, a sterilizing area, a 'sterile' or aseptic zone for carrying out the operation, and a disposal zone for used or dirty materials. This design has generally been continued, with small variations.

Bourdillon and Colebrook's studies on burn-dressing rooms showed that a positive-pressure (plenum) ventilation system (see Chapters 10 and 12) reduced bacterial air counts, and Lowbury showed later a reduction in infection with the same system. We mentioned in Chapter 10 that extractor fans in operating theatres can increase infection rates by drawing in contaminated air from the wards, so operating rooms were then provided with filtered air at a positive pressure at 20 or more changes per hour, with an outward flow from the operating room towards the periphery of the operating suite. Although this system was associated with reduced bacterial air counts, there is little evidence that it is associated with a reduction in sepsis.

Hart, in the USA, reported a reduction in wound infection rates following ultraviolet irradiation of the operating room.[20] A large study carried out by the National Research Council, also in the USA, in 1964 found that ultraviolet irradiation did not reduce the overall wound infection but that infections of clean wound were reduced slightly.[12] This improvement in clean wound infection rates was rather marginal, and ultraviolet irradiation was rarely used routinely in operating theatres, a mechanical ventilation system generally being preferred.

Bacterial air counts were shown to increase with the number of occupants in the theatre and with increased activity. Unnecessary activity was minimized for rational reasons, but no evidence of the effect of limited reductions in bacterial air counts on wound sepsis was obtained. Routine screening with air counts during general surgical operations did not appear to be predictive of potential hazard, but sampling could be useful when investigating an outbreak caused by a specific organism.

One of the major advances in surgery in the latter part of the twentieth century was the insertion of artificial implants (prostheses), such as hip and knee joints and cardiac valves, but these operations were sometimes associated with rather high infection rates, and the effects on the patient could be disastrous. These prostheses are particularly likely to be colonized with bacteria from the skin, and often clinical infection with coagulase-negative staphylococci and other low-grade pathogens followed colonization. A coagulase-negative staphylococcus, *Staph. epidermidis*, is a common cause of prosthetic infection and is the most frequently isolated organism found on human skin and in the air of operating theatres.

Sir John Charnley, in the Wrightington Hospital in the UK, was worried about the infection rate in prosthetic hip replacements in the late 1960s and introduced the ultraclean air system.[21] This system consists of an enclosure with a large turnover of filtered air (over 300 air changes per hour, compared with 20 air changes per hour in a conventional operating theatre). The operator and assistant are inside the enclosure, and they wear suits impermeable to bacteria and exhaust-ventilated helmets. The numbers of airborne bacteria within the enclosure during operations were very low, and there was a progressive reduction in wound infection rates from 9% to 1% over 9 years. Charnley introduced other improvements, but he also became a more skilful operator over the years, and doubt was cast by some surgeons on whether the improved results were due to the reduction in airborne organisms or to these increased surgical skills. A multi-hospital controlled trial was then organized in 1980 by Owen Lidwell and colleagues under the auspices of the British MRC, with 8000 patients. Patients whose prosthetic hip or knee joints had been inserted in an ultraclean air unit showed a deep-joint infection rate of 0.6% compared with 1.5% when these were inserted in a conventional operating theatre.[22] The reduction in infection corresponded with the reduction in airborne organisms. The results of this trial confirmed that airborne bacteria were a significant source of infection in this type of surgery, but not necessarily in other types of surgery. Ultraclean air systems have remained in use for hip and knee prostheses in the UK, but less so in other countries, especially the USA, where the conventional air systems usually

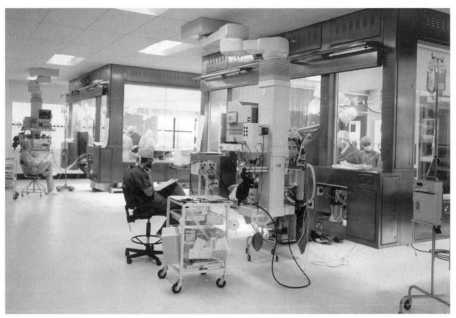

Figure 14.1   Ultraclean air units at Oswestry Orthopaedic Hospital. (Hospital Infection Research Laboratory, Birmingham.)

differ from the UK and similar reductions in wound infection could be obtained with antibiotic prophylaxis alone.

Another advantage of the Charnley enclosure system is that it is possible for more operations to be carried out at the same time in one room. A large theatre (barn) is in use in Oswestry in the UK, which contains four operating enclosures (cabins), allowing four operations to be carried out at the same time (Figure 14.1).[23] This arrangement could be introduced for other types of surgery, possibly with lower air flows, and although it is expensive, output could be increased.

Plastic isolators have also been used for enclosing the wound area or even the whole patient during the operation, separating the surgical team from the patient. These are as effective as the Charnley system and protect the patient from both contact and airborne spread, but they increase the difficulty of operating and are now used infrequently.

Aseptic operating theatre practices were improved over the years by surgeons such as Meleney,[24] Carl Walter[25] and Altemeier in the USA[26] and by workers in other countries. In 1968, the British MRC Subcommittee on Operating Theatres produced a useful report on aseptic and hygienic methods in operating theatres.[27] This classified methods as established, provisionally established, rational and ritual, depending on the strength of the available evidence. The recommendations included theatre clothing and masks, surgical hand disinfection and gloves, disinfection of the skin of the patient, the environment, sterilization of instruments, and cleaning and treatment of equipment. However, few major changes were introduced, but improvements occurred in sterilization and disinfection (see Chapter 11). It was shown that cotton operating theatre clothing allowed bacteria to pass through it, so bacteria-impermeable clothing was produced, but this was not used widely in general surgery until later in the century. Face masks were investigated more thoroughly bacteriologically, and filter-type disposable masks were introduced, although some evidence suggested that wearing masks during an operation did not influence infection rates in general surgery.[28,29] Others felt that the evidence for discontinuation of masks in theatres was inadequate. Disposable wound drapes and sterile disposable surgical gloves were also introduced, and nailbrushes were sterilized.

Cleaning the operating theatre floor after sessions and wearing special footwear were minor changes, although evidence indicated that the inanimate environment was of minimal importance in the spread of infection. Theatre walls and ceilings showed little bacterial contamination, and cleaning periods were reduced from daily or weekly to 3–6-monthly or even longer.[13,30]

Improvements occurred in hand disinfection by surgeons and in disinfection of the operating site. Scrubbing up with soap and water for 10 minutes followed by rinsing in alcohol continued as standard practice (see Chapters 8 and 11). Plain soap was replaced by hexachlorophene soap in the 1950s. The work of Lowbury and Lilly in the UK in the 1960s and 1970s led to a reduction in scrub-up times to 5 minutes, the cessation of the use of hexachlorophene, and the introduction of new antiseptics. German surgeons preferred the use of alcoholic disinfectant rubs for hand disinfection, but surgeons in the UK and countries outside Europe were slow to change (see Chapter 11). Despite the predominant use of aqueous disinfectants for scrubbing up, alcoholic solutions of chlorhexidine and povidone-iodine were used for disinfecting the operating site on the patient's skin. Povidone-iodine contained solubilized iodine and remained popular with surgeons because it still stained the skin brown but was less irritant or allergenic than iodine alone.

Prevention of infection in wards

It was well recognized after many years of experience with infectious diseases that the most effective measure for preventing the spread of infection in wards was the isolation of infected patients. This has been discussed in previous chapters. Isolation wards were used successfully in the early phases of the staphylococcal epidemic, but few hospitals had these facilities, and surgeons were unwilling to transfer infected postoperative patients to infectious-diseases units or hospitals even when they were available. Most wards had side rooms, but the same nurses looked after the uninfected and infected patients, and the existing side wards in the UK rarely had adequate facilities for barrier nursing. The numbers of side wards were usually inadequate to isolate all the carriers as well as infected patients, and the medical and nursing staff often did not recognize *Staph. aureus* or *P. aeruginosa* as being infectious. In addition, the nurses in surgical wards were often inexperienced in looking after infected patients. In a survey of 140 wards in 14 hospitals in the 1960s, Ayliffe and colleagues judged isolation facilities to be inadequate in 84 of the wards; of those found to be adequate, few were used for isolating infected patients. Side wards were often used for noisy, very ill or private patients rather than for infected patients.[31] Side wards were generally not mechanically ventilated, and precautions against contact transfer (wearing gowns and washing hands) were not always enforced sufficiently, especially with ancillary staff such as physiotherapists and laboratory staff. Medical staff did not always observe the aseptic methods laid down for nurses. Despite these findings, isolation facilities were not greatly increased in most new hospitals in subsequent years, and the same problems still remain. A few new hospitals were built in the UK in the mid-twentieth century with subdivided wards and more single rooms. In most countries, codes of practice for isolation were introduced in hospitals, and the system recommended in the USA was followed widely.[32] In particular, isolation rooms were labelled with coloured cards indicating the procedures required for a particular category of infection. A modified system was introduced in the UK.[13] Other systems followed in the USA, such as isolation for specific diseases rather than for a category, universal precautions and, later, body-substance isolation (see Chapter 17).[33]

Hospitals in some other countries, particularly in the USA and Europe, were often much better planned than those in the UK in terms of having smaller wards and more one- or two-bedded rooms, but they were not always better at controlling staphylococcal outbreaks. In the absence of side wards or isolation units, cohort nursing was sometimes introduced, particularly in neonatal units; that is, patients infected with the same organism were nursed together in one ward and no new patients were admitted until all the infected patients had been discharged. Alternatively, measures were introduced to prevent the spread of staphylococci in an open ward. A study in Bristol by William Gillespie and colleagues in the late 1950s in surgical wards showed that a series of special measures against sources and vectors reduced cross-infection of open wounds to about one-third of its former incidence. These measures included prophylactic application of neomycin and chlorhexidine cream to the noses of all patients, spraying all open or drained wounds with an antibiotic spray or covering them with gauze-containing chlorhexidine, disinfecting bedding, and disinfecting baths and bath water, urine bottles, crockery, nurses' hands and ward barber's equipment.[34] The improved results were obtained by using all measures together and demonstrated that individual measures may appear

to fail but can be successful in combination with others. It was also shown that
no precautions would succeed unless applied carefully and enthusiastically by all
staff. Daily visits were made to wards by the investigating team. Surprisingly, little
attention was paid to monitoring hand-washing, although hexachlorophene soap
was commonly used. Similar studies were made by others on nasal treatment or
prophylaxis. Rountree and colleagues in 1962 also reported a reduction in nasal
carriage on treating noses with neomycin-chlorhexidine cream and a reduction in
wound infection from 13% to 3.5%,[35] but Henderson and Williams found that nasal
carriage was reduced but wound sepsis was not.[36] Although recent studies suggest
that nasal carriage may be an important risk factor at least for some operations,[37]
it seemed likely at the time that nasal treatment alone did not necessarily reduce
the risk of wound sepsis. In Norway in the 1960s, Solberg demonstrated convincingly the effect of nasal and skin disinfection on reducing hand contamination and
organisms in the air, but he did not measure the effects on cross-infection.[38]

Removal of the infected patient from the surgical ward to isolation, or sending
the patient home, washing hands by staff after contact with the infected patient or
his or her immediate environment, and good aseptic techniques were identified as
the key control measures, and they have remained so.

No-touch techniques for wound dressings had been shown to reduce infection
in the streptococcal era by Miles and colleagues,[39] and these were continued with
some modifications. Other minor changes were introduced, such as wearing disposable plastic aprons instead of cotton gowns, using heat disinfection for the cotton
blankets that had replaced woollen blankets (which were rarely washed), dispos-
ing carefully of used linen and wound dressings, and using vacuum cleaners or
dust-attracting mops instead of sweeping brushes to clean the floors.[13]

Infections in baby units

The virulent type 80/81 staphylococci particularly affected baby units, and many
of the studies involved controlling outbreaks of this organism. The umbilicus and
skin as well as the nose were commonly colonized during outbreaks. In addition to
isolation, application of antiseptics to the skin and carriage sites of the infants and
hands of staff were the main measures (see Chapter 12).

Bathing with hexachlorophene detergent was introduced, but this was discontinued in the 1960s due to toxicity in neonates.[40,41] However, hexachlorophene
powder continued to be applied to the umbilicus and groin during outbreaks, as
toxic levels were not reached with the powder.[42] Chlorhexidine solutions were then
used if antiseptic baths were required.[13] Although neonatal skin sepsis continued
into the latter half of the century, the problem was much reduced. However, improved survival of premature babies introduced more problems of serious sepsis,
often with Gram-negative bacilli.

Prevention of urinary tract infection

Methods of prevention of infection in patients with indwelling catheters were introduced in the early twentieth century, of which the most effective was closed drainage (i.e. the catheter drained urine into a sterile, sealed bag or bottle). Dukes was probably the first to use this method.[43] Using similar methods, Pyrah and colleagues also showed a decrease in urinary tract infection,[44] but most of the controlled studies were carried out in Bristol in the 1950s and 1960s by Miller, Gillespie and colleagues[45] and in the USA by Kunin.[46] Miller and Gillespie initially used sterilized glass drainage bottles containing formaldehyde, but these were later replaced by disposable plastic bags without a disinfectant. In controlled trials, they obtained a significant reduction in infection rates when closed drainage was used instead of drainage into an open bucket. Even lower rates were obtained following disinfection of the urethra with chlorhexidine, by using plastic foam to anchor the catheter in female patients to prevent movement of the catheter, and by improving the disinfection of cystoscopes.[47] The cystoscopes were being disinfected inadequately in oxycyanide of mercury, and this was improved by the use of alcoholic chlorhexidine. Pasteurization was more effective but did not become popular, and 2% glutaraldehyde was used later in the century.[13] This series of controlled studies on closed drainage was one of the earliest to provide statistically significant clinical evidence for the effectiveness of a hospital infection preventive measure.

Additional measures, such as disinfection of the catheter-meatal junction and adding a disinfectant to a plastic drainage bag, failed to improve the results.[47] The use of a sterile container to empty drainage bags, the use of gloves (or hand disinfection without gloves) by staff to carry out the procedure, and the collection of samples from the catheter tubing with a syringe and needle were rational procedures supported by bacteriological evidence. Tanks of disinfectant used for decontamination of urine bottles or bedpans often became contaminated, particularly if the disinfectant was topped up and not replaced regularly. Disinfection of bedpans and urine bottles by heat eliminated this problem. However, infection still occurred if catheterization was prolonged, due to organisms spreading to the bladder, possibly in a biofilm between the catheter and the urethra. Isolation of patients with infections caused by antibiotic-resistant strains and with indwelling catheters was sometimes necessary to reduce cross-infection.[48]

Prevention of infection from respiratory equipment

The infections reported in the 1950s and 1960s led to the introduction of new methods of decontamination of respiratory equipment.[49] Anaesthetic face masks were cleaned and disinfected after use by each patient, and corrugated tubing was disinfected after each session. Humidifiers, especially nebulizers, were routinely changed and disinfected, usually with chemicals such as acetic acid, and were re-filled with sterile water. Mechanical ventilators represented a greater hazard than anaesthetic equipment, as they were used for several days or longer on one patient. They were decontaminated with low-temperature steam and formaldehyde, or neb-ulized hydrogen peroxide, but later autoclavable ventilators were introduced. Filters were included in the respiratory circuit to prevent contamination of the circuit from the patient, and vice versa,[13] and the ventilator circuits were replaced regularly at intervals of 2 or 3 days.[50] The face masks and much of the tubing were later replaced by disposable items. These measures virtually eliminated infection associated with contaminated equipment, and most of the remaining respiratory infections were then endogenous, caused by Gram-negative bacilli aspirated from the colonized mouth and throat. Prophylaxis for infection by means of selective decontamina-tion of the mouth, throat and stomach was introduced later.[51] This involved local applications of antibiotic pastes and the use of systemic treatment, usually with a cephalosporin. Respiratory infections were reduced by this regime, although mor-tality was often not affected. The emergence of antibiotic-resistant bacteria is a possible problem, and although the evidence has been variable, bacteriologists have never been enthusiastic about the technique.

Cross-infection between ventilated patients is a continuing hazard and still re-quires care in hand-washing after each patient contact and wearing gloves during all procedures.

Antibiotic policies and prophylaxis

The relationship between antibiotic usage and the emergence of bacterial resistance has been demonstrated clearly. The appearance of epidemics of penicillin-resistant staphylococci was described in the 1940s, and now most staphylococcal infections are caused by penicillin-resistant strains. Knight and Holzer in 1954 showed an increase in tetracycline-resistant staphylococci following treatment with the anti-biotic: the nasal carriage rate increased to over 90% within 4–5 days of receiving tetracycline.[52] This phenomenon was demonstrated with different antibiotics by many others. John McGowan from the Emory University, Atlanta, has been partic-ularly interested in the use of antibiotics and the emergence of resistance, and in the laboratory aspects of nosocomial infection.[53]

A number of factors have been involved in the increase in resistance. They include indiscriminate use of antibiotics by doctors around the world, use of antibiotics in animal feeds, over-the-counter sales of antibiotics to the general public in some countries, and cross-infection. In hospitals, nasal carriage of resistant strains of staphylococci was shown to be related to the age of patients and their length of stay in hospital, as well as to antibiotic usage.[54] Avoiding long stays in hospital by elderly patients would help to solve the problem, but this has often not proved possible due to an absence of suitable care facilities in the community.

Policies to prevent the emergence of resistance have met with limited success. Combinations of two or more agents have been successful in the treatment of tuberculosis, and a similar approach in the treatment of staphylococcal and Gram-negative bacillary infections was proposed by Chabbert at the Pasteur Institute in 1959. At the same time, Mary Barber and colleagues introduced a policy at Hammersmith Hospital, London,[55,56] involving the use of two agents (erythromycin and novobiocin) for treating staphylococcal infections and restricting the use of penicillin. This resulted in a reduction in isolates of antibiotic-resistant staphylococci and an increase in penicillin-sensitive strains, but strains resistant to both agents used in the combination gradually emerged. Lowbury also reported a delay in the emergence of resistance when the same two agents were used in combination for treating infected burns.[57]

There was a loss of interest in combinations for staphylococcal infections when methicillin was introduced in the 1960s. The discovery of R factors (see page 164) also limited the value of combination therapy for Gram-negative bacilli.

Restriction of the use of certain antibiotics was sometimes successful with Gram-negative bacilli. Price and Sleigh in 1970 obtained a marked reduction in antibiotic-resistant *Klebsiella* infections in a neurosurgical unit when prophylactic therapy was stopped.[58] Another approach was to avoid the use of new agents, such as amikacin, which meant that an antibiotic could be kept in reserve that would be effective against most Gram-negative bacilli. This was obviously not popular with manufacturers. Another method that was sometimes successful was the rotation of antibiotics, but this was difficult to carry out in practice.[59] Lawrence Garrod stated in 1963, 'Restriction of antibiotics to necessary indications to minimize the emergence of resistance seemed to be the most important principle in antibiotic usage', but apart from some successes in individual units, policies had little effect on the emergence of resistant staphylococci or Gram-negative bacilli by the end of the twentieth century.[55]

Antibiotic prophylaxis was expected to be a promising method for the prevention of certain infections, particularly contaminated postoperative wounds. John Burke in 1961 was the first to show experimentally in animals the importance of correct timing in the administration of prophylactic antibiotics,[60] and Bernard and Cole in 1964 demonstrated a marked reduction in wound infection with prophylaxis covering the operative period.[61] Prophylaxis was then used enthusiastically by surgeons, especially with penicillin and streptomycin or tetracycline, but it soon fell into disrepute by increasing the number of resistant strains in a ward.[59]

More recently, prophylaxis has again been shown to be effective provided that the antibiotics or other agents are known to be active against the potential pathogens and that antibiotic levels are highest during the operation to prevent bacteria from growing when they land on the operative site. However, the results may be less good if there are complicating factors. Simchen and colleagues in Israel in 1980 showed a reduction in infections in single operations on the colon from 27% to 16% following the use of prophylactic antibiotics, but this varied with the risk: those in the highest-risk group, for example patients with intestinal obstruction, showed little reduction.[62] Prophylaxis has now been extended to prosthetic operations as well as to potentially contaminated surgery, but for other clean operations it remains controversial. Prophylaxis was also improved when agents that were active against *Bacteroides* spp., such as metronidazole, were introduced for protection of contaminated operations.[13] Continuing prophylaxis for several days has been discouraged as not only is this no more effective than perioperative cover only but it also encourages the development of resistance. In surveys, it was found that prophylaxis was sometimes continued for weeks without review.

Topical applications of antibiotics were shown to be effective against infections in burns. Burn wounds are initially free from bacteria, but the layer of dead tissue and exudate soon becomes colonized with bacteria from the environment. An application of an antimicrobial agent is the most effective method of preventing colonization, in association with a good aseptic technique.

In the 1930s, haemolytic streptococci were the main causes of graft failure and sepsis (see Chapter 10). Colebrook and colleagues showed that penicillin cream applied to the burn prevented these infections, but the burns then became colonized with penicillinase-producing *Staph. aureus*.[63] These were less likely to cause sepsis, but there could still be a cross-infection problem. A greater hazard to the patient was *P. aeruginosa*, which although less virulent than the haemolytic streptococci could still cause graft failure and death, and infections were difficult to treat. In the 1950s, penicillin was replaced by Lowbury, Jackson and Cason at the Birmingham Accident Hospital Burns Unit with a broad-spectrum cream containing polymyxin, neomycin and chlorhexidine.[64,65]

Antibiotic resistance has always been a particular problem in the treatment of burns, and alternative agents, particularly with activity against *P. aeruginosa*, have been sought continuously.[65,66] Mafenide, a sulphonamide derivative, was introduced in the1960s, and Moyer in the USA followed with silver nitrate compresses, which were effective in reducing colonization with *P. aeruginosa* but were less effective against *Staph. aureus*. This was followed by silver sulfadiazine cream, suggested by MacMillan in the 1970s; this is still in use and its value was confirmed by Lowbury in the UK. There was also some controversy over the exposed treatment of burns or closed treatment with dressings, and this remains controversial today.[67]

The study of burns has been important in the overall prevention of infection. Colebrook's principles, described in 1950 (i.e. all burns should be dressed in clean air, that a strict aseptic technique should be used, and that topical antiseptics should be applied with changes of dressings), are, with small modifications, still valid.[63] Lowbury later expanded theses principles by describing the first line of defence consisting of topical application of antimicrobial agents, isolation of patients, early excision and grafting, and the second line of defence against invasion of tissues consisting of immunization, selective antibiotic therapy, and maintenance of natural defences.[13,64]

Topical use of antibiotics other than on burns has generally been discouraged, particularly if they are useful for treating more general infections, since resistance tends to emerge more rapidly to topical agents than to systemic agents, particularly in patients with widespread dermatitis.

Although antibiotics and other antimicrobial agents have revolutionized the treatment of infections, the failure to prevent emergence of resistance, despite the considerable effort to solve the problem over the past 50 years, has been disappointing.

The surveillance of infection and the organization of infection control

Surveillance was defined by Benenson as 'the continuing scrutiny of all aspects of occurrence and spread of disease that are pertinent to effective control'.[1] It consists of collection of data on infections, analysis of the results, and feedback to clinical staff. This enables outbreaks to be detected rapidly and preventive methods to be introduced. Longer-term collection of data and calculations of infection rates show changes over time and assist in the evaluation of existing preventive measures. Surveillance of infection has provided important evidence on the epidemiology of infectious diseases in the community in the past, and it seemed likely that it would have a similar role in the control of hospital infection.

Two methods of obtaining infection rates are used. Prevalence surveys record the number of cases of all infections present in a ward or hospital during a limited period of time (e.g. 1 week) or a specified point in time (e.g. 1 day). Patients are visited and assessed on one occasion only. Incidence surveys record the number of new cases of infection in a population over a defined period of time, usually at least several months. Prevalence surveys require less continuing resources than incidence surveys and provide a snapshot of the hospital. Prevalence rates tend to be higher than incidence rates, because infected patients are usually in hospital for longer than non-infected patients, but the value of prevalence surveys has been reduced in recent years due to the shorter stay of patients in hospital.

Studies in the nineteenth century usually provided statistics on mortality from all causes, and many hospitals also included numbers of infections in monthly or annual reports; however, hospital-acquired infections were rarely distinguished from those present on admission. William Farr, who was the first Director of the General Registrar's Office in England in 1837, classified death rates by age, disease and region, providing data for Florence Nightingale, who also proposed that ward sisters should keep detailed studies of mortality[2] (although how often this was carried out is unknown). Surgeons sometimes kept good records of wound infection in the early to mid-twentieth century, but not usually of other hospital-acquired infections (see Chapters 8 and 14). A few reports in the mid-twentieth century included all acquired infections, and two examples are noted here: Watkins and Lewis Faning in 1949 surveyed 14 children's hospitals using a questionnaire and reported that 7.1% of 10 000 children acquired an infection, of which 38% were of the respiratory tract, 23% were acute specific fevers, and 21% were of the gastrointestinal tract;[3] and Goodall in 1952 surveyed 5095 patients in 13 wards of eight hospitals and reported an acquired infection rate of 9.9%,[4] predominantly infections of the upper respiratory tract, surgical wounds and the urinary tract. The large number of upper-respiratory-tract infections was due to the inclusion of children's wards.

The staphylococcal outbreaks in the 1940s and 1950s demonstrated the necessity of recording infections in order to control existing outbreaks and to determine changes in incidence; studies on wound infection are described in Chapter 14. A limited amount of routine surveillance was carried out at this time in the UK and USA, where records of wound infections were sometimes kept in a wound book, but these records were often found to be inaccurate due to the absence of a single person responsible for keeping them up to date and also because of the lack of agreed definitions. Surgeons often disagreed on whether a wound was infected, and rounds of visits by bacteriologists or epidemiologists to patients on surgical wards commonly showed more infections than were recorded in the wound book. In the late 1950s, Brendan Moore, a medical microbiologist in Exeter, England, introduced a surveillance system in which an infection-control sister (infection-control nurse, ICN) regularly visited wards to detect staphylococcal infections and to deal with infection problems.[5] The ICN kept a record of infections and was supported by laboratory staff, who cultured samples from wounds and noses as necessary and phage-typed the staphylococci.

The Communicable Disease Center (later the Centers for Disease Control, CDC) in Atlanta, USA, collected information on staphylococcal infections in several hospitals in the 1950s. Later, it was felt by workers at CDC, mainly Theodore Eikhoff, Philip Brachman and John Bennett, that all hospital-acquired infections should be recorded, and they set up a pilot study in six community hospitals. The mean infection rate was low, at 1.4% with a range of 0.4–2.4%.[6] After the pilot study, an incidence study (National Nosocomial Infections Study, NNIS) was organized in 1969 in over 60 US hospitals. ('Nosocomial' is a word derived from the Greek and Latin words for hospital and was used in the USA for hospital infections, but the term 'hospital-acquired infection' continued to be used in the UK and many other countries until the end of the twentieth century.)

At the first International Conference on Nosocomial Infections held at Atlanta in 1970,[7] the preliminary results of the NNIS study were presented in talks by John Bennett, Julie Garner and William Scheckler of the Hospital Infections Section of the Epidemiology Program of CDC; the results of cross-sectional (prevalence) surveys carried out by the Hospital Infection Research Laboratory (HIRL) in England were also reported. However, there was disagreement between conference delegates on the validity of comparison of surveillance results between hospitals and the value of collecting data on all infections throughout the hospital. Brendan Moore believed, on the basis of studies by Owen Lidwell, that due to the multifactorial aspects of infection, calculation of incidence rates could give misleading results in individual hospitals at different times, and comparisons between hospitals would similarly be invalid. He felt that ICNs should spend as much time as possible on wards rather than recording large amounts of data that were of doubtful value in controlling infection.

Following the CDC conference, a trial was carried out in Dudley Road Hospital in Birmingham by an ICN, Ruth Challis, a research nurse, and the HIRL on the overall incidence of infection using modified NNIS criteria. The study showed that in a large hospital of 1000 acute beds, there was an overall infection rate of 5.0%, but collecting the data was very time-consuming and required the employment of a full-time ICN for that purpose only. In some wards, such as obstetrics, ophthalmology and gynaecology, most infections were endogenous and acquired infections were few. It was therefore decided to continue with restricted surveillance in high-risk wards, such as intensive care, and for surgical wound infections.[8] Brendan Moore's methods were continued, with modifications, in the UK for many years. Meanwhile, the NNIS scheme continued to expand in the USA, and over 250 hospitals had taken it up by 1986. Infection rates ranged from 1.7% in small community hospitals to 11.4% in large chronic hospitals, giving an average of about 5.0% per 100 discharged patients.[9]

As well as setting up the NNIS study, the CDC believed it was necessary to prove in a clinical trial that surveillance and the presence of trained infection-control personnel were necessary to control infection. A major retrospective study, the Study on the Efficacy of Nosocomial Infection Control (SENIC), was set up in 338 US hospitals chosen at random between 1975 and the early 1980s. Reductions in infection rates of 20–38% were reported for various types of infection under intensive surveillance, feedback to clinicians and an intensive control programme. The presence of ICNs and infection-control officers (epidemiologists) was also shown to influence infection rates; this will be discussed later.[10] This was an extremely expensive, statistically sound study, and the results were used to persuade hospital administrators of the necessity to set up surveillance programmes and to appoint infection-control personnel in all hospitals. Many CDC staff were involved in the project, but Robert Haley in particular played a major role in publicizing the results at conferences in many countries for some years. However, details of essential requirements remained uncertain, particularly the optimal amount of surveillance required to be cost-effective. Nevertheless, SENIC has remained a major influence on infection-control programmes around the world, although modifications have often been incorporated.

Prevalence surveys of hospital infection and antibiotic usage were carried out initially in Boston by Finland and colleagues in 1964 and then in 1967, giving a prevalence rate of 13.5%[11]. One of the first multi-hospital prevalence surveys was carried out by the HIRL in the West Midlands, England, in the 1960s, giving a prevalence rate of 10.4%.[7] Over the next 10 years, prevalence surveys were carried out in Norway (two surveys, 9.0% and 6.3%), Sweden (10.5%), Denmark (two surveys, 10.4% and 12.1%), Canada (8.2%) and the USA. A large survey in England and Wales in 1979, organized by Peter Meers, Director of the Division of Hospital Infection at the Public Health Laboratory Service (PHLS), and other colleagues, showed a national prevalence of 9.9%,[12] and a World Health Organization (WHO) survey of 47 hospitals in 1983–5 showed a prevalence rate of 8.4%, with a range of 3–21%.[13] Surveys were carried out, mainly in Europe, throughout the rest of the century, including in Italy (6.8%), Spain (two surveys, 8.5% and 8.1%), Belgium (two surveys, 9.3% and 7.2%), Czechoslovakia (6.1%), Greece (two surveys, 6.8 and 5.9%), Germany (3.5%), Australia, Thailand and Hong Kong.[14]

The second national prevalence survey in the UK was organized by Mike Emmerson and colleagues in 1994 and showed an overall rate of 9.0%.[15] A system of collecting data directly on the wards using laptop computers and a modified Epi-Info programme was introduced by M.C. Kelsey. Although the overall rate was unchanged, the data were not strictly comparable. However, surgical wound infection rates fell from 18.9% in the first survey to 12.3% in the second, but it is unknown how much of the reduction was due to earlier discharge of patients. The largest prevalence survey was carried out in France in 1996 (6.7%) and included 236 334 patients in 830 hospitals.[16] In most of the surveys, urinary infections were usually the most common type of infection, followed by infections of surgical wounds and infections of the respiratory tract.

Although there were many variations between surveys, the prevalence rates were mainly about 6–10% and did not change much between the 1960s and the end of the twentieth century. Improvements should be possible in most countries. Repeated surveys were sometimes useful in demonstrating changes in rates and often showed a reduction over time, but comparisons were difficult and changes between types of patient in the surveys and patient risk factors added further complications. Gary French and colleagues in Hong Kong in 1985 carried out a series of prevalence surveys and showed a reduction from about 9.0% to about 6.0% over 3 years. A significant reduction was also obtained in urinary tract infections.[17]

Following the publication of the SENIC study, incidence surveys were often introduced in other countries or individual hospitals using the NNIS scheme, usually with some modifications. However, as discussed already, the recording of all infections in a hospital was very time-consuming, especially in large acute hospitals. The community hospitals in the USA were usually smaller than general acute hospitals in many other countries.

The introduction of computers has had an important influence on surveillance. Computerization of laboratory results has become commonplace, and daily print-outs of reports enable infections caused by certain organisms, e.g. 'alert' organisms that require instant action, such as methicillin-resistant *Staphylococcus aureus* (MRSA) and *Streptococcus pyogenes*, and 'alert' infections, such as bacteraemia or meningitis, to be obtained easily every day. In the UK, the ICN visits the hospital laboratory every day and follows up any 'alert' organisms or infections in the wards. Visits are made to high-risk units, such as intensive care units, every day, irrespective of laboratory reports.[18] Often, the information available in the hospital or laboratory computer program is inadequate for infection control, and special programs have been produced. The Danop-Data system, for wound infections, was developed in Denmark by Kjaeldgaard and colleagues.[19] This was later modified to the WHOCARE system in the late 1980s by Anne Marie Worning of the WHO, Denmark and Ole Bent Jepson, who is in charge of the hospital hygiene department at the State Serum Institute in Copenhagen. The WHOCARE system can be used for collecting, analysing and reporting surgical wound infections and is available as a software or punch-card system.[20] A European multicentre nosocomial infection surveillance programme based on WHOCARE has been introduced in many hospitals, and English, Spanish, French, Italian and German versions have become available. Surveys have also been made of infections in intensive care units, including a large European prevalence study (EPIC) and a European Economic Community (EEC) study organized by Jacques Fabry from Lyons. Other countries, such as the UK and Belgium, have been introducing their own surveillance programmes in recent years (see Chapter 17).[21] Nevertheless, progress towards national and international collection of data in Europe and elsewhere remains slow.

The realization that collection of data on all infections in a hospital would rarely be possible, and the importance of correction for infection risks, had been recognized earlier by Simchen, Bibby and others (see Chapter 14), but the results and the large numbers of patients in the SENIC study changed the thinking in the USA.[10] Risk-correction formulae for wounds were produced by Haley and later by Culver and colleagues and are now in use in the NNIS system.[22] Initially, the risks to be considered included an operation on the abdomen, if the length of time of operation was over 2 hours, if a contaminated or dirty wound was involved, and if there were three or more underlying diagnoses. This formula was modified later to include a preoperative assessment of the patient and a length of time of operation depending on the type. Surveillance became focused increasingly on high-risk units, infections or procedures. In particular, Richard Wenzel in the USA carried out a number of studies in Charlottesville and then in Iowa on surveillance, risk factors, epidemiology and costs of infection. Despite the increased use of computers, he still remained a believer in the importance of 'shoe leather' epidemiology, particularly in the investigation of epidemics.[23]

In the UK, the optimal method of surveillance also became of increasing interest due to the high costs of surveillance of all infections in a hospital and the continuing support by many microbiologists of the simpler methods of Brendan Moore, the HIRL, and others. However, the National Health Service (NHS) wished to introduce routine and standardized surveillance methods in all hospitals. Helen Glenister and colleagues of the PHLS in the late 1980s compared various systems of collecting data including several risk factors with a 'gold standard' that aimed to identify all infections in the test populations.[24] Their reference method consisted of a review of nursing and medical notes, temperature charts, laboratory information, and liaison with nursing and medical staff. The survey showed that laboratory-based ward-liaison surveillance, which involved follow-up of positive microbiology reports and discussion of all patients with ward nursing staff twice weekly, showed the highest specificity of methods investigated (76%) when compared with the reference method. However, the method still required 45 hours per week in a 500-bed hospital compared with 126 hours using the reference method, and depended on samples being sent from a high percentage of infections as well as high-quality medical and nursing notes. Obtaining samples from infected lesions was probably more affordable in the UK than in many other countries, as the costs of laboratory tests were not borne by the patients, but the standard of medical records was often inadequate. The proposed method would be most appropriate for high-risk units rather than for units with low infection rates. The method, which was an extension of the method suggested by Lowbury and colleagues some years earlier, was then recommended by the NHS in England and Wales in the report of the Cooke committee in 1995,[25] and the PHLS set up trial surveillance studies in a selection of UK hospitals. Mary Cooke was Director of the PHLS Division of Hospital Infection at the time.

In the 1990s, the NNIS decided to discontinue reporting all infections but instead to report risk factor analyses.[9] Infection rates for urinary catheter infections, intravenous central-line-associated infections, ventilator pneumonias and isolates of micro-organisms were reported in intensive care units and also surgical site infections corrected for risks. Surveillance of infection methods continues to be developed in the twenty-first century and should help clinical staff to reach the 'irreducible minimum'. The historical perspective of surveillance was reviewed in 1987 by James Hughes from the CDC.[26]

A new difficulty in recording infections is the early discharge of patients from hospital in recent times and the emergence of hospital-acquired infections in the community. The political interpretation of infection rates remains a source of contention. Although popular with governments, the league-table approach is undesirable, and many infection-control workers feel that naming hospitals could be a source of frustration, mistrust, conflict and misleading results. Targeted surveillance is useful, but the results should remain the property of the individual hospital, although anonymous national results could be published, as in the USA.

Environmental surveillance (e.g. bacterial counts of air and surfaces) was popular in the USA and was discussed at the 1970 Atlanta meeting. George Mallison of the CDC felt that it provided useful information, but the UK delegates, and many delegates from the USA, believed that routine bacterial counts of the hospital environment were expensive, time-consuming and not predictive of infection risk. Since then, most countries, including the USA, have discontinued to recommend routine sampling, although some individuals continue to believe it to be worthwhile. Air sampling in operating theatres is increasingly being reintroduced as a measure of quality, but bacterial counts are influenced by many factors and are of little relevance to the acquisition of wound infection. Air sampling is now required in the UK as part of the commissioning process in operating theatres, and standards have been produced, although their scientific basis remains uncertain.

Organization of infection control

The pandemic of staphylococcal infections in hospitals after the Second World War led to the recognition that trained staff were required to take responsibility for prevention and control of infection at a local level. Consequently, in the 1960s and 1970s, hospitals appointed infection-control committees, infection-control officers (or hospital epidemiologists), and ICNs (or infection-control practitioners, ICPs).

In the UK during the Second World War, an Emergency Public Health Laboratory Service was set up to deal with any wartime infection problems, such as germ warfare, that might arise. This service consisted of a series of laboratories in different regions of the country directed by medically qualified bacteriologists. After the war, these laboratories were retained as the PHLS, and the regional laboratories were supported by central reference laboratories at Colindale. One of these reference laboratories was the Streptococcus, Staphylococcus and Air hygiene Laboratory directed by Robert Williams; the name was changed later to the Cross-infection Reference Laboratory when it was directed by Tom Parker. The PHLS in association with clinical bacteriologists in the new NHS and universities were therefore well equipped to investigate the staphylococcal outbreaks.

In the USA in the mid-1940s, the CDC in Atlanta carried out a similar task. In 1951, in collaboration with universities, medical institutes and public health laboratories, the CDC started to send out epidemiologists around the country to investigate outbreaks. Other countries also appointed medical bacteriologists or hospital epidemiologists and often set up a central laboratory for typing, for instance the Statens Seruminstitut (set up in 1955) in Denmark, directed by Kirsten Rosendal. Although the Hygiene Institutes in Germany were interested in disinfection, few were involved in studies on hospital infection; however, at a later stage, individuals such as Franz Daschner at Freiburg took an interest in infection control. Of the Hygiene Institutes in Austria, that attached to the University of Vienna under the direction of Professor Flamm started to take an interest in hospital hygiene in the early 1960s, an interest that has continued with Manfred Rotter, Walter Koller and others until the present time.

Maxwell Finland in Boston in the early 1950s realized the problem of absence from a hospital of any recognized authority with organized facilities for dealing with outbreaks. In 1955, Leonard Colebrook recommended that hospitals should appoint a full-time infection-control officer to review information on the incidence of sepsis and to co-ordinate preventive measures.[27] In 1959, this advice was followed, and the appointment of an infection-control committee and officer was recommended by the NHS Subcommittee on Control of Staphylococcal Infections in Hospitals (see Chapter 14). A few hospitals in the UK, such as Hammersmith Hospital, made part-time appointments of infection-control officers. In the early days, these were often surgeons or physicians, but later they were usually medical bacteriologists. In addition to the official memoranda, the first major book on hospital infection was produced by R.E.O. Williams and colleagues in 1960 and included a discussion on administration.[28] This was followed in the 1970s by the 'green book' on control of hospital infection by Edward Lowbury and colleagues[18] and *Hospital Infections* by John Bennett and Philip Brachman in the USA in 1979.[29]

Brendan Moore was responsible for infection control in several hospitals in south-west England. He found he was unable to visit regularly Torbay Hospital, 20 miles from his base at Exeter. Therefore in the late 1950s, he appointed a nurse to collect data on infections and deal with any infection problems in Torbay Hospital, where a surgeon was the infection-control officer.[5] It was also apparent to Brendan Moore that he did not have time to visit regularly wards in his own hospital, so he appointed another infection-control sister in Exeter. A nurse with similar duties was appointed in Jefferson Hospital in 1956 in the USA to work with Robert Wise, who was one of the earliest hospital epidemiologists.[30] Wise found that the presence of a nurse epidemiologist in the hospital wards had a stimulating influence on the staff, particularly for implementation of policies. Between 1956 and 1971, there was a reduction in staphylococcal bacteraemias in the Jefferson Hospital, and staphylococcal infections as a whole were reduced from 56% to 8%, demonstrating the value of an infection-control team and of definite policies for control.

In the 1950s, detailed recommendations on infection control were produced by the New York State Department of Health, but it was also realized that obtaining too much information often meant that little of value was obtained. Similar recommendations on organization, training and guidelines were made by the American Hospital Association and, in 1958, at the First National Conference on hospital-acquired staphylococcal infections in the USA.[31] ICNs or ICPs were appointed in the 1960s in increasing numbers in the UK, the USA and Canada, and in some other countries. Sweden had appointed two ICNs and a doctor by 1963. Denmark developed a team approach in which one team of nurses visited all the hospitals in the country and produced recommendations for infection-control measures in individual hospitals. In the Netherlands, many of the ICPs were microbiology-trained technical officers. In Canada, the Community and Hospital Infection Control Association (CHICA) was set up in 1976 as a multidisciplinary association. ICNs were appointed in the 1970s in South Africa and Australia, and by Dr Sabat Sabri in hospitals in Kuwait and Dr Danchaivijitr in Bangkok. Although the Council of Europe in 1972 recommended that hospitals should set up infection-control organizations, the response in most of Europe was slow.

In the West Midlands in England, the Regional Medical Officer was worried about the amount of hospital infection and set up the HIRL in association with the Medical Research Council (MRC) in 1964. The HIRL was directed by Edward Lowbury, and he was joined by one of the authors of this book (GA) and Barry Collins. Surveys of infection and of practices were made in the large hospitals of the region by a microbiologist and a research nurse (K. Brightwell). The HIRL has continued with studies on a range of relevant infection topics, such as surveillance, investigation of outbreaks, mode of spread of organisms, and disinfection, and provided early short courses for ICNs and other hospital personnel. The short education course for ICNs was developed later into a more comprehensive course by Marion Read of the Royal College of Nursing in Birmingham in collaboration with Lynda Taylor and the HIRL.

As ICNs increased in numbers and influence in the UK, it was decided to set up an association. The first meeting of the Infection Control Nurses Association was held in Bristol in 1970, with Brendan Moore as the first president, Henry Street as chairman, Annette Viant as secretary, and Kathy Brightwell as treasurer. Full members were all registered nurses, and others, including bacteriologists, could join as associate members.

In the USA, the CDC set up training courses for ICPs and also trained hospital epidemiologists, who took up posts in many of the university hospitals throughout the country. Hospitals in the USA were influenced particularly by guidelines produced by the hospital accreditation authorities and by the increasing numbers of claims for negligence. Since medical insurance paid for most of the medical care,

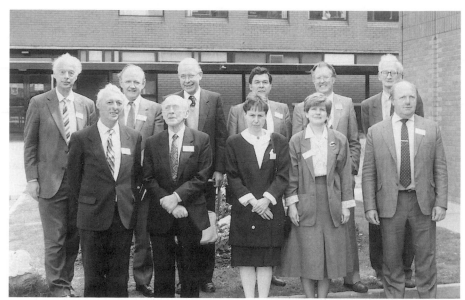

Figure 15.1   Staff and visiting speakers at the twenty-fifth anniversary of the Hospital Infection Research Laboratory, Birmingham in 1989. From left to right, back row: Bertil Nystrom, Richard Wise, Peter Cruse, E. Tikhomirov, John Babb, Graham Ayliffe; front row: David Williams, Edward Lowbury, Heike Langmaak, Elaine Josse, Ian Phillips. (Hospital Infection Research Laboratory, Birmingham.)

they were also influenced much more by costs of infection than the UK was at the time. Large numbers of ICPs were soon appointed, and they formed the Association of Practitioners for Infection Control (APIC) in 1972. This association is now the largest infection-control organization in the world. Infection-control associations in various countries were particularly interested in education and set up training courses, which have continued to develop.[32]

As discussed already, there was limited evidence on the effectiveness of infection-control programmes in the 1970s, and the conclusions of the SENIC project were implemented in many but not all hospitals in the USA. The results of this study showed that one ICN or ICP to 250 hospital beds was necessary in association with an effective surveillance and control programme to reduce hospital-acquired infection by 32%. The employment of a trained physician hospital epidemiologist was also associated with a reduction in wound infection.[10] This study had a major influence on appointments of infection-control personnel around the world, although the goal of one practitioner to 250 beds could rarely be met.

The infection-control officers in the UK felt the need for an organization to discuss their own problems, which were sometimes different from those of the ICNs. By 1980, most infection-control officers in the UK were medical microbiologists, and they decided to form the Hospital Infection Society (HIS), with Edward Lowbury as the first president, Graham Ayliffe as chairman, David Shanson as secretary, Peter Meers as treasurer, and Mark Casewell as meetings secretary. The hospital epidemiologists in the USA formed a similar organization, the Society for Hospital Epidemiologists of America (SHEA).[33] Both of these societies produced journals, the *Journal of Hospital Infection* in the UK and *Infection Control,* later renamed *Infection Control and Hospital Epidemiology,* in the USA. These two journals and the APIC's *American Journal of Infection Control,* which began in the 1970s, have had a major influence on progress in the subject and have since been joined by journals from other countries.

The training of infection-control officers in Europe differed from that in the USA, and a combined meeting of HIS and SHEA discussed and compared practices. The officers' duties and responsibilities were found to be very similar, although the Europeans mainly favoured a laboratory-based initiative in which a medically quali-fied microbiologist starts the epidemiological investigation, whereas the Americans often preferred to have a ward-based epidemiological approach from the outset.[34] The study found that infection-control officers in Europe were usually in charge of the laboratory and could more easily make decisions on bacteriological require-ments of investigations without further consultation, whereas those in the USA were better trained in epidemiology and infectious diseases but were often trained less well in microbiology. Most hospital microbiologists in the USA were not med-ically qualified. Since then, improved training has reduced the deficiencies of staff in both countries, and diplomas and university degrees in hospital infection are widely available for both ICNs or ICPs and doctors in many countries. Another combined conference of the HIS and SHEA was held in Arizona in 1986 on the 'irreducible minimum'. This conference concluded that although there was such a minimum in hospital infections, most hospitals had not yet reached it.[35]

The idea of the infection-control committee, team, officer and nurse (or practi-tioner) spread around the world, many countries making legislative requirements for them, and although there were variations, the duties were much the same.[25] Infection-control teams are responsible for day-to-day control activities; their du-ties are mainly surveillance of infection, investigation of problems, control of out-breaks, general hospital hygiene, decontamination of equipment, and formulation of policies. The ICN or ICP in particular provides advice on isolation of infected pa-tients, liaison with occupational health and other hospital staff, and especially with the microbiology laboratory, and the education of staff. The emergence of human immunodeficiency virus (HIV) infection has been associated with one of the major changes in infection control, the introduction of universal precautions or body substance isolation (see Chapter 17).[36] The implementation of these procedures, especially the avoidance of needlestick injuries, has become a time-consuming task of infection-control staff in all countries of the world. Another major change is the responsibility of the ICN for the expansion in risk assessment, which often extends beyond infection control. Other key duties, including quality assurance standards, clinical governance, and audit of infection-control procedures, have also become increasingly prominent.[18,25] Most of the infection-control tasks in hospital wards and departments are carried out by the ICN, who is usually the only person in the hospital employed full-time in infection-control, but ICNs now have a greater political/managerial role and there are increasing numbers of ICN consultants in the UK. Infection-control committees are sometimes large, involving clinicians, senior nurses, pharmacists, engineers, catering managers, occupational health staff, sterile services staff and a senior manager; others are much smaller, but all include a manager. The committees meet less frequently than the team and tend to make major recommendations on extra staff or funds as well as receiving reports and approving policies.

Doctors with responsibility for infectious diseases and public health were appointed in England and Wales at the end of the nineteenth century, but their responsibilities were mainly in the community. Although the posts were modified over the years, the medical officers of environmental health (MOEH) were not usually involved in hospital infection. However, a large outbreak of *Salmonella* food poisoning in a psychogeriatric hospital in 1984 and an outbreak of legionnaires' disease in 1984 were responsible for changes in infection-control administration in the UK. A public health report in 1988 recommended that the MOEH should be replaced by a consultant in communicable disease control (CCDC) who was well trained in epidemiology and microbiology and was made legally responsible for control of communicable diseases in a health district, including the hospitals, and was expected to collaborate with the infection-control officer in the hospital.[25] The other major change was the removal of crown immunity from hospitals. This meant that hospitals were now subject to the laws on hygiene from which they were previously exempt and could face legal action.

Another development was the appointment of infection-control link nurses. These nurses are on the staff of units such as intensive care units; they have part-time responsibilities in infection control in that unit only and report to the ICN. These posts are gradually being developed.[25]

From the 1980s onwards, contributions to control of hospital infection practices were made from many countries. An unofficial European working party with representatives from Denmark, Sweden, Finland, Germany, Italy, the UK, Norway, the Netherlands and Austria carried out various combined studies, such as the effect of preoperative bathing with an antiseptic on wound infection and on urinary tract and intravenous infections. Co-operative educational projects included a film on prevention of infection in intensive care units made in a Swiss hospital and organized by Franz Daschner (from Germany), with the collaboration of Bertil Nystrom (from Sweden) and Graham Ayliffe (from the UK). An international meeting was also held by the WHO in Denmark to discuss setting up an international federation, which resulted in the International Federation of Infection Control (IFIC) being set up in 1987, the members being organizations rather than individuals.[37] The first chairman of the IFIC was Shirley Bradley from the USA, who was followed by Graham Ayliffe from the UK and then by Anna Hambraeus from Sweden. The federation produced a handbook on basic concepts in infection control for educational purposes.[38] It is particularly interested in education and in providing help to developing countries. Meetings have been held in England, Slovenia, Turkey, South Africa, Croatia and Egypt, and members of the board have taken part in a number of other national and international meetings. Over 40 associations from 36 countries are members, and the federation is supported by a number of patron (commercial) members. In addition to IFIC, a number of infection-control workers have provided assistance to developing countries, including Donald Goldman and colleagues from Boston, Ole Bent Jepson from Denmark, and J. Ojajarvi from Finland.

In the 1980s and 1990s, international (and national) conferences on hospital infection became more popular, increasing the profile of the topic and the organizations, and industry was prepared to contribute to an increasing extent to fund these meetings.

In the 1990s, more governments took an interest in hospital infection. This was due mainly to political problems caused by antibiotic resistance and the increasing costs of infection. Costs of negligence claims in countries in addition to the USA and the emergence of variant Creutzfeldt–Jakob disease (vCJD) in the UK were causing increasing anxiety, and acquired immunodeficiency syndrome (AIDS) was causing major political problems in Africa (see Chapter 16). The early discharge of patients from hospital meant that many hospital infections appeared for the first time in the community, and community ICNs are now being appointed. The early discharge of patients to nursing homes requires expertise in aseptic procedures in these establishments. They can also be a reservoir for antibiotic-resistant bacteria, and admission of patients with resistant bacteria from long-term residential establishments to acute hospitals may be responsible for new outbreaks.

Some governments introduced legislation on infection control, and others produced more funding, and by the end of the twentieth century the profile of hospital infection had increased considerably. Improved quality assurance is now the general aim, and many hospital epidemiologists, particularly in the USA, are involved closely with all aspects of quality control as well as with hospital infection.

The approach to control is dynamic and should lead to change and improvement. However, the philosophy of infection control differs between countries, and developing countries usually still have to be more concerned with basic hygiene in the community. The effect of all these measures on infection rates remains uncertain, but the personal factor is still important and all staff (and patients) have a responsibility for preventing infection.

Emerging diseases at the end of the twentieth century

In the mid-twentieth century, the increased availability of antimicrobial agents, the availability of more effective vaccines, and the reduced morbidity and mortality from infectious diseases suggested that the latter were no longer a major problem when compared with cardiovascular diseases and cancer. Infectious diseases units were closed, fewer infectious diseases physicians were appointed, and funding for research on infection decreased. However, this attitude to infection changed later in the century, particularly with the emergence of human immunodeficiency virus (HIV) infection. The microbes fought back: new diseases appeared, and old infections re-emerged with increased virulence or with increased resistance to antimicrobial agents. Some diseases, such as malaria, mainly involved the community in tropical countries, but other organisms, such as the hepatitis viruses, enterococci and methicillin-resistant *Staphylococcus aureus* (MRSA), caused increasing problems in hospitals all over the world. Other infections, such as acquired immunodeficiency syndrome (AIDS), legionnaires' disease, some viral zoonoses and variant Creutzfeldt–Jakob disease (vCJD), the human form of bovine spongiform encephalitis, were identified for the first time.[1]

Emerging infections are infections whose incidence in humans has increased within the past two decades or threatens to increase in the near future;[1,2] they consist of:

- new or previously unrecognized diseases;
- well-recognized diseases that have become resurgent;
- diseases associated with the development of antimicrobial resistance in existing agents; these are responsible for the main problems in the control of hospital infection.

Viral hepatitis

Outbreaks of epidemic jaundice or liver inflammation have been described in the past. They were a major disease in armies, probably spread from contaminated water supplies. This disease was known as catarrhal or infective jaundice and was probably mainly hepatitis A, although it was commonly confused with serum hepatitis (hepatitis B) despite the different modes of spread.[3]

In this century, cross-infection with hepatitis A has been reported in patients and staff of long-term residential establishments; it is spread by the faecal-oral route. In acute hospital wards, cross-infection is infrequent since transmission is rare after the onset of jaundice, when viral shedding is much reduced. Patients with faecal incontinence and acute infection are a greater hazard. The development of a vaccine has reduced the spread of the disease amongst healthcare staff. Another virus, hepatitis E, has been shown recently to cause a similar infection and is endemic in some tropical countries, but hospital-acquired infection in developed countries appears to be rare.

An epidemic of serum hepatitis (hepatitis B) was described in 1885 in which 191 workmen developed jaundice after immunization against smallpox with human lymph. Other outbreaks were associated with injections of arsenic given as a treatment for syphilis between 1920 and 1940.[3] Hepatitis B acquired increasing importance in the Second World War when it occurred following yellow fever immunization, and there was also increasing evidence of transmission from blood, blood products and contaminated syringes. Efforts to isolate viruses from these infections initially failed. In 1967, an antigen was discovered by Blumberg and colleagues in the blood of an Australian aborigine; the antigen was associated with serum hepatitis and was known as the Australia antigen.[4] This antigen was later recognized as a virus particle (the Dane particle).[5] The differences between the two main hepatitis infections were defined by Krugman and colleagues by means of human experiments.[6] Serum from the disease with a short incubation period was termed MS-1 and was obtained from classical catarrhal or infective jaundice (type A); the serum from the disease with the longer incubation period, homologous serum jaundice (type B), was termed MS-2. It was shown later that serum from type B infections contained the Australia antigen. Viral hepatitis is now known to be caused by at least five agents: A, B, C, D and E.

The risks of acquisition of hepatitis B became increasingly prominent in hospitals at the time when HIV emerged in the 1980s. It was realized that hepatitis B was more infectious than HIV and could be transferred by the same routes.[7] Hepatitis B virus (HBV) and hepatitis D virus are DNA viruses. They are spread mainly in the blood in hospitals by transfusion or by 'sharps' injuries, although spread can occur following contamination of mucous membranes, and they can also spread sexually; airborne spread does not occur. Perinatal transmission is the most common mode of spread worldwide.[8] Hepatitis D is known as the delta agent and can cause infection only in the presence of HBV. Neither virus has been grown in tissue culture. There are 350 million carriers of hepatitis B in the world, mainly in Asia and sub-Saharan Africa.

The risks of infection of hospital staff from a contaminated needlestick injury from the blood of a carrier of the hepatitis e antigen is about 20%. The e antigen is associated with high infectivity.

Hospital outbreaks of hepatitis B were reported from renal dialysis units in the 1960s and 1970s, and infections have also been reported from capillary blood sampling in diabetics and from tattooing. Infection has been transferred from patients to staff, particularly in invasive surgery. Transmission from healthcare staff, for example surgeons and dentists, to patients is rare but has been reported, particularly from e antigen carriers. Another rare route of spread is via medical equipment, for example endoscopes. Transmission in transfusion blood and blood products is now rare since donor blood is screened and disposable needles are commonly used. Immunization of staff, introduced in 1974, has considerably reduced the risk of infection in healthcare workers, but this is still too expensive for routine use in developing countries.[8]

Hepatitis C virus was identified in 1989; there are about 100 million carriers worldwide. This infection was previously known as non-A, non-B hepatitis; it has not been grown in tissue culture. It is responsible for post-transfusion hepatitis and is common in haemophiliacs and drug addicts. Transmission in hospital is infrequent but can occur from needlestick injuries.[7,8] Acquisition by hospital staff also appears to be uncommon as the incidence is no higher than in the general population (0.5–2.0% in Europe). A report from Australia suggested that spread had occurred from contaminated anaesthetic equipment, but other modes of spread could not be excluded.

HIV infection and AIDS

In 1981, a mysterious illness occurring in San Francisco was reported to the Centers for Disease Control (CDC) in Atlanta. Five men, all homosexuals, developed pneumonia due to a rare protozoon, *Pneumocystis carinii*. This was usually associated with a potentially fatal breakdown in the immune system. Similar reports were soon received from other towns – reports that included Kaposi's sarcoma, another rare disease associated with immunodeficiency – and a viral infection was thought to be the underlying cause. Although this appeared initially to be a disease of homosexuals, it was later found to include intravenous drug users and haemophiliacs; in Africa, spread was mainly due to heterosexual intercourse.

After considerable research, a retrovirus (HIV-1) was identified in a patient by Barré-Sinoussi and other members of Luc Montagnier's team at the Pasteur Institute in 1983.[9] Soon afterwards, it was isolated from patients with AIDS and AIDS-related complex by Robert Gallo and his team at the National Cancer Institute, Bethesda, USA.[10] The disease is associated with destruction of certain white blood cells (CD4 + T-lymphocytes) in the immune system.[11] It spread rapidly, and over 500 cases were reported in the USA within 15 months and 21 000 worldwide by 1986, among which over half were in the USA. By the end of the twentieth century, it was present in all parts of the world. It was estimated that there were 34 million people carrying the virus in 1999 and that over 18 million had died since the disease was first diagnosed. Most cases are now in sub-Saharan Africa, where the disease remains out of control due mainly to the costs of treatment as well as to a failure to take adequate preventive precautions.[2] Possible cases were described in Uganda in the early 1950s, and it has been shown that the immediate predecessor of HIV-1 is probably the simian immunodeficiency virus (SIV) of the common chimpanzee. It may have been acquired initially by a hunter or market trader, possibly with cut hands, who butchered contaminated chimpanzee meat. However, this does not explain why it occurred at that particular time. There is recent evidence that the last common ancestor of all HIV variants was already present in 1931, plus or minus 10 to 20 years.

The virus has now developed resistance to commonly used drugs, and combinations of zidovudine with one or more other drugs are now often recommended. However, these combinations are usually too expensive for use in developing countries. Progress towards an effective vaccine is slow because of the ability of the virus to mutate, but preliminary vaccines are under trial in Africa.

The virus has low infectivity compared with most epidemic viruses. The risk of acquisition of infection from percutaneous contact is only 0.2–0.5% and is even lower following mucous membrane contact. The virus is killed readily by most disinfectants and by moist heat above 70 °C, but it can survive in dried blood for at least a week. It is transmitted mainly by sexual intercourse but also by inoculation of blood and blood products, by vertical transfer from mother to baby, and in breast milk. HIV is often transferred on the contaminated needles of drug addicts. Although present in saliva and tears, the virus is not transferred by these routes or in the air.[12] Transmission in hospitals is rare, but HIV can be acquired by staff from needlestick injuries (see above). Spread by blood transfusion and blood products has been almost eliminated in developed countries due to comprehensive screening programmes, but this route is still common in developing countries, particularly in Africa. Spread from a healthcare worker to a patient in developed countries is even more rare, and definite sources recorded have been only one dentist and one surgeon; however, unreported acquisitions are likely to have occurred. There is no evidence of transfer on endoscopes or other surgical instruments. Since it is difficult to predict who is likely to be a carrier, universal precautions (e.g. wearing gloves for all contact with blood or other body fluids) to reduce transmission risks have been introduced into healthcare establishments throughout the world (see page 228).[13]

Transmissible spongiform encephalopathies

Transmissible spongiform encephalopathies (TSEs) are fatal 'infections' mainly of the central nervous system and are associated with rapidly advancing dementia. They are probably caused by prions, self-replicating proteins that contain no detectable specific nucleic acids. The main diseases in the group are scrapie in sheep, Creutzfeldt–Jakob disease (CJD) in humans, and BSE in cows and humans.

Scrapie in sheep is associated with cerebral lesions and paralysis and has been recognized clinically for over 200 years. It was thought by Sigurdson in 1954 to be caused by a 'slow' virus, although no virus was detected, because of its transmissibility and long incubation period.[14] Similar diseases were recognized in other animals, for example mink, but there was no evidence that they were transmitted to humans. In humans, a similar disease with progressive dementia, spasticity and muscular weakness was first described histologically by Creutzfeldt in 1920 and by Jakob in 1921, and it became known as CJD.[3] This is a rare disease (0.5–1.0 cases per million population of the world per year). It develops in the elderly and can easily be confused clinically with senile dementia; many cases have a genetic component.

In 1959, a progressive neurological disease similar to scrapie occurring in cannabalistic tribes and known as kuru was reported in New Guinea. Deaths from the disease were mainly in women and young people, who sometimes ate infected human brain tissue. Hadlow, a vet, first drew attention to the similarity of scrapie and kuru.[15] The possible relationship between scrapie, kuru and CJD was investigated by Gajdusek and colleagues at the National Institutes of Health at Bethesda. They were able to transfer kuru to brain tissue in chimpanzees and to produce a spongiform encephalopathy (see below).[16]

In the 1980s, another similar disease, BSE, emerged in cattle in the UK and to a much lesser extent in other European countries; it was probably acquired from infected UK cattle feed. BSE appeared to be transmitted to humans probably by ingestion of contaminated beef; this transmissibility was confirmed in 1996 by the National CJD Surveillance Unit, based in Edinburgh. Although a large number of cattle were infected in the UK, the number of human infections has remained low, with 43 cases by July 1999 and over 70 cases by 2000. It seems likely that the species barrier is high, but owing to the long incubation period, a larger epidemic cannot be excluded yet. The new disease in humans is known as new vCJD.[17] It affects younger people than does classical CJD, it is rapidly fatal, and it has distinctive clinical and pathological features.

Normal prion proteins are found in the tissues of man and animals. An abnormal, partially protease-resistant form of the normal prion protein that accumulates mainly in the brain has been found in TSEs; this protein destroys normal tissue and gives the brain tissue a spongy appearance under the microscope. The protein has been demonstrated in lymphatic tissue (including the tonsil and appendix) of patients with early vCJD before neurological symptoms appear. Transmission in blood is a possibility, although there is no evidence that clinical infection has been acquired by this route. The agent does not stimulate any immunological response. The abnormal protein causes disease if injected into the brain of another animal. Prusiner in 1982[18] suggested that this protein, a prion, is the effective agent of TSEs, but others believe that another component, possibly a nucleic acid, is required that can trigger the change from normal to abnormal protein.

These prions have other unusual biological features. They are resistant to normal heat sterilization processes and to ethylene oxide, aldehydes, alcohols and most other chemical disinfectants, although they are inactivated by hypochlorites and sodium hydroxide, but at concentrations likely to damage medical equipment.[19]

The risks of transmission to healthcare workers are low. Possible infection from classical CJD in a neurosurgeon and two histology technicians has been reported. Transmission has been reported rarely on brain electrodes, on instruments used in neurosurgery, and on instruments used in operations for insertion of a dura mater implant and for transplantation of a cornea. Haematogenous spread has occurred from extracts of pituitary hormone in about 30 reported cases in several countries. No evidence of transmission of vCJD on equipment or from person to person has been reported, and studies are proceeding on early diagnosis and practical methods of inactivation of the protein.

Viral haemorrhagic fevers and other viral zoonoses

In recent years, several new viruses have been discovered that cause a potentially fatal haemorrhagic fever.[8,20] In 1967, 37 laboratory workers in Marburg and Frankfurt in Germany and in Belgrade became ill with high fevers and severe haemorrhages; seven died. This infection was traced to tissues from green monkeys from Uganda, and the causative organism was termed the Marburg agent, later shown to be a filovirus.[3] Sporadic cases have since been reported from Zimbabwe and Kenya.

Epidemics of a similar haemorrhagic disease were reported from the Sudan and Zaire in 1976, with a large number of deaths, including hospital staff. The disease was named Ebola haemorrhagic fever. In 1994, a Swiss zoologist acquired the disease when working with infected chimpanzees in west Africa, and another epidemic involving 316 cases and 245 deaths was reported in Zaire in 1996. Ebola virus has also been identified in monkeys in the USA and Italy. A few human cases infected with this strain occurred in the USA, but no fatalities occurred, possibly because of a less virulent virus. The monkeys were shipped in from the Phillipines, but any relationship with Africa is unknown. The Ebola virus is a filovirus similar to that causing Marburg disease.[20] The natural hosts of the virus remain unknown. It seems likely that monkeys and apes are victims rather than normal reservoirs, since the death rate in infected animals is very high.

In 1969, three missionary nurses working in Lassa and elsewhere in Nigeria developed a haemorrhagic fever, and two of them died. The same disease was also acquired by two laboratory workers, one of whom died, and the cause of both outbreaks was shown to be an arenavirus that naturally infects a rodent found in that part of Africa.[21] Epidemics of Lassa fever continued in localized areas of west Africa, with many deaths, including of hospital staff. Some cases were flown to Europe or the USA, but no infections from secondary cases occurred. Because of the high death rate and the absence of effective treatment, patients were usually nursed in plastic isolators in special infectious diseases units.[22]

The diseases are transferred by close person-to-person contact and in blood, urine, other body fluids and faeces. The risk of airborne spread appears to be slight, and plastic isolators are no longer thought to be necessary.[23] Spread to hospital staff from primary cases occurs frequently if barrier precautions are inadequate and if staff are trained inadequately. It also occurs if hygiene is poor, for example by using unsterile needles. It seems likely that infections in hospital staff acquired from secondary cases are less likely to be fatal and that spread can be controlled by good basic isolation precautions. Nevertheless, the high mortality in the outbreaks of zoonoses (animal diseases) in Africa could present a possible future threat to the world, and careful surveillance and control measures are necessary.

Other viral zoonoses can cause severe infections varying in their death rates, for example rabies, hantavirus, dengue, Congo-Crimean haemorrhagic fever, encephalitis caused by arboviruses, and yellow fever.[3,8] Rabies is carried by many animals, including dogs, foxes, bats and raccoons, and is usually transferred to humans by a bite from an infected animal. It is a fatal disease of the nervous system, but it can be prevented by immunization. Rabies has been transmitted to humans rarely by an implanted cornea.

Hantavirus infection is a potentially fatal disease acquired from rodents. It has been acquired by laboratory workers from infected cell lines. Dengue, a common disease of tropical regions, is transmitted by mosquitoes; it is usually mild, but a severe haemorrhagic form can occur.

Person-to-person transmission is not usually a problem with these infections and they are not usually a nosocomial risk, but care may be necessary in handling contaminated secretions, such as saliva in rabies. Isolation is often recommended because of the high death rate rather than due to the risk of transmission.

Legionnaires' disease

This is caused by aerobic Gram-negative bacilli, *Legionella pneumophila* and other *Legionella* spp., which were not identified as a cause of disease until 1976 by McDade and colleagues at the CDC.[24] They were found to be ubiquitous and can be isolated from most water supplies, lakes and other areas of standing water.[25,26] They were first identified as a cause of a pneumonia-like illness in delegates at a meeting of the American Veterans of the American Legion in Philadelphia, and the disease was thus named legionnaires' disease. The source appeared to be the hotel air-conditioning system. The first recorded hospital outbreak occurred in a psychiatric hospital in Washington in 1965; *Legionella* were not identified, but the diagnosis was confirmed later by serology.

Since 1976, many other hospital outbreaks have been reported around the world, often with a large number of cases. An outbreak in a Stafford hospital in the UK associated with a cooling tower was followed by a public inquiry and new government regulations on control of infectious diseases.

The disease is now identified regularly in association with contaminated aerosols. It mainly affects elderly males, heavy smokers and immunocompromised patients. It does not spread from person to person. Sources of infection in hospitals are usually aerosols from cooling towers, but showers and jacuzzis and even mechanical respiratory ventilators are potential sources, particularly in units for immunosuppressed patients. Although sporadic cases are not uncommon, outbreaks in hospitals and elsewhere, for example hotels and large office blocks, are still relatively rare and are usually prevented by careful management of cooling towers and water supplies by regular cleaning, regular disinfection and good design.[26]

Helicobacter pylori infection

This is another recently described organism. *H. pylori* is found in the stomachs of normal people. It was first isolated in Australia by Barry Marshall and can be a cause of gastritis and gastric ulcer. It is presumably transferred from person to person, but the mechanism is unknown. It has been isolated from gastroscopes, although there is no good evidence of disease transmisssion by this route.[27]

Listeria monocytogenes infection

This is a Gram-positive bacillus found ubiquitously in man, animals and the environment.[28] Soft cheeses and pâté are common sources of infection. It can cause bacteraemia or meningitis in newborn babies or immunocompromised patients. It is uncommonly a hospital-acquired infection, although it may be introduced into a ward by a pregnant mother, who may infect her own baby, with subsequent transfer to other babies in the neonatal unit.[29]

Cryptosporidia infection

Protozoa are infrequent causes of hospital infection, but *Cryptosporidium* was identified in 1976 as a cause of diarrhoeal disease.[30] Major outbreaks of infection are mainly in the community but can involve hospitals; they are usually acquired from contaminated water supplies. Person-to-person spread, although uncommon, can occur, particularly in units for immunocompromised patients, where it can be severe in patients with AIDS.[31] *Cryptosporidia* have been isolated from gastro-intestinal endoscopes and could be transmitted from these instruments, but there is no evidence of outbreaks arising from these sources.

Tuberculosis and other mycobacterial infections

Pulmonary tuberculosis (see also Chapter 9) decreased rapidly in the developed world during the twentieth century due to improvements in hygienic conditions and later to the use of streptomycin and other antituberculosis agents.[3] Most of the sanitoria built in the early 1900s were closed by the 1960s. Nevertheless, in 1997 there were over seven million cases in the world, of which three million died. The number of cases in developing countries has continued to increase.

Spread between patients and staff in hospitals has presumably always been a problem, but in view of the high incidence in the community and the absence of a typing method, evidence of hospital-acquired infection has rarely been obtained. There were reports in the second half of the twentieth century of hospital staff, particularly doctors, nurses and those working in pathology laboratories and mortuaries, acquiring infection. Outbreaks have been reported in chronic care and paediatric wards and in immunocompromised patients, particularly those with AIDS. Molecular typing now enables outbreaks to be traced more readily.

There is surprisingly little documented evidence of *Mycobacterium tuberculosis* spreading on medical equipment and causing infection.[32] The organism has been isolated from anaesthetic masks and bronchoscopes, and infection in only one or two patients has been reported following bronchoscopy with inadequately decontaminated equipment despite the many thousands of people that are bronchoscoped every year.

An emerging problem is the increasing development of antibiotic resistance of *M. tuberculosis* to the commonly used antituberculosis agents. These resistant organisms, along with antibiotic-sensitive strains, are often brought into developed countries by immigrants from the developing world. Although occurring mainly in countries with limited resources, especially where the incidence of HIV infection is high, the organisms are also becoming a major problem in certain areas and in certain groups in the richer countries, for example drug addicts and homeless people in the USA and some other countries in the developed world.[33,34] The reserve antimicrobial agents are more expensive, are more toxic, and require longer periods of treatment, so that they often cannot be afforded in developing countries and treatment may be discontinued before the course is completed. New, inexpensive agents are urgently required.

Many other nontuberculous mycobacteria, such as *M. chelonei*, *M. fortuitum* and *M. avium-intracellulare*, have been described that have caused more infections in recent years, usually in immunocompromised patients and especially those with AIDS, but person-to-person spread is rare.[35] Some mycobacteria grow in biofilms in water tanks, pipework and the rinse water of endoscope washing machines.[32] They cause various diseases, including pulmonary, skin and surgical wound infections, injection site abscesses, and endocarditis. They have been transmitted on items of equipment, such as dialysis machines, bronchoscopes, porcine heart valves and other implants. They may also contaminate bronchoscope washings, giving rise to 'pseudoinfections' and infrequently to clinical infections. 'Pseudoinfections' refer to isolates of bacteria obtained from patients' samples that are of environmental origin and not from clinical infections.

Fungal infections

Hospital-acquired fungal infections have increased over the past 50 years due mainly to selection by antibiotics and the greatly increased number and improved survival of immunocompromised patients. Only a few species of fungi cause human systemic disease and are likely to be acquired in hospital. The most important is *Candida albicans* (originally known as *Monilia albicans*).[36] This is a yeast-like organism that forms buds and pseudomycelia; it is a normal inhabitant of the mouth, vagina and intestinal tract, although it can cause severe local infections. Invasive infections can involve the oesophagus and gastrointestinal tract, the lungs and the urinary tract; such infections are usually in immunocompromised patients, such as leukaemics or post-transplant patients. Invasion of the bloodstream may be associated with abscesses in other organs, for example the brain, liver or kidney, and rarely endocarditis. Cross-infection in hospital is uncommon, but outbreaks have been identified, particularly in neonates, by the use of various typing methods. Spread on the hands of staff would seem to be the most likely route of spread.[37] Molecular typing methods should increase the number of reported outbreaks.

Other *Candida* spp., for example *C. tropicalis* and *C. parapsilosis*, are infrequent causes of hospital infection. An outbreak of *C. tropicalis* was reported in wounds of patients undergoing cardiac surgery in 1991, where the organism was probably acquired from a member of staff with colonized hands and nose. This source was identified by the use of DNA typing.[36] *Candida* spp. from contaminated fluids, especially parenteral feeds, have caused bloodstream infections.

The genus *Aspergillus* contains a number of species, but *A. fumigatus* and to a lesser extent *A. flavus* and *A. niger* are the most common causes of human aspergillus infections. Systemic infection, rare in hospitals, commonly involves the lungs of immunocompromised patients, particularly in liver, bone marrow and heart transplant units.[38] Spread may occur from the lungs to other organs, such as the kidney, liver and brain. Spores are normally present in the air, but person-to-person transmission either does not occur or, if it does, is very rare and is likely only in highly immunosuppressed people. *A. fumigatus* is a common saprophyte growing on many substrates. Its spores are airborne and are released by any slight air movement, with the result that they are ubiquitous in the atmosphere but are concentrated particularly close to a recently disturbed source.[39] Adjacent building sites may be a source, but inadequately sealed service ducts in transplant units are especially dangerous. An appropriate filter in high-risk units should reduce the risk of infection. Since *Aspergillus* spores are ubiquitous, sporadic infections are always likely to be acquired in the community.

The continuing emergence of antibiotic-resistant hospital organisms

Several organisms that are part of the normal human bacterial flora have increased in incidence as causes of infection, have developed antibiotic resistance, and are now major problems in infection control. These include *Clostridium difficile*, multi-resistant Gram-negative bacilli, vancomycin-resistant enterococci (VRE) and MRSA.

Antibiotic-associated diarrhoea

This is a disease of the twentieth and twenty-first centuries. It occurs mainly in hospitals for the elderly. In the 1950s, it was considered to be due to replacement of the normal bowel flora with antibiotic-resistant, toxin-producing *Staph. aureus* during antibiotic treatment, usually following a surgical operation. Patients developed severe watery diarrhoea, mortality was high, and large numbers of staphylococci were found in the faeces. A number of outbreaks were described, but it is possible that the original 'staphylococcal' disease was due to undetected *C. difficile* toxin and that the staphylococci were colonizers also selected by antibiotic therapy. Following the emergence of methicillin- and other penicillinase-resistant penicillins and cephalosporins, the staphylococcal toxin disease apparently disappeared.

C. difficile was identified as part of the normal gut flora of infants in 1935, but its significance was not recognized until the early 1970s, when it was described as a cause of a rather similar illness to staphylococcal enterocolitis, ranging in severity from mild diarrhoea to severe pseudomembranous colitis. It was initially reported after surgical operations, usually during treatment with clindamycin, but it is now associated with other antibiotics.[40] It occurs mainly in the elderly and occasionally in neonates.

The causal organism is a Gram-positive sporing bacillus found in the normal intestinal tract, but the disease is actually caused by toxins and the organisms are selected by antibiotics and multiply considerably in the intestinal tract. The spores survive well on drying and can be found in large numbers in the environment, for example on bedding, floors and other surfaces, toilets and bedpans, when disseminated by patients with profuse diarrhoea or incontinence.[41] Transmission on endoscopes or rectal thermometers can occur, but the main route of spread is probably on the hands and clothing of staff. The presence of many carriers makes control difficult, but good hygienic practices, such as hand-washing, are important. Isolation of heavy dispersers should be considered in an outbreak, and thorough routine cleaning of the environment is necessary. The organism is resistant to most disinfectants and no effective noncorrosive agent for environmental disinfection is available, although hypochlorites are often recommended. The disease can be treated by vancomycin or metronidazole.

Cross-infection can be identified by various typing methods, but the newer molecular methods are the most useful. Many hospital outbreaks are caused by a single type, and occasionally spread between hospitals has been reported. One type is particularly common in the UK, and collaborative studies are taking place with other countries to determine whether some types occur internationally as epidemic strains. One of the largest outbreaks reported was in Manchester, England in the early 1990s, in which 175 cases were identified in three hospitals. Most patients were elderly, and infection was considered to have contributed to 17 deaths.[42]

Gram-negative bacilli

Although MRSA and VRE have attracted most attention in recent years, treatment of severe infections caused by these has usually been possible. However, some Gram-negative bacilli are entirely resistant to available nontoxic antibiotics but differ from MRSA in that outbreaks tend to be confined to special units, with spread between wards and hospitals being less frequent.

Improvements in the control of Gram-negative outbreaks have occurred, and single-source outbreaks from contaminated fluids or cross-infection with antibiotic-resistant strains in urology wards have now decreased considerably.

The opportunists (see Chapter 13) have continued to cause severe infections in high-risk units such as burns, intensive care and neonatal units, and in units for immunosuppressed patients, such as leukaemic or transplant patients. The most resistant organisms tend to be acinetobacters, among which the most extreme have acquired resistance to the new cephalosporins, carbapenems and quinolones; occasionally, they are sensitive only to polymyxins, which are not very effective agents.[43] In contrast to MRSA, there appears to be little prospect of effective new agents in the near future.

Pseudomonas aeruginosa and other pseudomonads are still frequent causes of infection in these units, and they remain some of the most common causes of bacteraemia in immunocompromised patients. *P.* (now *Burkholderia*) *cepacia* is a common cause of infection and colonization in patients with cystic fibrosis. The pseudomonads have supplemented natural antibiotic resistance with acquired resistance to newer agents, although rather less so than acinetobacters.[44]

Another problem group consists of the enterobacters, citrobacters and klebsiellas, which are usually part of the normal intestinal flora as well as the moist inanimate environment. The klebsiellas acquired resistance to gentamicin in the 1970s, but they are now often resistant to the new cephalosporins and penicillins as well. This group of organisms, in particular the enterobacters, has acquired resistance to the new cephalosporins by a mutation of existing beta-lactamases producing extended-spectrum beta-lactamases (ESBLs); they are often resistant to all drugs except carbapenems.[45]

The organisms spread through cross-infection and transfer of plasmids, but cross-infection remains the major route. Control of infection has already been discussed (see Chapter 14), but in recent years decontamination of equipment has increased in importance and has generally been improved, although problems still remain. Isolation of patients with highly resistant strains is commonly advised, although airborne spread is rare, and hand disinfection with alcohol has been used increasingly.

Streptococcus pneumoniae (pneumococci)

This is a Gram-positive coccus occurring in pairs. It has always been, and still is, an important cause of community-acquired infection, especially in developing countries. Before the discovery of sulphonamides and penicillin, the pneumococcus was the most common cause of death from bacteraemia and pneumonia in hospitals and the community. Hospital outbreaks were reported occasionally throughout the twentieth century, but since the 1940s little attention has been paid to it as a cause of hospital-acquired infection because it remained highly susceptible to penicillin for many years.

The first penicillin-resistant strains were reported in New Guinea in 1967 and soon after in South Africa, but it was not until the 1980s that reports of resistance to penicillin and occasionally to other antibiotics started to appear in other countries. Molecular typing methods have now suggested that a global spread is occurring from an original resistant clone.[46] It differs from enterococci and MRSA in that it has remained mainly a community organism and spread in wards is less frequent, but new typing methods are demonstrating that outbreaks are more common than thought previously. The incidence of infection by resistant strains varies between different hospitals and countries, but increasing resistance could still create major problems in the future, both in hospitals and in the community.

Enterococci

Enterococci are Gram-positive cocci occurring in pairs or short chains. They are part of the normal intestinal flora. They commonly cause urinary tract or wound infections, usually in association with Gram-negative bacilli such as *Escherichia coli*. They are generally of low virulence, and infections are usually endogenous in origin. The properties and problems of enterococci were reviewed by Murray,[47] and resistance to antibiotics was reviewed by Moellering.[48]

Although they showed a low-level natural resistance to penicillins and amino-glycosides, such as gentamicin, enterococci were not a major clinical problem until recently, apart from rare cases of endocarditis; spread from person to person was infrequent.

Since the 1970s, a number of reports have shown an increase in the incidence of serious infection, and an increase in resistance to penicillins, aminoglycosides and vancomycin started to cause concern. These strains produced a beta-lactamase similar to that of *Staph. aureus*. The first outbreak of VRE was reported in London by Uttley and colleagues in the late 1980s,[49] and further reports appeared from the USA and other countries, particularly in high-risk units such as intensive care and dialysis units. Enterococci survive well in the environment, and spread can occur on equipment, such as bedpans, urinals and electronic thermometers.[50] Infections may be associated with medical-device procedures, such as urinary and vascular catheterization. Contaminated endoscopes, such as colonoscopes and sigmoido-scopes, are also potential sources, although evidence of spread is lacking.

Enterococci have become a source of concern because of their acquisition of multiresistance, especially to vancomycin, which is the main agent for treating severe enterococcal and MRSA infections. This means that effective treatment is sometimes not available for seriously ill patients. These untreatable patients are still infrequent, but with resistant strains increasing slowly they could be a future problem. The other source of anxiety is the possibility of transferring vancomycin resistance to MRSA. Plasmids and transposons have been isolated in enterococci, and vancomycin resistance has been transferred to staphylococci in the laboratory.

The origin of vancomycin resistance remains unknown, but one possibility is that it might have been acquired from other bacteria in the food chain. Agents similar to vancomycin have been used as food additives for animals, an example of the potential hazards of treating or feeding animals with agents used for treating humans.

Techniques for the control of enterococcal cross-infection are similar to those used for MRSA, except that carriage sites are different, i.e. the intestinal tract rather than the nose or skin. In the USA, the Hospital Infection Control Practices Advisory Committee (HICPAC)[51] and John Boyce and colleagues[52] produced useful guidelines for control. Isolation of infected patients and carriers has been successful, and hand-washing with alcoholic preparations is commonly recommended. The main problem, as with MRSA, is the early detection and treatment of carriers; for instance, in one study, 47% of residents in a nursing home were colonized with resistant strains.

Careful decontamination of equipment is also required. The role of the inanimate environment in spread remains uncertain, but the ability of enterococci to survive well suggests that it may be of relevance and some believe that clean hospitals will help to reduce enterococcal cross-infection.

Restriction of antibiotics, especially vancomycin, would probably be effective, and it is possible that other antibiotics, such as third-generation cephalosporins, may have a selective role.

Coagulase-negative staphylococci

These were originally known as *Staph. albus* but in recent years they have been subdivided into different species, the most common being *Staph. epidermidis* (see Chapter 12).[53] They are the predominant aerobic organisms in the skin flora and are of low virulence, but they have increased as causes of hospital infection over the past 20–30 years.[54] For instance, in the National Nosocomial Infections Study (NNIS) in the USA, they were isolated from 4% of infections in the 1970s, increasing to 11% in the 1990s; in the national prevalence survey of hospitals in England and Wales in 1980, staphylococci other than *Staph. aureus* were 3.0% of isolates compared with 10.6% *Staph. aureus*; and in the 1994 national survey, they had increased to 7.7%, whereas *Staph. aureus* had shown a much smaller increase to 14.7%.

The increase in coagulase-negative staphylococci was associated with more cardiac and joint prostheses operations being undertaken and a considerable increase in intravascular catheterization and combined ambulatory peritoneal dialysis (CAPD). Coagulase-negative staphylococci now form one of the most common causes of bacteraemia during intravenous catheterization (see Chapter 14) and are third in the numbers of isolates of organisms causing all hospital infections after *E. coli* and *Staph. aureus*.[54]

The staphyloccci produce a slime that, with enzymes, enables them to adhere to prostheses and catheters, so protecting them from antibiotics and antibodies. Many strains are now multiresistant, and more than 50% of hospital strains are resistant to methicillin; resistance continues to increase. Most infections are endogenous or acquired from the hands of staff. Outbreaks appear to be rare but have been reported in cardiac surgery, intensive care units and neonatal units. Investigations of outbreaks have been difficult because of the absence of useful typing methods, but possibly more outbreaks will be identified with the newer molecular typing methods.

Intravenous fluids were probably given for the first time by Thomas Latta in Edinburgh in the 1830s for treating cholera, but now almost all patients undergoing major surgery are given intravenous solutions during and after operation, usually only for a short time. Central venous catheters are now used commonly for long-term therapy and the administration of drugs. Millions of central venous catheters are used every year and, due to their longer time in situ, are more susceptible to infection. Most infections are acquired from the patient's own skin flora, but they can also be acquired from the hands of staff. Contaminated intravenous fluids have been responsible for major outbreaks due to deficiencies in sterilization (see Chapters 11 and 14). Many of the controlled studies on prevention of infection in central venous catheterization have been carried out by Dennis Maki and colleagues at the University of Wisconsin, and this is one of the few areas in infection control where good clinical evidence of effective measures has been obtained.[55]

Control of infection depends on good aseptic techniques, skin disinfection and staff hand-washing or disinfection. Antibiotic prophylaxis in surgery can also be effective, but the presence of increasing numbers of multiresistant strains has also increased the requirement for prophylactic vancomycin, which is undesirable as vancomycin use may select resistant enterococci and possibly in the future vancomycin-resistant MRSA.

MRSA

A surprising decline in MRSA in the UK, Denmark and some other European countries in the 1970s suggested that the epidemic strains present at the time were facing possible eradication.[56] The reason for this was uncertain, but it seemed likely that they were selected by tetracycline and streptomycin, and that the decline was due to a reduction in the use of these agents. The increased numbers and activity of infection-control staff was probably also an associated factor. However, sporadic strains of MRSA continued to be isolated, often of similar phage types, in the 1970s, but usually they did not spread.

The improvement in all countries did not last, and a second wave emerged initially in Australia, the USA and Ireland in the late 1970s and early 1980s. A large outbreak in Melbourne was reported by Robin Pavillard and colleagues in the early 1980s, and spread continued to other hospitals in eastern but not western Australia.[57,58] Epidemic strains were also being reported by Conor Keane and colleagues in Ireland at about the same time.[59] In 1981, a similar strain emerged in the London Hospital and was described by Georgia Duckworth, David Williams and colleagues.[60] It soon spread to other hospitals in south-east England and gradually to hospitals around the country, and since then similar strains have emerged in most countries in the world. It was originally shown that MRSA was present in some countries before methicillin was used clinically, and although strains in different countries appeared to be similar, it is unlikely that a single clone spread around the world, as seemed to occur with penicillin-resistant pneumococci.[61] It seems more probable that existing transmissible strains were selected by antibiotics, and that spread then occurred mainly in the hospitals of the country concerned, although there are reports of inter-country spread. The reason for a pandemic at this time remains unknown, but possibly the increased use of cephalosporins and other newly available antibiotics may have provided the selective influence. It is also possible that there is an as yet unidentified transmissibility factor.

The increase in outbreaks was demonstrated clearly in the USA in the NNIS, in which isolates of MRSA increased from 2.4% in 1975 to 29% in 1991.[62] A study by Voss and colleagues of 200 isolates from 43 hospitals in ten European countries in 1994 showed that the frequency of MRSA ranged from less than 1% to 30%; the incidence was highest in southern Europe.[63] Many other similar studies have been reported. Figure 16.1 shows the number of isolates in a large hospital in Birmingham, UK, from 1968 to 1993. The decline and re-emergence is evident

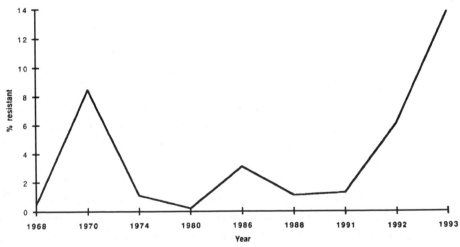

Figure 16.1   MRSA from wounds or lesions in a large general hospital in Birmingham, UK, 1968–93. (Hospital Infection Research Laboratory, Birmingham.)

after some initial control in the 1980s. Despite the same control methods being used throughout the period, including the isolation of patients in a special unit, spread of MRSA continued throughout the 1990s. The reason for failure of established methods of control remains unknown, but probably the spread of the strain into community residential establishments for the elderly was a major factor in Birmingham, as elsewhere.[64] These elderly people often returned to hospital as emergencies and were not usually screened for MRSA. Contributing factors in the UK were overcrowded hospitals, understaffing, movement of patients from ward to ward, and failure to discharge elderly patients from the hospital back into the community at the end of treatment. Attempts at cost reduction by governments were responsible for many of these deficiencies and defeated the efforts of enthusiastic but limited numbers of infection-control staff.

Scandinavian countries and the Netherlands did not have the same problems. Rosdahl and colleagues in Denmark in 1991 reported that only 0.2% of isolates were resistant to methicillin since 1984.[65,66] The suggested explanation in the Netherlands and Denmark is that control was maintained by rapid detection and isolation of infected or colonized patients. They also seemed to have more effective control over antibiotic use, especially the third-generation cephalosporins. However, they are relatively small countries and may have been less exposed to the same pressures of highly transmissible strains. John Pearman and others in Western Australia successfully kept out MRSA by screening patients and staff entering from eastern Australia and elsewhere, and promptly isolating and treating those found to be infected or colonized.[58]

Although the epidemiology of the 'new' strains of MRSA has been well studied, few good microbiological studies have been carried out. It is likely that their properties are similar to the organisms in the earlier outbreaks of the 1960s. However, it has been suggested that survival in the environment is better in the new strains, that the inanimate environment now has a greater role in spread, but that airborne spread is less relevant, apart from in burns wards. MRSA has been isolated from stethoscopes, blood-pressure cuffs and pens, but the role of the environment as a source is still doubtful and more evidence is required. Although clean hospitals are certainly important as far as the morale of patients and staff is concerned, it is generally agreed that spread on the hands of staff is the major route and that people are the main sources.

Although the principles for controlling epidemics of infectious disease have been known for at least 100 years, most hospitals found established outbreaks of MRSA throughout the hospital difficult to control without using considerable resources. Guidelines and recommendations for control were developed in many countries. In the USA, advice was provided by the CDC, by individuals such as Richard Wenzel and John Boyce, and by consensus panels.[67,68] In the UK, a working party from several infection societies published detailed guidelines in 1998, which were followed by a controversy over whether it was always necessary to eradicate MRSA from the hospital or, if there were no clinical problems, whether it was acceptable to do nothing other than to maintain good standards of hygiene.[69] It was shown in some burns units that the endemic strain of MRSA appeared to be of low virulence and rarely caused clinical infection, but it was generally agreed that eradication was desirable in high-risk conditions. This system of establishing priorities for isolation had been suggested by Spicer in Australia as far back as 1984 (he introduced the term 'seek and destroy'), and this system was later recommended by the World Health Organization (WHO).[70,71] These priorities were often established in hospitals in which eradication procedures were introduced into high-risk units, such as intensive care. Patients admitted to these units were screened on admission, as were patients admitted from other hospitals. It is probable that screening of all admissions to a hospital, and treatment and isolation of all with positive isolates, would be an effective method of eradication,[72] but this would be very expensive and isolation facilities are still likely to be inadequate unless new hospital-building policies are introduced (see Chapter 17). Nevertheless, there is some evidence that appropriate hand disinfection of staff will reduce cross-infection.[73]

Treatment of skin and nasal carriage sites with topical agents or antiseptics was often effective in the 1960s and 1970s, but recurrence of the colonizing strain was still common. Mupirocin (pseudomonic acid) cream was introduced as a topical agent in 1983 and mainly replaced neomycin and chlorhexidine. Controlled studies by Mark Casewell and colleagues showed it to be one of the most effective agents in removing staphylococci from noses,[74] but resistant strains have since emerged. Barry Cookson, who at the time of writing is the Director of the Hospital Infection Laboratory at Colindale, has been particularly involved in the mechanisms of mupirocin resistance and in data collection on MRSA.[75]

A greater hazard was the emergence of vancomycin-resistant strains described by Hiramatsu and colleagues in Japan in 1997[76] and more recently in other countries. New antibiotics have recently become available, but resistance has already been reported.

Staph. aureus has acquired resistance to all clinically useful antibiotics usually soon after their introduction, and the present pandemic of MRSA shows no sign of abating. Although global control measures are required, including international surveillance to deal with antibiotic resistance, developing countries have more urgent problems such as AIDS and malaria, and hospital infection at present has a much lower priority.

The past, present and future

The past

Although hospitals have existed from the time of ancient civilizations,[1] postoperative and other hospital-acquired infections, as distinct from infectious diseases, were reported infrequently until the numbers and complexity of operations increased after the introduction of anaesthesia in the nineteenth century. Infections such as erysipelas, pyaemia and hospital gangrene could not be prevented adequately until surgeons possessed an understanding of bacteriology and of the sources of infection.

One of the earliest 'scientific' theories (the miasmic theory) in the Middle Ages accounted for the spread of epidemic disease by corruption of the air induced by extremes in weather and more locally by the putrid miasmas arising from decaying organic matter, cesspools, corpses and marshes. This theory lasted until the end of the nineteenth century and was responsible for most of the recommended control measures. Nevertheless, many realized that it did not cover all situations and believed that contagion (contact between patients) was responsible for the spread of some infections, such as leprosy, smallpox and plague. Girolama Fracastoro in 1546 suggested that contagion was caused by 'seeds' (seminaria) specific for each disease; he recognized that infection could be spread by these seeds both by direct contact and fomites and by infection at a distance through the air. Although this idea was accepted initially, the old theory of miasmas soon crept back. However, others such as Kircher and Redi supported Fracastoro's theory and demonstrated that diseases could probably spread by 'seeds' or living organisms. Anthony van Leeuwenhoek, one of the best-known microscopists of the time, identified such living organisms under the microscope but failed to associate them with disease.

Despite the difficulties of understanding infective processes without a knowledge of bacteriology, some surgeons, such as Paré, had made significant advances centuries earlier. Theodoric, in Bologna in 1266, did not accept the general surgical opinion at the time that 'laudable pus' in a wound indicated that it was a healthy wound, believing that it should be clean and dry and that general cleanliness, including the hands of the surgeon, was necessary when operating. Theodoric could probably be called the founder of aseptic surgery.[2]

John Pringle, an army surgeon in the 1700s, was one of the earliest surgeons to recognize that hospitals were potentially dangerous places, writing in 1752 the first scientific account of the epidemiology and prevention of hospital cross-infection. He recommended adequate ventilation of wards and wide spacing between beds, fumigation of wards when necessary, separation of patients with different diseases, and high standards of cleanliness. Although he still believed in miasmas, he obviously identified the importance of contagion as well. He also introduced the term 'antisepsis' and was the first to develop tests on chemical agents against 'putrefaction', which occurred following contagion.

His younger colleague in the navy, James Lind, made similar recommendations, including the disinfection or destruction of the contaminated clothes and bedding of typhus patients. He stated that 'filthiness was a chief source of infection' and realized that miasmas were unimportant in the spread of typhus.

Many physicians in the 1700s believed contagion to be responsible for the spread of infection. John Gregory, Professor of Medicine in Edinburgh, wrote in 1788 that measles and scarlet fever were produced by contagion, although he still thought that 'a certain state of the air is necessary to render the contagion active and the diseases epidemic'.

The next advances in the realization of the importance of contagion were mainly made by obstetricians. Among these was Alexander Gordon of Aberdeen, who in 1795 demonstrated unequivocally the contagious nature of puerperal fever. He stated that 'nurses and physicians, who have attended patients affected with puerperal fever, ought carefully to wash themselves and get their apparel fumigated, before it be put on again'. Oliver Wendell Holmes in 1843 stated that the hands should be disinfected and clothing changed after contact with a case of puerperal fever, and Ignaz Semmelweiss was the first to demonstrate in a clinical trial the importance of hand disinfection in reducing the transmission and mortality of puerperal fever. However, the work of Semmelweiss and the other obstetricians had surprisingly little influence on surgical practice for many years, despite the recognition by James Simpson that puerperal fever was a similar infection to erysipelas. Surgeons were loathe to believe that they could be responsible for killing their patients, and some retained this attitude throughout most of the twentieth century.

Postoperative mortality in hospitals was recorded in the nineteenth century by Farr, and his results were used by Florence Nightingale to demonstrate the hazards of operating in the large and overcrowded hospitals of the major cities.[3] However, this difference between large and small hospitals was considered to be invalid by Bristowe and Holmes, who concluded that large hospitals were as safe as small ones. Sir James

Simpson produced data on amputation wounds supporting Farr's results, but again these were criticized by Holmes. These arguments continued, demonstrating the difficulty of comparing infection rates in different hospitals, which is still with us today. Nevertheless, the idea of small wards without overcrowding, and with good ventilation and high standards of cleanliness, proposed by Florence Nightingale and James Simpson, despite the fact that they remained believers in miasmas, still have some relevance in preventing the spread of infection today, in addition to demonstrating the importance of data collection to support an argument.

The discovery of bacteria and their properties by Pasteur, Koch and colleagues, and the description of staphylococci in acute abscesses by Alexander Ogston at the end of the nineteenth century, had the greatest influence on the understanding and prevention of infection and led within a few years to the aseptic principles in use today. Lister used this knowledge to reduce wound infection and postoperative mortality and to eradicate hospital gangrene, demonstrating that by the use of a phenolic disinfectant applied on a dressing, organisms could be kept out of a wound. He was not aware of the work of Semmelweiss and was not particularly concerned with hand disinfection, although he did immerse his hands and his instruments in a disinfectant solution before operating. He did not wear gloves or clean clothes for operating, nor did he clean or disinfect the theatre environment, other than experimenting with the use of a carbolic acid spray during his early work, a study that demonstrated that the environment had only a minor role in the spread of hospital infection. Lister's work was described in detail by a colleague, W. Watson-Cheyne, who in 1882 summarized the knowledge of pyogenic wound infections and discussed the importance of inoculum size and depressed vitality of tissues as factors associated with infection. He demonstrated that *Staphylococcus aureus* could be isolated from the air of surgical wards, from the surface of the body, and from the healthy nasopharynx, and that organisms could enter the operation wound from the air, from surgical instruments, from the skin surrounding the wound, and from the hands of the surgeon.

Lister's methods were taken up enthusiastically in Europe, but often less so in the USA and Britain. Lawson Tait of Birmingham stated that his operation results without disinfectants were as good as Lister's with them, but he did pay attention to the cleanliness of hands and instruments.

Lister's antiseptic technique was then replaced to some extent by aseptic techniques, although antiseptics continued to be used on the skin. A major figure at this time was Curt Schimmelbusch, who worked in Von Bergman's clinic in Berlin. He and his colleagues believed that the first step in every disinfection process was good cleaning, and in his book he described many aspects of the aseptic treatment of wounds. He used a steam sterilizer for sterilizing surgical dressings and indicated the importance of not stirring up dust when dressing wounds. He also avoided admitting patients with septic wounds to wards containing patients with clean wounds. He commented that the 'surgeon's hands should be regarded with suspicion', and he disinfected nailbrushes as he considered them to be sources of infection. Furbringer in the same department described the scrubbing of surgeons' hands with soap and water followed by wiping with gauze soaked in 80% volume alcohol for 1 minute, and Neuber from Kiel introduced clean caps and gowns for operating, as well as cleanable surgical instruments and surfaces in the operating room. Rubber gloves were introduced by William Halsted and colleagues in the USA, and von Mikulicz-Radedecki, who was initially an assistant of Bilroth, was probably the first to use a face mask when operating. Although Bilroth was a distinguished surgeon, he carried out much of the early work on the bacteriology of wounds. The aseptic techniques described at the beginning of the twentieth century have remained in use, with some modifications, until the present time.

Another major figure at the beginning of the twentieth century was Charles V. Chapin, a public health physician from Rhode Island, USA, whose thinking was far ahead of his time. He believed that infection was spread by direct contact, that air, dust, fomites and walls were not of great importance, and that terminal disinfection (disinfection of a room after discharge of the patient) was of little value; his statements were usually backed up with evidence. He stated that the effectiveness of isolation of patients in controlling an epidemic varied inversely with the numbers of missed cases and carriers, and isolation in an extreme outbreak was unlikely to be successful: 'A spark in the dry grass should be stamped out at any cost, but it is useless to waste time in extinguishing the smouldering flame left here and there as the line of fire is sweeping across the prairie.' Chapin also saw 'the degree of emphasis change from law enforcement to community education as the primary concern of public health administration', and the 'last nail in the coffin of the "filth" theory of disease'. Unfortunately, the change of emphasis at the end of the twentieth century seems to be reverting towards increasing law enforcement, especially in Europe, although education is also improving.

The twentieth century proceeded with more surgeons using the new aseptic techniques, with a considerable reduction in mortality and postoperative infection. However, with new surgical techniques emerging, there was less interest in infection over the next 50 years, although some surgeons (such as Brewer and Meleney) retained an interest in recording infection rates in response to improvements in technique.

The use of the new bacteriologically based control of infection methods by Colebrook and colleagues, especially the introduction of typing methods to detect carriers of epidemic strains of haemolytic streptococci (*Streptococcus pyogenes*) and to assess cross-infection, reduced the problems with this organism in puerperal infection and burns. However, it was not known how much of this reduction was due to the measures taken or to a reduction in virulence of the organism.

Some other improvements in hygiene also emerged, such as hand disinfection, in which new agents such as hexachlorophene and chlorhexidine were introduced. Alcohol continued to be used by surgeons as a surgical hand disinfectant after scrubbing with soap and water, and as a preoperative skin disinfectant, but only the other European countries (i.e. not the UK) used it alone for disinfection of hands in wards (hygienic hand disinfection) until well into the second half of the twentieth century.

The introduction of sulphonamides in the 1930s and penicillin in the 1940s was seen as the probable beginning of the end of common bacterial infections. Good aseptic techniques were considered unnecessary and often ignored, but after a few years' use of penicillin in hospitals, outbreaks of penicillin-resistant *Staph. aureus* were reported. Other antibiotics were introduced, and staphylococci and Gram-negative bacilli acquired resistance to almost all of them. Despite the early warnings by workers in the UK, Europe and the USA, antibiotics continued to be overused throughout the century. However, the outbreaks of staphylococcal infections from the 1950s were investigated thoroughly, particularly by British workers.

Phage typing allowed epidemics to be followed, and it was found that epidemic strains waxed and waned. The virulent type 80/81 of the 1940s and 1950s was replaced by other, less virulent phage types. Methicillin-resistant *Staph. aureus* (MRSA) appeared in the 1960s and declined in the 1970s, only to return in the 1980s and spread around the world. Staphylococcal carriers or infected patients who shed large numbers of the organisms into the environment on skin scales were usually responsible for spread within a ward, and removal of these patients to isolation often ended the epidemic. Multiple containment measures in wards without isolation facilities were often effective in reducing colonization rates, but isolation in single rooms was the preferred measure.

The Gram-negative bacilli had less publicity than MRSA, but they continued to develop resistance to antibiotics and some now presented an even greater treatment problem. Outbreaks were often from common sources, usually contaminated fluids. Removal of containers of disinfectant or other fluids from wards and improved control of sterilization processes have almost eliminated these outbreaks, but infections continue to occur in wounds, burns and the urinary tract.

The present

Many changes have occurred in medical and surgical practice in the past 20 years, and these have often influenced the risks of patients acquiring infections. Surgical operations are now frequently carried out using minimally invasive techniques involving endoscopy, with very small surgical incisions. This type of surgery generally causes less tissue damage and results in a shorter hospital stay than more traditional

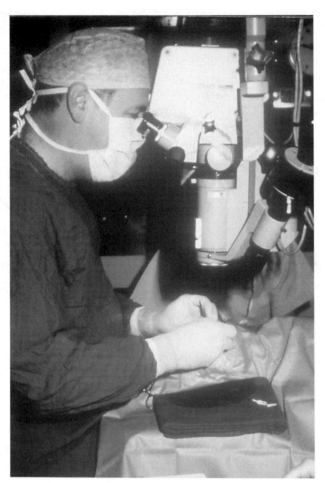

Figure 17.1   Surgical operations with an operating microscope. (Wellcome Library, London.)

surgery. Other types of day surgery are becoming increasingly common, and the length of time spent in hospital after all types of surgery has generally decreased. These procedures are likely to have reduced the risks of postoperative infection and of cross-infection with antibiotic-resistant bacteria.

However, the increased age of patients undergoing surgery, the increased complexity of other operations such as extensive open cardiac surgery, and the use of artificial implants have all tended to increase infection risks. Many more hip and knee replacement implants are now carried out, and considerable improvements in reducing the risk of infection in these have been made following the use of the ultraclean air system and correctly administered antibiotic prophylaxis. The requirements for surgery have also tended to change; for instance, thyroidectomies, gastrectomies and incisions of appendix and mastoid abscesses have decreased

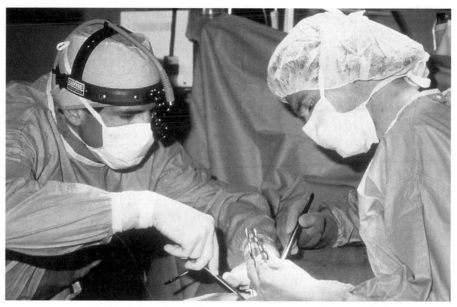

Figure 17.2   Cardiac surgery: opening the chest. (Wellcome Library, London.)

considerably in frequency. Wound infection rates have generally shown a reduction over the past 30 years – for instance, open cholecystectomies (removal of the gallbladder) have shown a reduction from 20% in the 1960s to 2.6% in 1997–8 – but infection rates after some operations can still be as high as 10.8% in high-risk colonic surgery despite the use of prophylactic antibiotics.[4] Prophylactic antibiotics have had more influence than any other procedure in reducing infection rates in contaminated operations and for the insertion of artificial implants, but their use in other types of clean surgery remains controversial since rates are already low. A study reported by Raf Mertens and colleagues comparing infections following hernia operations in Belgium and Holland showed mean rates of 1.2% and 0.4%, respectively.[5] Although the rates were both low, the lower rates in Holland were probably due to differences between the countries in discharge policy and post-operative surveillance in the community rather than to techniques at operation. The reduced hospital stay of most patients means that a higher percentage of hospital infections is being detected initially in the community, thus increasing the responsibilities of community health staff and necessitating the appointment and training of community infection-control nurses. However, the community service is not always able to cope adequately with all these new problems, since official convalescent homes are no longer available in the UK and care for elderly patients at home is often not sufficient, with the result that the number of patients requiring readmission to hospitals after discharge has also increased.

Developments in new techniques to improve the survival of patients with organ failure have led to the emergence of intensive care units (ICUs). These tend to be small, highly equipped units with a high nurse/patient ratio and supervised by specialists in intensive care; the patients are all severely ill, often with respiratory failure associated with traumatic accidents, severe burns or severe infection after major surgery. Patients are predominantly elderly, immunocompromised and particularly susceptible to infection; they are likely to have indwelling catheters, central venous catheters and invasive recording equipment, and they are usually being treated with mechanical respiratory ventilation. Some patients may require haemodialysis or peritoneal dialysis. In addition to the high risk of device-associated infection, cross-infection is likely to occur due to frequent handling of patients. The need for urgent treatment often reduces the time available for hand-washing and aseptic procedures by staff.

Patients are admitted to an ICU from any ward in the hospital and often from other hospitals or directly from the community. A variety of micro-organisms will be introduced, and there is often inadequate time for screening for hazardous strains. It is not surprising that infection rates in ICUs are higher than in other wards and units in the hospital[6] and that the high use of antibiotics encourages the emergence of resistant strains of staphylococci (e.g. MRSA) and Gram-negative bacilli (e.g. *Pseudomonas aeruginosa*), which cause therapeutic problems, requiring new and expensive antibiotics. The ICU is also unavoidably responsible for spreading resistant strains around the hospital when patients are transferred to other wards. Similar problems occur in neonatal ICUs, where very premature babies with low immunity are especially at risk of acquiring infection.

Infection rates arising from treatment with medical devices have been reduced, usually by improved aseptic and decontamination techniques. The use of gloves, effective skin antisepsis and good aseptic techniques have reduced infection from intravascular procedures. Closed drainage has had the greatest effect on acquired urinary tract infection, but good asepsis and possibly the use of catheters impregnated with antimicrobial agents are producing further reductions. However, if antibiotics are used for impregnating catheters, then resistance may be a problem. The use of antibacterial filters and the routine changing of respiratory circuits have helped to reduce respiratory tract infections during mechanical ventilation, but colonization of the mouth and throat with antibiotic-resistant bacteria remains a major problem, and topical antibacterial prophylaxis to the mouth and throat to prevent infection with these organisms remains controversial.

Fibre-optic endoscopes are now used widely for surgery and for diagnostic purposes. Nonflexible instruments are used for operative endoscopy and can usually be sterilized by heat, but the flexible endoscopes used for gastroscopy, bronchoscopy and colonoscopy are long, with narrow lumens, and are difficult to clean. Infection used to be a common complication, but it has been almost eliminated by thorough cleaning and disinfection with an automated machine.

Endogenous sources are responsible for most device-associated infections, but cross-infection with resistant organisms, especially on the hands of staff, still plays a major role.

The employment of single-use items has increased considerably, and reuse of medical devices is discouraged or in some cases banned by health authorities; this is due to some extent to the emergence of prions, which are resistant to routine sterilization processes, although the infection risk of these agents on medical devices appears to be very low. Single use of certain items, such as respiratory tubing and suction equipment, is probably not cost-effective and there is little evidence of a reduction in infection. In fact, there is very little evidence that single-use items, with some exceptions, have influenced infection rates when compared with correctly processed reused items. The main problem with reuse is the design of devices that cannot be cleaned adequately. However, central sterilizing services have continued to develop in recent years and provide a high-quality service able to carry out safe reprocessing.

The numbers of immunosuppressed or immunocompromised patients in hospitals have increased considerably; they include transplant patients, leukaemics, patients with other malignant conditions and acquired immunodeficiency syndrome (AIDS) patients. For patients with such conditions, specialized units have been designed to prevent organisms entering from elsewhere, i.e. to provide protective isolation, but most of these infections are endogenous and some workers believe that simple protective isolation is unnecessary. This remains controversial since the risk varies with the degree of immunosuppression, and infections with opportunist organisms, such as *P. aeruginosa*, can still be a hazard and may be fatal. Bone marrow and liver transplants are particularly susceptible to *Aspergillus* infections, and units with appropriate air filters are commonly recommended for these patients. Immunocompromised patients are also particularly susceptible to *Legionella*, which have caused outbreaks in transplant units, and to viruses such as varicella and *Herpes simplex*.

The emergence of human immunodeficiency virus (HIV) infection and AIDS in the early 1980s has led to widespread changes in hygienic techniques. The problems arose with the realization that patients could be HIV carriers without clinical evidence of infection or any indication of being in a high-risk group. Many workers believed that blood and secretions from all patients, irrespective of whether they were colonized or infected, should be treated as potentially infective.

Despite the low rate of transmission to other patients or staff in hospitals, staff became extremely anxious about the risks of catching the disease, and excessive precautions are now taken since treatment controls the disease but does not cure it and no vaccine is available. Needlestick injuries are the main risk, and procedures such as non-capping of needles after use and transfer of needles to puncture-proof boxes have been introduced. Eye protection when there is a danger of splashing blood is also advised. These procedures, along with wearing gloves, are part of the universal precautions introduced in the USA in the 1980s and are used for all procedures involved in the handling of blood and certain secretions, especially if bloodstained. Universal precautions are now used all over the world. The costs are extremely high (assessed as $269 million in the USA) and often cannot be afforded by developing countries, where the need is greatest. The emergence of AIDS drew attention to viral hepatitis. It was realized that hepatitis B was more infectious than HIV, and that they were transmitted by the same routes. However, an effective vaccine for hepatitis B has been introduced that prevents infection in healthcare workers. A number of other hepatitis viruses have now been described, of which hepatitis C is the most important. This is less infectious than hepatitis B and as yet no vaccine is available.

Universal precautions have been expanded to include the wearing of gloves for all procedures necessitating contact with mucous membranes, lesions, body fluids, excretions and secretions; this is known as body substance isolation. A few studies have demonstrated a reduction in hospital infection following its use, but none have shown that it is more effective than hand-washing or disinfection without using gloves.[7] The potential hazards of blood have also been responsible for new regulations on the handling and containing of clinical waste, but there is no evidence that infection has been acquired from waste, except perhaps from needlestick injuries.

The main anxiety among hospital infection workers in developed countries is the increasing incidence of antibiotic-resistant organisms, as discussed already. Although there are similar or greater problems in developing countries, the high infection rate and mortality from other diseases such as AIDS, tuberculosis and malaria give these a greater priority.

Outbreaks of strains of *Clostridium difficile*, vancomycin-resistant enterococci (VRE) and highly resistant Gram-negative bacilli are now often reported in hospitals, especially in high-risk units, but these are less likely to spread between hospitals than MRSA.

MRSA has now spread to hospitals in most countries of the world and is difficult to control. It is a strain of *Staph. aureus* that has acquired resistance to methicillin and related antibiotics, such as cloxacillin (methicillin is no longer used, but the name remains since the organism was first reported in 1961), and usually also to several other antibiotics. In some countries, such as the UK, serious infections have increased considerably over the past few years and are a continuing problem for most infection-control teams. The reason why MRSA exists in so many hospitals at the present time is due partly to changes in hospital practice. Epidemic staphylococci, including MRSA, are especially likely to colonize elderly people, particularly if they are treated with antibiotics, and are increasingly acquired with prolonged hospital stay. They are also more likely to spread in overcrowded conditions and when there are staff shortages. Hospitals have often reduced considerably the number of beds for both acute and chronic patients over the past 30 years, and most hospitals are now overstretched. The result of this is that colonized patients are transferred, after blocking beds in an acute hospital possibly for some weeks, to residential establishments for the elderly, but they may return to the acute hospital at a later date still carrying the organism. Specialist or referral hospitals are particularly likely to have MRSA problems, as many of their patients are transferred directly from other hospitals. The other problems of control are the considerable and expensive requirements for extensive screening for healthy carriers, and the lack of isolation facilities in most hospitals. Although all these factors are relevant, the extraordinary ability of epidemic MRSA to spread remains a mystery since there is no laboratory test for transmissibility. The other factor in the rise in epidemic MRSA is the role of antibiotics in selecting it. Excessive antibiotic use is clearly important, but whether specific antibiotics such as cephalosporins are the main selecting agents remains uncertain. MRSA, enterococci and *Clostridium difficile* survive well in the dry environment, and inadequate cleaning of hospitals has sometimes been blamed for their spread. MRSA is commonly spread by heavy dispersers who contaminate the environment, but cleaning will be effective for only a short time if the disperser remains in the ward because it is bedding and clothing, not floors, that will contaminate the hands of staff. The role of the environment in the spread of VRE and *C. difficile* is also uncertain, but thorough cleaning of a ward after discharge of patients colonized or infected with these organisms is usually considered to be necessary, even though people and their immediate environment are the main sources. Gram-negative bacilli do not survive well in the dry environment, but some infections caused by these organisms are highly resistant to antibiotics and are difficult to treat.

Another group of illnesses that emerge occasionally in hospitals are gastrointestinal infections. These tend to be self-limiting, such as rotavirus in infants, and they are controlled by good hygiene and isolation or cohort nursing. However, food poisoning can be responsible for large outbreaks with occasional deaths, particularly in the elderly. Food hygiene standards in hospitals have improved by the use of a quality-control system, such as hazard analysis of critical control points involving defining microbiological or other hazards at certain critical points during the processing of food. This system is sometimes used to monitor other potentially hazardous processes in hospitals.

It is important to know the extent of infection in a hospital. Most hospitals have a surveillance method, such as the recording of specific pathogens and antibiotic-resistant organisms ('alert' organisms). Such methods have been sim-plified by the computerization of laboratory results, although other data of value in infection control are often not included. Surveillance has been extended since the Study on the Efficacy of Nosocomial Infection Control (SENIC) project showed that effective surveillance and control could reduce infection. A system for national recording of infections has been in use in the USA for many years, and modifica-tions are now in use in other countries. It seems likely that a targeted system, such as device-associated infections, will continue at least in high-risk units. Owing to the multifactorial nature of hospital infections, it is inadvisable for surveillance results to be incorporated in national league tables, as is now becoming popular with many governments, because the results can be misleading.

The potential risks to staff and patients of HIV and hepatitis virus infections, recent reports on the high numbers of hospital infections (i.e. one in ten patients in hospital acquires an infection), the increase in antibiotic-resistant organisms, and the escalating costs of infection have all led to a demand for evidence-based guidelines[8] and audits of infection-control procedures. However, as stated above, infections are multifactorial and controlled trials of individual factors are often not practical or cost-effective. Control of infection is an art as well as a science. It requires well-trained staff and bacteriological studies in addition to national guidelines if good decisions are to be made.

The future

Infectious diseases have always depended very much on social conditions. In recent years, large increases in populations, particularly in cities, inadequate sanitation, local wars, natural disasters and increased antibiotic resistance of bacteria have been responsible for the re-emergence of diseases, such as tuberculosis and malaria, that were thought to have been under control. Respiratory infections, gastrointestinal infections and AIDS are responsible for a large number of illnesses and a high mortality in the developing world. It has been estimated in a United Nations study that 70 million people will have died of AIDS by 2010. In addition, health resources of both poor and richer countries have also been reduced or have become inadequate to cope with the increasing costs of modern healthcare.

Increased international travel enables infections to be carried rapidly around the world and could initiate a new major epidemic, for instance of a viral haemorrhagic fever or influenza, at any time. Most of these infections are spread primarily in the community, but many require admission to hospital. Cross-infection to other patients and staff may occur with hazardous virus diseases, such as Ebola fever, and infections such as dysentery and rotavirus can spread to other patients unless standards of hygiene are high. The potential hazards of spread of viral infections, such as smallpox, have increased with the threat of biological warfare. Although there have also been some successes in international control of diseases, such as the eradication of smallpox and considerable reductions in poliomyelitis and measles by means of vaccines, other projects, such as the elimination of malaria and AIDS, have so far been less successful and effective vaccines have yet to be discovered. The costs of vaccines and new antimicrobials are often too high for developing countries to afford, and consideration needs to be given by the developed world and manufacturers to provide more financial support for the World Health Organization (WHO).

Whether prions will be an increasing problem remains uncertain, but it seems unlikely that the numbers of bovine spongiform encephalitis (BSE) cases will be high. However, research is now being well funded and methods of detection of the disease and of inactivating prions should be improved.

The incidence of the typical hospital-acquired infections in surgical wounds and in catheterization of the urinary tract, the vascular system and the respiratory tract has changed little over the past 30 years, with a mean of about 5–10%; such infections are very costly. There has been a reduction in infection rates in some procedures, such as clean wound infection, but rates have remained high in intensive care units for reasons discussed already. Future reductions are possible, with more use of endoscopic operative procedures and intravascular surgery, the impregnation of catheters with antimicrobial agents, and improved staffing and hygiene. However, with the increasing age and thus the susceptibility of patients, an irreducible minimum is likely to be reached soon with most procedures. The need for conventional operating theatres will need reassessment, and new designs are likely to be considered since airborne risks are low with many of the new surgical techniques.

However, the main anxiety in all countries is the development of resistance to antibiotics. Antibiotics have been in use for only about 60 years and some organisms have demonstrated considerable versatility in developing resistance to each clinically useful antibiotic soon after it has begun to be used.[9] Some organisms, such as the beta-haemolytic streptococci, have remained sensitive to penicillin throughout this period, and others, such as the pneumococci, have so far developed only limited resistance, although penicillin-resistant pneumococci are now spreading around the world. Highly resistant pneumococci could present a major therapeutic problem in the community and in hospitals. We have now reached the stage where few new antibiotics are being discovered, and the possibility of untreatable infections could well occur within the next 50 years.

Resistant organisms in hospitals are a product of a combination of antibiotic use and cross-infection. Restriction in the use of antibiotics has been recommended since penicillin first appeared, but apart from a few instances, usually in special units, a restriction policy has rarely been shown to work. Doctors are obviously unwilling to avoid using an antibiotic if there is a good clinical indication for its use, and the treatment of a single sick patient will always have priority over consideration for the community as a whole. Policies for whole hospitals have been tried rarely, and although sometimes successful, it seems likely that restriction of antibiotics will not be used on a large scale unless the clinical situation in the world becomes desperate. The other major problem in controlling antibiotic use is over-the-counter selling without a prescription. Changing the law, usually in poorer countries, would be politically unpopular since it is cheaper to buy the antibiotics directly rather than to visit a doctor. Education of hospital doctors in the correct use of antibiotics may help, but this is unlikely to influence the incidence of resistant strains in hospitals. Although most antibiotics are used in the community, often excessively, the hospital remains the main source of highly resistant strains.

The other possibilities for overcoming the problem of resistance are the development of new antimicrobial agents designed specifically to inhibit enzymes responsible for resistance, or the use of vaccines for prevention or treatment of infection. It could be many years before these approaches are available on the market, and then they may still be too expensive for poorer countries. Effective vaccines against organisms that are part of the normal flora are difficult to produce, although a vaccine against *P. aeruginosa* produced in the past was discontinued because it would only be of value in developing countries where the funds to buy it would be inadequate. On the optimistic side, resistant strains may reach a plateau in which most will remain sensitive to certain agents and the problem of the untreatable patient will occur only rarely. Or epidemic resistant strains may decline naturally, as has occurred with staphylococci with the disappearance of type 80/81 strains and the first epidemic of MRSA. However, the present hospital epidemic strains are still spreading and may only be replaced by different resistant strains in the future. At some stage, we may have to introduce widespread and expensive eradication procedures.

The other source of resistant strains is from animals. These strains may emerge following veterinary treatment or the use of antibiotics as food additives. Transfer of resistant strains, such as some *Salmonella* spp. and possibly VRE to humans can occur. Legal restrictions are possible with food additives, but the problems of restriction of agents for therapeutic use are similar to those in human medicine.

Few organisms become resistant during the treatment of a single patient, but the offspring of a single resistant organism may spread throughout a hospital. Spread of resistance from one organism to another may be by transfer of plasmids, but cross-infection by organisms is the main mode of spread between patients. Control of cross-infection should therefore be a more practical proposition than the restriction of antibiotics in reducing resistant strains in hospitals. For the purposes of control,

MRSA will be considered here, but similar principles apply to other organisms, such as Gram-negative bacilli and VRE,[10] although carriage sites are mainly different.

Possible methods of control of MRSA (see also Chapter 16) are:

1 *Nonspecific procedures*, especially the improvement of general hygiene, such as hand disinfection and wearing gloves and gowns for contact with infected patients, but the problem that has been with us since the time of Semmelweiss is the implementation of hand-washing by staff. Although reports from individual hospitals have indicated some success in reducing MRSA by the use of alcoholic hand rubs,[11] education has usually had only a temporary success. Although it is possible to select priorities for hand-washing/disinfection, there may be insufficient time to wash hands after every patient contact. Taking a pulse or moving a pillow can contaminate the hands, and one mistake can undo days of careful technique. The use of an alcoholic hand rub on a bedside table can save time by eliminating the need to go to a sink, and this is likely to be the cheapest and most effective method of control.

2 *High-risk units.* Isolation of the infected patient or carrier is probably the most effective control measure, but eradication measures in priority areas such as intensive care may be an important compromise. The latter involves screening all new patients, followed by isolation and treatment with topical antimicrobial agents, such as mupirocin, of nasal carriers and infected patients.

3 *Lower-risk units*, such as general surgical wards. Isolation of carriers and infected patients, particularly heavy dispersers, in association with hygienic measures may be effective in removing the strain from the ward, but if the numbers of infected or colonized patients are high, then a separate MRSA ward may be necessary. If sufficient isolation facilities are not available and the outbreak must be stopped, then other measures may be tried, such as prophylactic treatment with topical mupirocin or another agent of the noses of all patients, daily antiseptic baths, impermeable antiseptic dressings to wounds, and general hygienic measures.

In addition to the adoption of one of the above procedures, other measures should be introduced, such as adequate staffing, the avoidance of overcrowding, and the transfer of patients from an 'infected' to a 'non-infected' ward.

The present pandemic of MRSA continues, and existing control methods have not worked as they did in previous epidemics. These methods will limit the spread of MRSA, but they appear to be inadequate to eradicate the organism from a hospital with epidemic strains in several wards. As Chapin indicated 100 years ago, an outbreak can be prevented if treated early, but it becomes extremely difficult if a hospital has a large number of cases. The success of prompt identification of carriers and infected patients and subsequent action by means of good surveillance and hygiene, isolation of carriers and infected patients, and control of the use of antibiotics has been demonstrated in several places, including the Netherlands, Denmark and Western Australia. However, similar techniques in some of these countries have been less effective in the control of antibiotic-resistant Gram-negative infections. It is also possible that these countries were not faced with the same shortage of hospital beds and isolation facilities as in countries where prevention methods failed.

The main problem with the present epidemic of MRSA is the admission of carriers to the hospital from other hospitals in the same or another country, or from residential establishments for the elderly. If there are many carriers in the community, then the only way to eradicate the strain would be to screen all patients in the hospital for carriage and then to screen all patients on admission. Screening of patients in long-term residential establishments and their subsequent treatment would be a major and probably undesirable task. The hospital eradication programme would involve sampling several sites on each patient and, if positive, isolating the patient for treatment until clear of the organism. To achieve this, more isolation facilities would be required, together with the development of a simple and rapid diagnostic test, a programme that would require more staff in laboratories and would be very expensive. However, it could be introduced in certain hospitals as a controlled study, perhaps comparing it with a hospital using only hygienic measures. As recognized for many years, hospitals with small wards and an ample number of single rooms suitable for isolation are required to cope with any future epidemic situation. The reintroduction of convalescent establishments would relieve the pressures on acute hospitals.

National and international surveillance of resistant strains has been recommended, and ascertainment of the numbers of carriers and infections, such as the present collection of data on bacteraemias in the UK, would be useful, but the number of patients at risk and the incidence would not be known unless hospitals had a screening programme of all patients and possibly staff as well. Prevalence surveys of nasal carriers in a number of hospitals have been carried out in the past, showing that many had no MRSA and that these organisms were mainly a problem in large or tertiary referral hospitals. These surveys could be repeated in certain key hospitals.

An important part of controlling hospital infection is the education of staff and the appointment of trained infection-control staff. The numbers of infection-control nurses are increasing around the world, and link nurses with responsibilities on the ward where they are working will improve the situation. However, nursing and medical students are often not trained well in microbiology and infection control due to the many extra topics they are being taught. This is surprising since problems of infection will continue to take up much of their time when they qualify as nurses or doctors.

Since the future cannot be predicted, surveillance and implementation of an effective hygienic programme with the introduction of eradication in high-risk areas should be instituted in all hospitals. The present epidemic may continue to increase or it may decline, but meanwhile research on the transmissibility of MRSA, on design of purpose-designed antibiotics, and on vaccines for all relevant organisms, including enterococci and Gram-negative bacilli, should have a high priority. If it is considered to be too expensive to introduce a complete MRSA eradication programme, then research into the effectiveness of the method in several hospitals should also be an immediate priority in case it is needed in the future, irrespective of the cost. The increasing incidence of resistant strains is an added expense in that the new, more expensive antibiotics are required for treating severe clinical infections, and these are being paid for directly over the counter in some countries. This practice should be stopped and prescription-only antibiotics provided for both human and veterinary use.

Several other topics will indirectly affect the control of infection in the future. The increasing use of nonbiodegradable disposables is causing problems in the disposal of clinical (and other) waste. Suitable waste-disposal sites are disappearing in many countries, while incineration is expensive and produces toxic products. The trend, therefore, should be to reduce the use of single-use medical devices wherever possible. Manufacturers must be persuaded to produce reusable devices that can be cleaned and sterilized efficiently in central service units in hospitals. This change in policy would be particularly valuable in developing countries.

Legal requirements for processing devices and procedures associated with control of infection are becoming increasingly restrictive and not based on an assessment of infection risk, especially in Europe. Appropriate studies should be made before such requirements are introduced.

The multiplication of claims for negligence is taking increasing amounts of funds away from patient care, and risk analysis is now a major consideration in hospital administration. Some training in risk analysis for the public is also required, and more court cases should be defended. Nevertheless, a quality assurance system with good written records of procedures must be in place to ensure standards remain high and to reduce the chances of errors. The acquisition of infection is usually not due to negligence, and it is necessary for patients to understand that some infections are inevitable and that there is an irreducible minimum.[12] Alternative methods of compensation are needed for no-blame situations.

Many of the proposed possible measures described above are expensive and would not be possible in poorer countries. Much more support is required in these countries for future control of hospital and community infection, but good education and implementation of cost-effective hygienic procedures will remain the key requirements for future improvements.

References

Preface

1 Meleney, F.L. (1948). *Treatise on Surgical Infections.* New York: Oxford University Press.

2 Jones, J. (1866–7). Notes upon the history of hospital gangrene. *South. Med. Surg. J.*, **1**, 55–71.

3 Selwyn, S. (1991). Hospital infection: the first 2500 years. *J. Hosp. Infect.*, **18** (Suppl. A), 5–64.

Chapter 1

1 Bell, W.G. (1924). *The Great Plagues in London in 1665.* London: Bodley Head.

2 Copeman, W.S.C. (1960). *Doctors and Disease in Tudor Times.* London: Dawson.

3 Howe, G.M. (1972). *Man, Environment and Disease in Britain. A Medical Geography through the Ages.* Newton Abbott: David and Charles.

4 Bonser, W. (1963). *The Medical Background of Anglo-Saxon England.* London: Wellcome.

5 Rosen, G. (1958). *A History of Public Health.* New York: MD Publications.

6 Stubbs, S.G.B. and Bligh, E.W. (1931). *Sixty Centuries of Health and Physick.* London: Sampson Low, and Marston and Co.

7 Block, S.S. (2001). *Disinfection, Sterilization and Preservation*, 5th edn. Philadelphia and London: Lippincott Williams and Wilkins.

8 Winslow, C.E.A. (1944). *The Conquest of Epidemic Disease. A Chapter in the History of Ideas.* Princeton, NJ: Princeton University Press.

9 Clay, R.M. (1909). *The Medieval Hospitals of England.* London: Methuen.

10 Gasquet, F.A. (1893). *The Great Pestilence (A.D. 1348–9).* London: Simpkin Marshall.

11 Wain, H. (1970). *A History of Preventive Medicine.* Springfield, IL: Thomas.

12 Creighton, C. (1891, 1894). *A History of Epidemics in Great Britain.* Cambridge: Cambridge University Press.

13 Bullock, W. (1938). *The History of Bacteriology.* New York: Dover Publications.

14 Dobell, C. (1932). *Anthony van Leeuwenhoek and His 'Little Animals'.* New York: Harcourt Brace.

15 Bates, D.G. (1981). Thomas Willis and the fevers literature of the 17th century. In *Theories of Fever from Antiquity to the Enlightenment*, ed. W.F. Bynum and V. Nutton, pp. 45–70. London: Wellcome Institute.

16 Cunningham, A. (1981). Sydenham versus Newton. In *Theories of Fever from Antiquity to the Enlightenment*, ed. W.F. Bynum and V. Nutton, pp. 71–98. London: Wellcome Institute.

17 Smith, F.B. (1979). *The People's Health, 1830–1910*. London: Croom Helm.

18 Cassar, P. (1964). *Medical History of Malta*. London: Wellcome.

19 Cipolla, C.M. (1981). *Fighting the Plague in Seventeenth Century Italy*. Wisconsin: University of Wisconsin Press.

Chapter 2

1 Neuberger, M. (1921). *History of Medicine*. Oxford: Oxford University Press.

2 Browne, E.G. (1921). *Arabian Medicine*. Cambridge: Cambridge University Press.

3 Talbot, C.H. (1967). *Medicine in Medieval England*. London: Oldbourne.

4 Rosen, G. (1958). *A History of Public Health*. New York: MD Publications.

5 Rubin, S. (1974). *Medieval English Medicine A.D. 500–1300*. London: David and Charles.

6 Garrison, F.H. (1929). *An Introduction to the History of Medicine*. Philadelphia and London: Saunders.

7 Wain, H. (1970). *A History of Preventive Medicine*. Springfield, IL: Thomas.

8 Howe, G.M. (1972). *Man, Environment and Disease in Britain. A Medical Geography through the Ages*. Newton Abbott: David and Charles.

9 Thompson, J.D. and Goldin, G. (1975). *The Hospital: A Social and Architectural History*. New Haven and London: Yale University Press.

10 Dainton, C. (1961). *The Story of England's Hospitals*. London: Museum Press.

11 Parsons, F.G. (1932). *A History of St Thomas' Hospital*, Vol. 1.

12 Bell, W.G. (1924). *The Great Plague in London in 1965*. London: Bodley Head.

13 Cipolla, C.M. (1981). *Fighting the Plague in Seventeenth Century Italy*. Wisconsin: University of Wisconsin Press.

14 Copeman, W.S.C. (1960). *Doctors and Disease in Tudor Times*. London: Dawson.

15 More, T. (1965). *Utopia*, transl. P. Turner. London: Penguin Books.

16 Porter, R. (1987). *Disease, Medicine and Society in England 1550–1860*. London: Macmillan Education.

17 Bradford, E. (1972). *The Shield and the Sword. The Knights of St John*. London: Hodder and Stoughton.

18 Park, K. (1991). Healing the poor. Hospitals and medical assistance in Renaissance Florence. In *Medicine and Charity before the Welfare State*, ed. J. Barry and C. Jones. London: Routledge.

19 Henderson, J. (1989). The hospitals of late-medieval and Renaissance Florence: a preliminary survey. In *The Hospital in History*, ed. L. Granshaw and R. Porter. London: Routledge.

20 Trexler, B.J. (1971). Hospital patients in Florence: San Paolo 1567–1568. *Bulletin of History of Medicine and Allied Sciences*, **48**, 41–59.

21 Selwyn, S. (1991). Hospital infection: the first 2500 years. *J. Hosp. Infect.*, **18** (Suppl. A), 5–64.

22 Paget, S. (1897). *Ambroise Paré and His Times*. New York: Putnam.

23 Rutkov, I.M. (1993). *Surgery. An Illustrated History*. St Louis: Mosby.

Chapter 3

1 Woodward, J.H. (1974). *To Do the Sick No Harm. A Study of the British Voluntary Hospital System to 1875*. London: Routledge and Kegan Paul.

2 Garrison, F.H. (1929). *An Introduction to the History of Medicine*. Philadelphia: Saunders.

3 Steele, J.C. (1877). The mortality of hospitals, general and special, in the United Kingdom, in times past and present. *J. R. Stat. Soc.*, **40**, 177–261.

4 Pringle, J. (1750). *Observations on the Nature and Cure of Hospital and Jayl Fevers*. London: Millar Wilson and Payne.

5 Foster, E. (1768). *An Essay on Hospitals, or, Succinct Directions for the Situation, Construction and Administration of Country Hospitals*. Dublin.

6 Aikin, J. (1771). *Thoughts on Hospitals*. London.

7 Cherry, S. (1980). The hospitals and population growth. 1. The voluntary general hospitals, mortality and local populations in the English provinces in the eighteenth and nineteenth centuries. *Popul. Stud. (Camb.).*, **34**, 59–75, 251–65.

8 Eade, P. (1900). *The Norfolk and Norwich Hospital, 1770–1900*. London: Jarrold.

9 Howard, J. (1789). *An Account of the Principal Lazerettos in Europe with Various Papers Relative to the Plague Together with Further Observations on some Foreign Prisons and Hospitals; and Additional Remarks on the Present State of those in Great Britain and Ireland*. London: Warrington, Cadell and Johnson.

10 Thompson, J.D and Goldin, G. (1975). *The Hospital: A Social and Architectural History*. New Haven and London: Yale University Press.

11 Clark, J. (1802). *Collection of Papers Intended to Promote an Institution for the Cure and Prevention of Infectious Fevers in Newcastle and Other Populous Towns, Together with the Communications of the Most Eminent Physicians Relative to the Safety and Importance of Annexing Fever Wards to the Newcastle and Other Infirmaries*. Newcastle.

12 Gooch, B. (undated, but 1772 or later). *Medical and Chirurgical Observations*. London: Robinson.

13 Tenon, M. (1788). *Mémoires sur les Hôpitaux de Paris*. Paris: Ph-D Pierres.

14 Richmond, P.A. (1961). The Hôtel-Dieu of Paris on the eve of the revolution. *J. Hist. Med. Sci.*, **16**, 335–53.

15 Lesky, E. (1977). Hospital acquired infections – a historical survey. *Hexagon Roche*, **5**, 1–10.

Chapter 4

1 Wain, H. (1970). *A History of Preventive Medicine*. Springfield, IL: Thomas.

2 Zinsser, H. (1935). *Rats, Lice and History*. Boston: Little Brown.

3 Murchison, C. (1873). *A Treatise on the Continued Fevers of Great Britain*. London: Longman, Green.

4 Douthwaite, A.W. (1892). *A Treatise on Fevers*. Office of Shanghai Mercury.

5 Selwyn, S. (1966). Sir John Pringle: hospital reformer, moral philosopher and pioneer of antiseptics. *Med. Hist.*, **10**, 266–74.

6 Pringle, J. (1750) *Observations on the Nature and Cure of Hospital and Jayl-fevers*. London: Millar and Wilson.

7 Pringle, J. (1752). *Observations on the Diseases of the Army in Camp and Garrison*. London: Miller, Wilson and Payne.

8 Brocklesbury, R. (1764). *Oeconomical and Medical Observations in Two Parts. From the Year 1758 to the Year 1763 Inclusive. Tending to the Improvement of Military Hospitals, and to the Cure of Camp Diseases, Incident to Soldiers (With Appendix)*. London: Becket and De Hondt.

9 Pringle, J. (1750). Some experiments on substances resisting putrefaction. *Phil. Trans. R. Soc.*, **46**, 550–58.

10 Selwyn, S. (1979). Early experimental models of disinfection and sterilization. *J. Antimicrob. Chemother.*, **5**, 229–30.

11 Lind, J. (1757). *An Essay on the Most Effectual Means of Preserving the Health of Seamen, in the Royal Navy.* London: Millar.

12 Monro, D. (1780). *Observations on the Means of Preserving the Health of Soldiers and of conducting Military Hospitals.* London: Murray.

13 Smyth, J.C. (1795). *Description of Jail Distemper.* London: Johnson.

14 Smyth, J.C. (1796). *An Account of the Experiment Made at the Desire of the Lords Commissioners of the Admiralty on Board the Union Hospital Ship to Determine the Effect of the Nitrous Acid in Destroying Contagion.* London: Johnson.

15 Guyton-Morveau, L.B. (1802). *Treatise on the Means of Purifying Infected Air, of Preventing Contagion and Arresting its Progress,* transl. R. Hall. London: Hurst.

16 French Council of Health (1795). Instructions for maintaining cleanliness and purifying air of hospital wards, transl. 1804. *Med. Phys. J.*, **11**, 97–111.

17 Winslow, C.E.A. (1944). *The Conquest of Epidemic Disease. A Chapter in the History of Ideas.* Princeton, NJ: Princeton University Press.

18 Howard, J. (1789). *An Account of the Principal Lazerettos in Europe with Various Papers Relative to the Plague Together With Further Observations on Some Foreign Prisons and Hospitals; and Additional Remarks on the Present State of those in Great Britain and Ireland.* London: Johnson, Dilly and Cadell.

19 Tenon, M. (1788). *Mémoires sur les Hôpitaux de Paris.* Paris: Ph-D Pierres.

20 Ackerneknecht, E.H. (1967). *Medicine at the Paris Hospital, 1794–1845.* Baltimore, Johns Hopkins.

21 Buer, M.C. (1926). *Health, Wealth and Population in the Early Days of the Industrial Revolution.* London: Routledge.

22 Woodward, J. (1974). *To Do the Sick No Harm. A Study of the British Voluntary Hospital System to 1875.* London: Routledge and Kegan Paul.

23 Good, J.M. (1795). *Dissertation on the Diseases of Prisons and Poor-Houses.* London: Dilly.

24 Beddoes, T. (1803). *Hygeia, or Essays Moral and Medical on the Causes Affecting the Personal State of our Middling and Affluent Classes,* Vol. 3. London: Phillips.

25 Hudson, A. (1868). *Lectures on the Study of Fever.* Dublin: McGee.

26 Simon, J. (1887). *Public Health Reports I and II.* London: Churchill.

27 O'Malley, J.B. (1931). *Florence Nightingale. 1820–1856. A Study of Her Life Down to the End of the Crimean War.* London: Thornton Butterworth.

Chapter 5

1 Grimek, M.D. (1983). *Les maladies a l'aube de la civilisation occidentale.* Paris: Paget.

2 Peckham, C.H. (1935). A brief history of puerperal infection. *Bull. Inst. Hist. Med.*, **3**, 187–212.

3 Thompson, J.D. and Goldin, G. (1975). *The Hospital: A Social and Architectural History.* New Haven and London: Yale University Press.

4 Tenon, M. (1788). *Memoires sur les Hôpitaux de Paris.* Paris: Ph-D Pierres.

5 Gunn, A. (1964). Maternity hospitals. In *The Evolution of Hospitals in Britain*, ed. Poynter. London: Pitman.

6 DeLacy, M. (1989). Puerperal fever in eighteenth century Britain. *Bull. Hist. Med.*, **63**, 521–56.

7 Adami, G. (1922). *Charles White of Manchester (1738–1813) and the Arrest of Puerperal Fever.* London: Hodder and Stoughton.

8 Nightingale, F. (1871). *Introductory Notes on Lying-in Institutions.* London: Longman Green.

9 Clarke, J. (1849). Observations on the puerperal fever. In *Essays on the Puerperal Fever*, ed. F. Churchill, pp. 363–443. London: Sydenham Society.

10 McKeown, T. and Brown, R.G. (1955). Medical evidence related to English population changes in the eighteenth century. **9–10**, 119–41.

11 Steele, J.C. (1877). The mortality of hospitals, general and special, in the United Kingdom, in times past and present. *J. R. Stat. Soc.*, **40**, 177–261.

12 Leake, J. (1849). On the childbed fever. In *Essays on the Puerperal Fever*, ed. F. Churchill, pp. 117–204. London: Sydenham Society.

13 Gordon, A. (1849). A treatise on the epidemic of puerperal fever of Aberdeen. In *Essays on the Puerperal Fever*, ed. F. Churchill, pp. 445–500. London: Sydenham Society.

14 Youngson, A.J. (1979). *The Scientific Revolution in Victorian Medicine.* London: Croom Helm.

15 Armstrong, J. (1814). *Facts and Observations Relative to the Fever Commonly Called Puerperal.* London and Edinburgh: Longman.

16 Loudon, I. (1986). Deaths in childbed from the eighteenth century to 1935. *Med. Hist.*, **30**, 1–41.

17 Selwyn, S. (1965). Sir James Simpson and hospital cross-infection. *Med. Hist.*, **9**, 241–8.

18 Shepherd, J.A. (1969). *Simpson and Syme of Edinburgh.* Edinburgh: Livingstone.

19 Donnison, J. (1977). *Midwives and Medical Men.* New York: Schocken.

20 Collins, R. (1992). Reducing maternal mortality in childbirth. In *Irish Masters of Medicine* ed. D. Coakley. Dublin: Town House.

21 Holmes, O.W. (1843). The contagiousness of puerperal fever. *N. Engl. Q.J. Med. Surg.*, **1**, 503–30.

22 Colebrook, L. (1954). Puerperal infection, 1800–1950. In *Historical Review of British Obstetrics and Gynaecology*, ed. J.M.M. Kerr, R.W. Johnstone and M.H. Phillips, pp. 202–25. Edinburgh: Livingstone.

23 Newsom, S.W.B. (1993). Ignaz Semmelweiss. *J. Hosp. Infect.*, **23**, 175–87.

24 Rotter, M.L. (1997). 150 years of hand disinfection – Semmelweis heritage. *Hyg. Med.*, **22**, 332–9.

25 Wain, H. (1970). *A History of Preventive Medicine.* Springfield, IL: Thomas.

26 Le Fort, L. (1866). *Des maternités. Etude sur les maternités et les institutions charitables accouchement a domicile dans les principaux états de l'Europe.* Paris: Masson et Cie.

Chapter 6

1 Chevalier, A.G. (1941). Hygienic problems of the Napoleonic armies. *CIBA Found. Symp.*, **3**, 974–80.

2 Rutkov, I.M. (1993). *Surgery. An Illustrated History.* St Louis: Mosby.

3 Richardson, R.G. (1974). *Larrey: Surgeon to Napoleon's Imperial Guard.* London: Murray.

4 Meleney, F.L. (1948). *Treatise on Surgical Infections*. New York: Oxford University Press.

5 Howard, M.R. (1988). British medical services at the battle of Waterloo. *Br. J.*, **4**, 1653–6.

6 Erichsen, J.E. (1874). Lectures on hospitalism: and the causes which determine the mortality after amputations. *Lancet*, **1**, 84–6, 122–6, 151–4, 221–4.

7 O'Malley, J.B. (1931). *Florence Nightingale. 1820–1856*. London: Thornton Butterworth.

8 Woodham-Smith, C. (1951). *Florence Nightingale*. New York: McGraw Hill.

9 Donahue, M.P. (1996). *Nursing the Finest Art. An Illustrated History*, 2nd edn. St Louis and Baltimore: Mosby.

10 Lesky, E. (1977). Hospital-acquired infections – a historical survey. *Hexagon Roche*, **5**, 1–10.

11 Jones, J. (1871). Investigations upon the nature, causes and treatment of hospital gangrene as it prevailed in the Confederate armies 1861–1865. In *Surgical Memoirs of the War of the Rebellion*, ed. J. Jones. New York: U.S. Sanitary Commission.

12 Miller, F.T. ed. (1957). *Prisons and Hospitals. The Photographic History of the Civil War*. New York: Castle Books.

13 Linder, F. (1981). Alexander Ogston. In *The Staphylococci*, ed. A. Macdonald and G. Smith. Aberdeen: Aberdeen University Press.

14 Jones, J. (1866–7). Notes upon the history of hospital gangrene. *South. Med. Surg. J.*, **1**, 55–71.

15 Pouteau, C. (1793). *Oeuvres posthumes*. Paris: Pierres.

16 Thomson, J. (1813). *Lectures on Inflammation*. London: Ballantyne.

17 Blackadder, H.H. (1818). *Observations on Phagedaena Gangraenosa*. Edinburgh: Brown.

18 Meleney, F.L. (1924). Hemolytic streptococcus gangrene. *Arch. Surg.*, **9**, 317–64.

19 Strasberg, S.M. and Silver, M.S. (1968). Haemolytic streptococcal gangrene. An uncommon but frequently fatal infection in the antibiotic era. *Am. J. Surg.*, **115**, 763–8.

20 Cherry, S. (1980). The hospitals and population growth. 1. The voluntary general hospitals, mortality and local populations in the English provinces in the eighteenth and nineteenth centuries. *Popul. Stud. (Camb.).*, **34**, 59–75, 251–65.

21 Griffith, G.T. (1926). *Population Problems in the Age of Malthus*. Cambridge.

22 McKeown, T. and Brown, R.G. (1955). Medical evidence related to English population changes in the eighteenth century. *Pop. Studies*, **9–10**, 119–41.

23 Sigsworth, E. (1966). A provincial hospital in the eighteenth and early nineteenth centuries. *R. Coll. Gen. Prac. Yorks Faculty J.*, 24–31.

24 Woodward, J. (1974). *To Do the Sick No Harm. A Study of the British Voluntary Hospital System to 1875*. London: Routledge and Kegan Paul.

25 Alanson, E. (1782). *Practical Observations on Amputation and the After Treatment*. London: Johnson.

26 Bell, J. (1801). *The Principles of Surgery*, Vol. 1. Edinburgh: Cadell and Davies.

27 Tait, L. (1877). *An Essay on Hospital Mortality. Based upon the Statistics of the Hospitals of Great Britain for Fifteen Years*. London: Churchill.

28 Eade, P. (1900). *The Norfolk and Norwich Hospital, 1770–1900*. London: Jarrold.

29 Beverley, M. (1874). Hospital hygiene illustrated by references to the Norfolk and Norwich Hospital in the present, past and future. *Br. Med. J.*, **2**, 314–16.

30 Sympson, T. (1878). *A Short Account of the Old and of the New Lincoln County Hospitals*. Lincoln: Williamson.

31 Bristowe, J.S. and Holmes, T. (1863). On the Hospitals of the United Kingdom, in the *Sixth Report of the Medical Officer*, pp. 463–74. London.

32 Birmingham General Hospital. Annual reports, 1852–81.

33 Nunnelly, T. (1841). *A Treatise on the Nature, Causes and Treatment of Erysipelas*. London: Churchill.

34 Nightingale, F. (1863). *Notes on Hospitals*, 3rd edn. London: Longman.

35 Selwyn, S. (1965). Sir James Simpson and hospital cross-infection. *Med. Hist.*, **9**, 241–8.

36 Simpson, J. (1869). Some propositions on hospitalism. *Lancet*, **2**, 295–7, 332–5, 431–3, 475–8, 535–8.

37 Simpson, J. (1870). Some propositions on hospitalism. *Lancet*, **2**, 698–700.

38 Simpson, J. (1869). Hospitalism and its effects. *Edinburgh Med. J.*, **14**, 1084–115.

39 Holmes, T. (1864). Mortality in hospitals. *Lancet*, **1**, 338–9.

40 Holmes, T. (1869). On 'hospitalism'. *Lancet*, **2**, 194–6, 229–30.

41 La Force, F.M. (1997). The control of infections in hospitals: 1750–1950. In *Prevention and Control of Hospital Infections*, ed. R.W. Wenzel, pp. 3–17. Baltimore: Williams and Wilkins.

42 Lesky, E. (1977). Hospital-acquired infections – a historical survey. *Hexagon Roche*, **5**, 1–10.

43 Wangensteen, O.H., Wangensteen, S.D. and Klinger, C.F. (1972). Surgical cleanliness, hospital salubrity, and surgical statistics, historically considered. *Surgery*, **71**, 477–93.

Chapter 7

1 Bynum, W.F. and Nutton, V. eds. (1981). *Theories of Fever from Antiquity to the Enlightenment*. London: Wellcome Institute.

2 Winslow, C.E.A. (1944). *The Conquest of Epidemic Disease. A Chapter in the History of Ideas*. Princeton, NJ: Princeton University Press.

3 Mead, R.D. (1720). *A Short Discourse Concerning Pestilential Contagion and the Methods to be Used to Prevent it*. London: Buckley and Smith.

4 Pye, G. (1771). *A Discourse on the Plague. Wherein Dr Mead's Notions are Considered and Rejected*. London: Darby.

5 Pringle, J. (1810). *Observations on the Diseases of the Army*. London: Stockdale.

6 Pringle, J. (1750) *Observations on the Nature and Cause of Hospital and Jayl-fevers*. London: Millar and Wilson.

7 Lind, J. (1757). *An Essay on the Most Effectual Means of Preserving the Health of Seamen, in the Royal Navy*. London: Millar.

8 Alexander, W. (1771). *An Experimental Enquiry Concerning the Causes Which Have Generally Been Said to Produce Putrid Diseases*. London: Becket, DeHondt and Cadell.

9 Guyton-Morveau, L.B. (1802). *Treatise on the Means of Purifying Infected Air, of Preventing Contagion and Arresting its Progress*, transl. R. Hall. London: Hurst.

10 Beddoes, T. (1803). *Hygeia, or Essays Moral and Medical on the Causes Affecting the Personal State of our Middling and Affluent Classes*, Vol. 3. London: Phillips.

11 Gordon, A. (1849). A treatise on the epidemic of puerperal fever etc. In *Essays on the Puerperal Fever*, ed. F. Churchill, pp. 445–500. London: Sydenham Society.

12 Youngson, A.J. (1979). *The Scientific Revolution in Victorian Medicine*. London: Croom Helm.

13 Ackerneknecht, E.H. (1948). Anticontagionism between 1821 and 1867. *Bull. Hist. Med.*, **22**, 562–93.

14 Bulloch, W. (1938). *The History of Bacteriology.* New York: Dover Publications.

15 Murchison, C. (1873). *A Treatise on the Continuing Fevers of Great Britain.* London: Parker, Son and Bourne.

16 Wangensteen, O.H. and Wangensteen, S.D. (1978). *The Rise of Surgery. From Empiric Craft to Scientific Discipline.* Minneapolis: University of Minnesota Press.

17 Wangensteen, O.H., Wangensteen, S.D. and Klinger, C.F. (1972). Surgical cleanliness, hospital salubrity, and surgical sepsis, and surgical statistics historically considered. *Surgery*, **71**, 477–93.

18 Thomson, J. (1813). *Lectures on Inflammation.* London: Ballantyne.

19 Blackadder, H.H. (1818). *Observations on Phagedaena Gangraenosa.* Edinburgh: Brown.

20 Erichsen, J.E. (1874). Lectures on hospitalism, and the causes which determine the mortality after amputations. *Lancet*, **1**, 84–6, 122–6, 151–4, 221–4.

21 Wainwright, M. (2001). Microbiology before Pasteur. *Microbiol. Today*, **28**, 19–21.

22 Rutkov, I.M. (1993). *Surgery. An Illustrated History.* St Louis: Mosby.

23 Foster, W.D. (1970). *A History of Medical Bacteriology.* London: Heinemann.

24 Lesky, E. (1977). Hospital-acquired infections – a historical survey. *Hexagon Roche*, **5**, 1–10.

25 Kolmos, H.J. (1993). Salomonsen og hans bakteriologiske bedrift på Kommunehospitalet i 1873. *Bibliotek for Laeger*, **185**: 232–49.

26 Smith, G. (1981). Ogston the bacteriologist. In *The Staphylococci. Proceedings of the Alexander Ogston Centennial Conference*, ed. A. Macdonald and G. Smith, pp. 9–21. Aberdeen: Aberdeen University Press.

27 Ogston, A. (1880). Über abscesse. *Arch. Klin. Surg.*, **25**, 588–600.

28 Watson-Cheyne, W. (1882). *Antiseptic Surgery: Its Principles, Practice, History and Results.* London: Smith and Elder.

29 Spink, W.W. (1978). *Infectious Diseases. Prevention and Treatment in the Nineteenth and Twentieth Centuries.* Folkestone: Dawson.

Chapter 8

1 Wangensteen, O.H. and Wangensteen, S.D. (1978). *The Rise of Surgery: From Empiric Craft to Scientific Discipline.* Minneapolis: University of Minnesota Press.

2 Hugo, W.B. (1978). Phenols: a review of their history and development as antimicrobial agents. *Microbios*, **23**, 83–5.

3 Rutkow, I.M. (1993). *Surgery. An Illustrated History.* St Louis: Mosby.

4 Godlee, R.J. (1917). *Lord Lister.* London: Macmillan.

5 St Clair Thomson (1927). Lister: A house surgeon's memories. *Br. Med. J.*, **1**, 659–62.

6 Lister, J. (1867). On the antiseptic principle in the practice of surgery. *Br. Med. J.*, **2**, 246–8; *Lancet*, **2**, 353–6, 668–9.

7 Lister, J. (1875). The effect of the antiseptic treatment upon the general salubrity of surgical hospitals. *Br. Med. J.*, **2**, 769–71.

8 Kapadia, H.M. (2002). Sampson Gamgee: a great Birmingham surgeon. *J. R. Soc. Med.*, **95**, 96–100.

9 Lesky, E. (1977). Hospital-acquired infections – a historical survey. *Hexagon Roche*, **5**, 1–10.

10 Schimmelbusch, C. (1893). *The Aseptic Treatment of Wounds.* Transl. 1894, A.T. Rake. London: H.K. Lewis.

11 Watson-Cheyne, W. (1882). *Antiseptic Surgery: Its Principles, Practice, History and Results.* London: Smith and Elder.

12 Meleney, F.L. (1948). *Treatise on Surgical Infections.* New York: Oxford University Press.

13 Price, P.B. (1938). The bacteriology of normal skin: a new quantitative test applied to study of bacterial flora and disinfectant action of mechanical cleansing. *J. Infect. Dis.*, **63**, 301–18.

14 Halsted, W.S. (1913). Ligature and suture material. *J. Am. Med. Soc.*, **60**, 1119–26.

15 Lynn Thomas, J. (1905). Modern fashions in surgery. *Br. Med. J.*, **2**, 1628–30.

16 Walter, C.W. (1958). *The Aseptic Treatment of Wounds.* New York: Macmillan.

17 Block, S.S. (2001). *Disinfection, Sterilization and Preservation*, 5th edn. Philadelphia: Lippincott Williams and Wilkins.

18 Papin, D. (1681). *A New Digester or Engine for Softening Bones.* Paris: Pierre J. Duplein.

19 Bullock, W. (1938). *The History of Bacteriology.* New York: Dover Publications.

20 Henry, W. (1832). Further experiments on the disinfecting powers of increased temperatures. *Philosph. Mag.*, **11**, 22–3.

21 Magath, T.B. (1937). The history of steam sterilization. *Ann. Med. Hist.*, **9**, 338–44.

22 Ayliffe, G.A.J. and Lowbury, E.J.L. (1982). Airborne infection in hospital. *J. Hosp. Infect.*, **3**, 217–40.

23 Flugge, C. (1897). Uber Luftinfektion. *Z. Hyg. Infektionskr.*, **25**, 179–224.

24 Mikulicz, J. (1897). Das operieren in sterilisierten zwimhandschuhen und mit mundbinde. *Zentralbl. Chir.*, **24**, 713–17.

25 Belkin, N.L. (1997). The evolution of the surgical mask: filtering efficiency versus effectiveness. *Infect. Control Hosp. Epidemiol.*, **18**, 49–57.

26 Chapin, C.V. (1910). *The Sources and Mode of Infection.* New York: John Wiley and Sons.

27 Wells, W.F. and Wells, M.W. (1936). Airborne infection. *J. Am. Med. Assoc.*, **107**, 1698–703, 1805–9.

28 Robb, H. (1909). The air of the operating theatre as a possible factor in the infection of wounds. *Am. J. Obstet. Dis. Women Child.*, **40**, 451–63.

29 Brewer, G.E. (1915). Studies on aseptic technic with a report of recent observations at the Roosevelt Hospital, N.Y. *J. Am. Med. Assoc.*, **64**, 1369–72.

30 Meleney, F.L. (1935). Infection in clean operating wounds: a nine-year study. *Surg. Gynecol. Obstet.*, **60**, 264–75.

31 Howe, C.W. (1954). Postoperative wound infections due to *Staphylococcus aureus*. *N. Engl. J. Med.*, **251**, 411–17.

32 Howe, C.W. (1956). The problem of postoperative wound infections caused by *Staphylococcus aureus*. *Ann. Surg.*, **146**, 384–96.

Chapter 9

1 Nightingale, F. (1863). *Notes on Hospitals*, 3rd edn. London: Longman.

2 Thompson, J.D. and Goldin, G. (1975). *The Hospital: A Social and Architectural History.* New Haven and London: Yale University Press.

3 Poynter, F.N.L., ed. (1964). *The Evolution of Hospitals in Britain.* London: Pitman.

4 Gainsborough, H. and Gainsborough, J. (1964). *Principles of Hospital Design.* London: Architectural Press.

5 Williams, R.E.O., Blowers, R., Garrod, L. and Shooter, R.A. (1966). *Hospital Infection. Causes and Prevention*, 2nd edn. London: Lloyd Luke.

6 Whyte, W., Howie, J.G.R. and Eakin, J.A.E. (1969). Bacteriological observations in a mechanically ventilated experimental ward and in two open-plan wards. *J. Med. Microbiol.*, **2**, 335–45.

7 Ayliffe, G.A.J. and Lowbury, E.J.L. (1982). Airborne infection in hospital. *J. Hosp. Infect.*, **3**, 217–40.

8 Selwyn, S. (1991). Hospital infection: the first 2,500 years. *J. Hosp. Infect.*, **18** (Suppl. A), 5–64.

9 Wright, D.W. (1967). A short history of isolation accommodation in Bristol. *Bristol. Med. Chir. J.*, **83**, 35–8.

10 Gray, J.A. (1999). *The Edinburgh City Hospital.* East Linton, Scotland: Tuckwell Press.

11 Chapin, C.V. (1910). *The Sources and Mode of Infection.* New York: John Wiley and Sons.

12 Rundle, C. (1912). The bed isolation of infectious diseases. *Proc. R. Soc. Med.*, **5**, 171–82.

13 Harries, E.H.R. (1935). Infection and its control in children's wards. *Lancet*, **2**, 173–8, 233–9.

14 McKendrick, G.D.W. and Emond, R.T.D. (1976). Investigation of cross-infection in isolation wards of different design. *J. Hyg. (Lond.)*, **76**, 23–31.

15 Parker, M.T., John, M., Emond, R.T.D. and Machacek, K.A. (1965). Acquisition of *Staphylococcus aureus* by patients in cubicles. *Br. Med. J.*, **1**, 1101–5.

16 Creighton, C.A. (1984). *A History of Epidemics.* Cambridge: Cambridge University Press.

17 Fairbrother, R.W. (1934). *Handbook of Filterable Viruses.* London: Heinmann.

18 Collier, L.H. (1990). Virology. In *Topley and Wilson's Principles of Bacteriology, Virology and Immunology*, ed. L. Collier, A. Balows and M. Sussman, pp. 1–19. London: Arnold.

19 Zuckerman, A.J., Banatvala, J.E. and Pattison, J.R., eds. (1994). *Principles and Practice of Clinical Virology*, 3rd edn. Chichester and New York: John Wiley and Sons.

20 Spink, W.W. (1978). *Infectious Diseases. Prevention and Treatment in the Nineteenth and Twentieth Centuries.* Folkestone: Dawson.

21 Gale, A.H. (1959). *Epidemic Diseases.* London: Penguin Books.

22 Birmingham General Hospital. Annual reports, 1852–1881.

23 Smith, W., Andrewes, C.H. and Laidlaw, P.P. (1933). A virus obtained from influenza patients. *Lancet*, **255**, 66–8.

24 Landsteiner, K. and Popper, E. (1909). Uebertragung der poliomyelitis acuta affen. *Z. Immunitätsdforsch*, **2**, 377–85.

25 Sabin, A.B. and Olitsky, P.K. (1936). Cultivation of poliomyelitis virus in vitro in human embryonic nervous tissue. *Proc. Soc. Exp. Biol. Med.*, **34**, 357–9.

26 Enders, J.F., Weller, T.H. and Robbins, F.C. (1949). Cultivation of the Lansing strain of poliomyelitis virus in cultures of various human embryonic tissues. *Science*, **109**, 85–7.

27 Christie, A.B. (1980). *Infectious Diseases, Epidemiology and Clinical Practice.* Edinburgh and London: Churchill Livingstone.

28 Winslow, C.E.A. (1944). *The Conquest of Epidemic Disease. A Chapter in the History of Ideas.* Princeton, NJ: Princeton University Press.

29 Pringle, J. (1810). *Observations on the Diseases of the Army*. London: Stockdale.

30 Pringle, J. (1750). *Observations on the Nature and Cure of Hospital and Jayl-fevers*. London: Millar and Wilson.

31 Lind, J. (1757). *An Essay on the Most Effectual Means of Preserving the Health of Seamen, in the Royal Navy*. London: Millar.

32 World Health Organization (1997). *Infectious Diseases: Global Alert, Global Response*. Geneva: World Health Organization.

33 Ayliffe, G.A.J. (1979). Trends in resistance and their significance in primary pathogenic bacteria. In *Recent Advances in Infection*, ed. D. Reeves and A.M. Geddes, pp. 2–18. Edinburgh and London: Churchill Livingstone.

34 Hobbs, B.C. and Roberts, D. (1993). *Food Poisoning and Food Hygiene*, 6th edn. London: Arnold.

35 Kitasato, S. (1889). Ueber den Tetanusbacillus. *Z. Hyg.*, **7**, 225–7.

36 Robinson, D.T., McCleod, J.W. and Downie, A.W. (1946). Dust in surgical theatres as a possible source of post-operative tetanus. *Lancet*, **1**, 152–4.

37 Sevitt, S. (1949). Source of two hospital-infected cases of tetanus. *Lancet*, **2**, 1075–8.

38 Eikhoff, T.C. (1962). An outbreak of surgical wound infections due to *Clostridium perfringens*. *Surg. Gynecol. Obstet.*, **114**, 102–8.

39 Ayliffe, G.A.J. and Lowbury, E.J.L. (1969). Sources of gas gangrene in hospital. *Br. Med. J.*, **2**, 333–7.

40 World Health Organization (1993). *Tuberculosis: A Global Emergency*. Geneva: World Health Organization.

41 Garrison, F.H. (1929). *An Introduction to the History of Medicine*. Philadelphia and London: Saunders.

42 Riley, R.L. and O'Grady, F. (1961). *Airborne Infection*. New York: Macmillan.

43 Hansen, G.A. (1875). On the aetiology of leprosy. *British and Foreign Medico-Chirugical Review*, **55**, 459–89.

44 Bulloch, W. (1938). *The History of Bacteriology*. New York: Dover Publications.

45 Zinsser, H. (1935). *Rats, Lice and History*. Boston: Little Brown.

46 Roncali, R.A. (1987). The history of scabies in veterinary and human medicine from biblical to modern times. *Vet. Parasitol.*, **25**, 193–8.

47 Friedman, R. (1947). *The Story of Scabies*. New York: Froben Press.

48 Herridge, C.F. (1963). Norwegian scabies. *Br. Med. J.*, **1**, 239–40.

Chapter 10

1 Spink, W.W. (1978). *Infectious Diseases. Prevention and Treatment in the Nineteenth and Twentieth Centuries*. Folkestone: Dawson.

2 Domagk, G. (1935). Ein Beitrag zur Chemotherapie der Bacteriellen Infektionen. *Dtsch. Med. Wochenschr.*, **61**, 250–53.

3 Colebrook, L. and Kenny, M. (1936). Treatment of human puerperal infections and of experimental infections in mice with prontosil. *Lancet*, **1**, 1279–86.

4 Lancefield, R.C. (1933). A serological differentiation of human and other groups of haemolytic streptococci. *J. Exp. Med.*, **57**, 571–95.

5 Griffith, F. (1934). The serological classification of *Streptococcus pyogenes*. *J. Hyg. (Camb).*, **34**, 542–84.

6 Allison, V.D. and Brown, W.A. (1937). Reinfection as a cause of complications and relapses in scarlet fever wards. *J. Hyg. (Camb).*, **37**, 153–71.

7 Williams, R.E.O., Blowers, R., Garrod, L. and Shooter, R.A. (1966). *Hospital Infection. Causes and Prevention*, 2nd edn. London: Lloyd Luke.

8 Gregory, J. (1788). *Elements of Practice of Physic*, vol. 4. London: Strahan and Cadell.

9 Colebrook, L. (1954). Puerperal infection in 1800–1950. In *Historical Review of British Obstetrics and Gynaecology, 1800–1950*, ed. M. Kerr *et al.*, pp. 202–25. Edinburgh: Livingstone.

10 Parker, M.T. (1994). Leonard Colebrook and his family. *J. Hosp. Infect.*, **28**, 81–90.

11 Williams, R.E.O. (1994). Sir Ashley Miles. *J. Hosp. Infect.*, **27**, 161–6.

12 Miles, A.A. (1944). Epidemiology of wound infection. *Lancet*, **1**, 809–14.

13 McKissock, W., Wright, J. and Miles, A.A. (1941). The reduction of cross-infection of wounds. A controlled experiment. *Br. Med. J.*, **2**, 375–7.

14 Cruikshank, R. (1935). The bacterial infection of burns. *J. Pathol. Bacteriol.*, **41**, 367–9.

15 Bourdillon, R.B. and Colebrook, L. (1946). Air hygiene in dressing rooms for burns or major wounds. *Lancet*, **1**, 561–5, 601–5.

16 Strasberg, S.M. and Silver, M.S. (1968). Haemolytic streptococcus gangrene. An uncommon but frequent fatal infection in the antibiotic era. *Am. J. Surg.*, **115**, 763–8.

17 Hamburger, M., Jr, Green, M.J. and Hamburger, V.G. (1945). The problem of the 'dangerous carrier' of haemolytic streptococci. 1. Number of haemolytic streptococci expelled by carriers with positive and negative nose cultures. *J. Infect. Dis.*, **77**, 68–81, 96–108.

18 Wright, J., Cruikshank, R. and Dunn, W. (1944). The control of dustborne streptococcal infections in measles wards. *Br. Med. J.*, **1**, 611–14.

19 Rammelkamp, C.H., Morris, A.J. and Catanzaro, F.J. *et al.* (1958). Transmission of group A streptococci. (3). The effect of drying on the effect on the infectivity of the organism for man. *J. Hyg. (Lond.).*, **56**, 280–87.

20 Crossley, K.B. (1999). Streptococci. In *Hospital Epidemiology and Infection Control*, ed. C. Glen Mayhall, pp. 385–93. Baltimore: Williams and Wilkins.

Chapter 11

1 Bowie, J.H. (1955). Modern apparatus for sterilization. *Pharm. J.*, **174**, 473, 489–92.

2 Howie, J.H. and Timbury, M. (1956). Laboratory tests of operating theatre sterilizers. *Lancet*, **2**, 669.

3 Nuffield Provincial Hospitals Trust (1958). *Present Sterilizing Practices in Six Hospitals.* London: Nuffield Provincial Hospitals Trust.

4 Medical Research Council Reports (1959, 1960, 1964). Sterilization by steam under increased pressure. *Lancet*, **1**, 425–35; **2**, 1243–5; **2**, 193–5.

5 Perkins, J.J. (1956). *Principles and Methods of Sterilization.* Springfield, IL: Charles. C. Thomas.

6 Walter, C. (1948). *The Aseptic Treatment of Wounds.* New York: Macmillan.

7 Hansford, J. (1998). Sterile services – the first fifty years of the NHS. *Institute of Sterile Services Journal*, **3**, 18–22.

8 Alder, V.G. and Gillespie, W.A. (1957). The sterilization of dressings. *J. Clin. Pathol.*, **10**, 299–6.

9 Knox, R. and Penikett, E.J.K. (1958). Influence of initial vacuum on steam sterilization of dressings. *Br. Med. J.*, **1**, 680–82.

10 Bowie, J.H., Kelsey, J.C. and Thompson, G.R. (1963). The Bowie and Dick autoclave tape test. *Lancet*, **1**, 586–7.

11 Newsom, S.W.B. (1998, 1999). Sterilisers and the development of sterile services, parts 1 and 2. *Institute of Sterile Services Journal*, **3**(2), 13–15; **3**(4), 11–16.

12 Darmady, E.M., Hughes, K.E.A. and Tuke, W. (1957). Sterilization of syringes by infra-red radiation. *J. Clin. Pathol.*, **10**, 291–8.

13 The Nuffield Provincial Hospitals Trust (1957). *The Planning and Organisation of Central Syringe Services*. London: The Nuffield Provincial Hospitals Trust.

14 Clothier, C.M. (1972). *Report of the Committee Appointed to Inquire into the Circumstances, Including the Production, which Led to the Use of Contaminated Infusion Fluids in the Devonport Section of Plymouth General Hospital*. London: HMSO.

15 Phillips, C.R. and Kaye, S. (1949). The sterilizing action of gaseous ethylene oxide. *Am. J. Hyg.*, **50**, 270–79.

16 Nordgren, C. (1939). Investigation on the sterilization efficacy of gaseous formaldehyde. *Acta. Pathol. Microbiol. Scand. Suppl.*, **40**, 1–165.

17 Alder, V.G. (1987). The formaldehyde/low temperature steam sterilizing procedure. *J. Hosp. Infect.*, **9**, 194–200.

18 Line, S.J. and Pickerill, J.K. (1973). Testing a steam-formaldehyde sterilizer for gas penetrating efficiency. *J. Clin. Pathol.*, **26**, 716–19.

19 Spach, D., Silverstein, F.E. and Stamm, W.E. (1993). Transmission of infection by gastro-intestinal endoscopy and bronchoscopy. *Ann. Intern. Med.*, **118**, 117–28.

20 Ayliffe, G.A.J., Babb, J.R. and Bradley, C.R. (1992). 'Sterilization' of arthroscopes and laparo-scopes. *J. Hosp. Infect.*, **22**, 265–9.

21 Hanlon, G.W. (1999). Re-use of disposables. In *Principles and Practice of Disinfection, Preservation and Sterilization*, ed. A.D. Russell, W.B. Hugo and G.A.J. Ayliffe, pp. 777–86. Oxford: Blackwell Science.

22 Ayliffe, G.A.J., Coates, D. and Hoffman, P.N. (1993). *Chemical Disinfection in Hospitals*. London: Public Health Laboratory Service.

23 Rutala, W.A. (1996). APIC guideline for selection and use of disinfectants. *Am. J. Infect. Control*, **24**, 313–42.

24 Wangensteen, O.H. and Wangensteen, S.D. (1978). *The Rise of Surgery from Empiric Craft to Scientific Discipline*. Minneapolis: University of Minnesota Press.

25 Block, S.S. (2001). *Disinfection, Sterilization and Preservation*, 5th edn. Philadelphia: Lippincott Williams and Wilkins.

26 Russell, A.D., Hugo, W.B. and Ayliffe, G.A.J. (1999). *Principles and Practice of Disinfection, Preservation and Sterilization*, 3rd edn. Oxford: Blackwell Science.

27 Brewer, J.H. (1939). The antibacterial effects of the organic mercurial compounds with special reference to their use as germicides for sterilization of surgical and dental instruments. *J. Am. Med. Assoc.*, **112**, 2009–18.

28 Ayliffe, G.A.J., Fraise, A.P., Geddes, A.M. and Mitchell, K. (2000). *Control of Hospital Infection. A Practical Handbook*, 4th edn. London: Arnold.

29 Alder, V.G. and Gillespie, W.A. (1961). Disinfection of woollen blankets in steam at sub-atmospheric pressure. *J. Clin. Pathol.*, **14**, 515–18.

30 Domagk, G. (1935). Eine neue Klasse von disinfektionsmitteln. *Dtsch. Med. Wochenschr.*, **61**, 829–32.

31 Davies, G.E., Francis, J., Martin, A.R., *et al.* (1954). 1:6-Di-4-chlorophenyl-diguanidohexane ('Hibitane'): laboratory investigation of a new antibacterial agent of high potency. *Br. J. Pharmacol.*, **9**, 192–6.

32 Lowbury, E.J.L. and Lilly, H.A. (1973). Use of 4% chlorhexidine detergent solution (Hibiscrub) and other methods of skin disinfection. *Br. Med. J.*, **1**, 510–15.

33 Lowbury, E.J.L., Lilly, H.A. and Ayliffe, G.A.J. (1974). Pre-operative disinfection of surgeon's hands: use of alcoholic solutions and effect of gloves on the skin flora. *Br. Med. J.*, **4**, 369–72.

34 Newsom, S.W.B. (1999). Special problems in hospital antisepsis. In *Principles and Practice of Disinfection, Preservation and Sterilization*, ed. A.D. Russell, W.B. Hugo and G.A.J. Ayliffe, 4th edn, pp. 416–37. Oxford: Blackwell Science.

35 Public Health Laboratory Service (1965). Use of disinfectants in hospitals. A report by the Public Health Laboratory Service Committee on the testing and evaluation of disinfectants. *Br. Med. J.*, **1**, 408–13.

36 Larson, E. (1988). A causal link between handwashing and risk of infection? Examination of the evidence. *Infect. Control Hosp. Epidemiol.*, **9**, 28–36.

37 Beck, E.G., Borneff, J., Grun, L., *et al.* (1977). Empfehlungen für die Prüfung und Bewertung der Wirksamkeit Chemischer Disinfektionsverfahren. *Zentralbl Bakteriol. [B]*, **165**, 335–80.

38 The 2nd international colloquium about the evaluation (classification) of disinfectants in Europe (1973). English translation. *Zentralbl. Bakteriol. [B]*, **157**, 411–551.

39 Reybrouk, G. (1999). Evaluation of the efficacy of antimicrobial agents. In *Principles and Practice of Disinfection, Preservation and Sterilization*, ed. A.D. Russell, W.B. Hugo and G.A.J. Ayliffe, 4th edn., pp. 124–44. Oxford: Blackwell Science.

40 Rotter, M.L. (1999). Hand washing and hand disinfection. In *Hospital Epidemiology and Infection Control*, ed. C. Glen Mayhall, pp. 1339–55. Baltimore: Williams and Wilkins.

41 Ayliffe, G.A.J., Babb, J.R. and Taylor, L.J. (1999). *Hospital-acquired Infection. Principles and Prevention*, 3rd edn. Oxford: Butterworth Heinemann.

42 Hugo, W.B. (1978). Early studies in the evaluation of disinfectants. *J. Antimicrob. Chemother.*, **4**, 489–94.

43 Bullock, W. (1938). *The History of Bacteriology*. New York: Dover Publications.

44 Brock, T.D. (1961). *Milestones in Microbiology*. London: Prentice Hall.

45 Reddish, G.F. (1927). Examination of disinfectants. *Am. J. Public Health*, **17**, 320–29.

46 Rideal, S. and Walker, J.T.A. (1903). The standardization of disinfectants. *Journal of the Royal Sanitary Institute*, **24**, 424–41.

Chapter 12

1 Meleney, F.L. (1948). *Treatise on Surgical Infections*. New York: Oxford University Press.

2 Loeb, L. (1903). The influence of certain bacteria on the coagulation of the blood. *J. Med. Res.*, **10**, 407–19.

3 Elek, S.D. (1959). *Staphylococcus pyogenes and its Relation to Disease.* Edinburgh and London: Livingstone.

4 Fleming, A. (1929). On the antibacterial action of cultures of a Penicillium, with special reference to their use in the isolation of *B. influenzae. Br. J. Exp. Pathol.*, **10**, 226–36.

5 Chain, E., Florey, H.W., Gardner, A.D., *et al.* (1940). Penicillin as a chemotherapeutic agent. *Lancet*, **2**, 226–8.

6 Barber, M. (1947). Staphylococcal infections due to penicillin-resistant strains. *Br. Med. J.*, **2**, 863–5.

7 Lowbury, E.J.L. and Ayliffe, G.A.J. (1974). *Drug Resistance in Antimicrobial Therapy.* Springfield, IL: Charles C. Thomas.

8 Spink, W.W. (1978). *Infectious Diseases: Prevention and Treatment in the Nineteenth and Twentieth Centuries.* Folkestone: Dawson.

9 Fisk, R.T. (1942). Studies on staphylococci-2. Identification of *Staphylococcus aureus* strains by means of bacteriophage. *J. Infect. Dis.*, **71**, 161–5.

10 Wilson, G.S. and Atkinson, J.D. (1945). Typing of staphylococci by the bacteriophage method. *Lancet*, **1**, 647–8.

11 Blair, J.E. and Williams, R.E.O. (1961). Phage typing of staphylococci. *Bull. World Health Organ.*, **24**, 771–84.

12 Rountree, P.M. and Freeman, B.M. (1955). Infections caused by a particular phage type of *Staphylococcus aureus. Med. J. Aust.*, **2**, 157–60.

13 Williams, R.E.O., Blowers, R., Garrod, L.P. and Shooter, R.A. (1966). *Hospital Infection. Causes and Prevention*, 2nd edn. London: Lloyd-Luke.

14 Shooter, R.A., Smith, M.A., Griffiths, J.D., *et al.* (1958). Spread of staphylococci in a surgical ward. *Br. Med. J.*, **1**, 607–13.

15 Gillespie, W.A., Alder, V.G. and Ayliffe, G.A.J. (1959). Staphylococcal cross-infection in surgery Effects of some preventive measures. *Lancet*, **1**, 781–4.

16 Barber, M. and Garrod, L.P. (1963). *Antibiotic and Chemotherapy.* Edinburgh and London: Livingstone.

17 Shanson, D.C. (1981). Antibiotic-resistant *Staphylococcus aureus. J. Hosp. Infect.*, **2**, 11–36.

18 Rolinson, G.N., Stevens, S., Batchelor, F.R., *et al.* (1960). Bacteriological studies on a new penicillin BRL 1241. *Lancet*, **11**, 564–7.

19 Tansey, E.M. and Reynolds, L.A. (2000). *Wellcome Witnesses to Medicine, vol. 6. Post Penicillin Antibiotics from Acceptance to Resistance.* London: Wellcome Trust.

20 Jevons, M.P. (1961). 'Celbenin'-resistant staphylococci. *Br. Med. J.*, **1**, 124–5.

21 Barber, M. (1961). Hospital infection yesterday and today. *J. Clin. Pathol.*, **14**, 2–10.

22 Ayliffe, G.A.J. (1997). The progressive intercontinental spread of methicillin-resistant *Staphylococcus aureus. Clin. Infect. Dis.*, **24** (Suppl. 1), S74–S79.

23 Brachman, P.S. and Eikhoff, T.S., eds. (1970). *Proceedings of the International Conference on Nosocomial Infections, Centers for Disease Control, August 3–6.* Chicago: American Hospital Association.

24 Duguid, J.P. and Wallace, A.T. (1948). Air infection with dust liberated from clothing. *Lancet*, **2**, 845–9.

25 Hare, R. and Thomas, C.G.A. (1956). Transmission of *Staphylococcus aureus*. *Br. Med. J.*, **2**, 840–44.

26 Davies, R.R. and Noble, W.G. (1962). Dispersal of bacteria on desquamated skin. *Lancet*, **2**, 1295–7.

27 Solberg, C.O. (1965). A study of carriers of *Staphylococcus aureus*. *Acta. Med. Scand.*, **175** (Suppl. 436), 1–96.

28 Blowers, R., Hill, J. and Howell, A. (1973). Shedding of *Staphylococcus aureus* by human carriers. In *Airborne Transmission and Airborne Infection*, ed. J.F.P. Hers and W.C. Winkler, pp. 432–4. Utrecht: Oosthoek.

29 Ayliffe, G.A.J., Babb, J.R. and Collins, B.J. (1973). Dispersal and carriage of staphylococci in healthy male and female subjects and patients with skin disease. In *Airborne Transmission and Airborne Infection*, ed. J.F.P. Hers and W.C. Winkler, pp. 435–7. Utrecht: Oosthoek.

30 White, A. (1961). Relation between quantitative nasal cultures and the dissemination of staphylococci. *J. Lab. Clin. Med.*, **58**, 273–7.

31 Ayliffe, G.A.J. and Lowbury, E.J.L. (1982). Airborne infection. *J. Hosp. Infect.*, **3**, 217–40.

32 Hare, R. and Cooke, E.M. (1961). Self-contamination of patients with staphylococcal infections. *Br. Med. J.*, **2**, 333–6.

33 Selwyn, S. and Chambers, D. (1965). Dispersal of bacteria from skin lesions: a hospital hazard. *Br. J. Dermatol.*, **77**, 349–56.

34 Eichenwald, H.F., Kotsevalov, O. and Fasso, L.A. (1960). The 'cloud baby' an example of bacterial-viral interaction. *Am. J. Dis. Child.*, **100**, 161–73.

35 Mortimer, E.A., Jr, Lipsitz, P.J., Wolinski, E., *et al.* (1966). Transmission of staphylococci between newborns. Importance of the hands of personnel. *Am. J. Dis. Child.*, **104**, 289–95.

36 Mortimer, E.A., Jr, Wolinski, E., Gonzaga, A.J. and Rammelkam, C.H., Jr (1966). Role of airborne transmission in staphylococcal infections. *Br. Med. J.*, **1**, 319–22.

37 Williams, R.E.O. (1966). Epidemiology of airborne staphylococcal infection. *Bacteriol. Rev.*, **30**, 660–72.

38 Ayliffe, G.A.J., Brightwell, K.M., Collins, B.J., *et al.* (1977). Surveys of hospitals in the Birmingham region. 1. Effect of age, length of stay and antibiotic use on nasal carriage of tetracycline-resistant *Staphylococcus aureus* and on post-operative wound infection. *J. Hyg. (Lond.).*, **79**, 299–314.

39 Colebrook, L., Duncan, J.M. and Ross, W.P.D. (1948). The control of infection in burns. *Lancet*, **1**, 893–9.

40 Lowbury, E.J.L. (1954). Air conditioning with filtered air for dressing burns *Lancet*, **1**, 292–4.

41 Ayliffe, G.A.J. and Beard, M.A. (1962). A system of air recirculation and antibacterial surface treatment in a surgical ward. *J. Clin. Pathol.*, **15**, 242–6.

42 Parker, M.T., John, M., Emond, R.T.D. and Machacek, K.A. (1965). Acquisition of *Staphylococcus aureus* by patients in cubicles. *Br. Med. J.*, **1**, 1101–5.

43 Maki, D.G., Alvarado, C.J., Hassemer, M.L., *et al.* (1982). Relation of the inanimate environment to endemic nosocomial infection. *N. Engl. J. Med.*, **307**, 1562–6.

44 Van Griethuysen, A.J.A., Spies-van Rooijen, N.H. and Hoogenboom-Verdegaal, A.M.M. (1996). Surveillance of wound infections and a new theatre: unexpected lack of improvement. *J. Hosp. Infect.*, **34**, 99–106.

45 Williams, R.E.O., Noble, W.C., Jevons, M.P., *et al.* (1962). Isolation for the control of staphy-lococcal infection in surgical wards. *Br. Med. J.*, **2**, 275–82.

46 Brachman, P.S. and Eikhoff, T.S., eds. (1970). *Proceedings of the International Conference on Nosocomial Infections, Centers for Disease Control, August 3–6.* Chicago: American Hospital Association.

47 Lidwell, O.M. (1981). Some aspects of the transfer and acquisition of *Staphylococcus aureus* in hospitals. In *The Staphylococci. Proceedings of the Alexander Ogston Centennial Conference,* ed. A. Macdonald and G. Smith, pp. 175–202. Aberdeen: Aberdeen University Press.

48 Burke, J.F. (1963). Identification of the sources of staphylococci contaminating the surgical wound during operation. *Ann. Surg.*, **158**, 898–904.

49 Bengtsson, S., Hambraeus, A. and Laurell, G. (1979). Wound infections after surgery in a modern operating suite: clinical, bacteriological and epidemiological findings *J. Hyg. (Lond.).*, **83**, 41–57.

50 Ayliffe, G.A.J. (1991). Role of the environment in the operating suite in surgical wound infection. *Rev. Infect. Dis.*, **13** (Suppl. 10), S800–S804.

51 Humphreys, H. and Taylor, E.W. (2002). Operating theatre ventilation standards and the risk of post-operative infection. *J. Hosp. Infect.*, **50**, 85–90.

52 Rountree, P.M. and Beard, M.A. (1968). Hospital strains of *Staphylococcus aureus* with particular reference to methicillin-resistant strains. *Med. J. Aust.*, **2**, 1163–8.

53 Ayliffe, G.A.J., Collins, B.J., Lowbury, E.J.L., *et al.* (1967). Ward floors and other surfaces as reservoirs of hospital infection. *J. Hyg. (Lond.).*, **65**, 515–36.

54 Hambraeus, A. (1973). Transfer of *Staphylococcus aureus* via nurses' uniforms. *J. Hyg. (Lond.).*, **71**, 799–814.

55 Ayliffe, G.A.J., Babb, J.R. and Taylor, L. (1999). *Hospital-acquired Infection. Principles and Prevention.* Oxford: Butterworth Heinmann.

56 Wypkema, W. and Alder, V.G. (1962). Hospital cross-infection and dirty walls. *Lancet*, **2**, 1066–8.

Chapter 13

1 Finland, M., Jones, W.F. and Barnes, M.W. (1959). Occurrence of serious bacterial infections since introduction of antibacterial agents. *J. Am. Med. Assoc.*, **170**, 2188–97.

2 McCabe, W.R. and Jackson, G.C. (1962). Gram-negative bacteraemias. *Arch. Intern. Med.*, **110**, 847–55.

3 McHenry, M.C., Martin, W.J. and Wellman, W.F. (1962). Bacteraemia due to Gram-negative bacilli. *Ann. Intern. Med.*, **56**, 207–19.

4 French, G. (2000). Nosocomial Gram-negative infections. *Br. J. Infect. Control*, **2**, 9–12.

5 Watanabe, T. (1963). Infectious drug resistance in enteric bacteria. *Bacteriol. Rev.*, **27**, 87–115.

6 Lowbury, E.J.L. and Ayliffe, G.A.J. (1974). *Drug Resistance in Antimicrobial Therapy.* Springfield, IL: Charles C. Thomas.

7 Datta, N. (1962). Transmissible drug resistance in an epidemic strain of *Salmonella typhimurium. J. Hyg. (Camb.).*, **60**, 301–10.

8 Lowbury, E.J.L., Kidson, A. and Lilly, H.A., *et al*. (1969). Sensitivity of *Pseudomonas aeruginosa* to antibiotics: emergence of strains highly resistant to carbenicillin. *Lancet*, **2**, 448–52.

9 Greenwood, D. (1989). *Antimicrobial Chemotherapy*. Oxford: Oxford University Press.

10 Ayliffe, G.A.J., Babb, J.R. and Taylor, L.J. (1999). *Hospital-acquired Infection. Principles and Prevention*, 3rd edn. Oxford: Butterworth Heinemann.

11 Gould, J.C. (1963). *Pseudomonas pyocyanea* infections in hospitals. In *Infection in Hospitals. Epidemiology and Control*, ed. R.E.O. Williams and R.A. Shooter, pp. 119–30. Oxford: Blackwell Scientific Publications.

12 Russell, A.D., Hugo, W.B. and Ayliffe, G.A.J. (1999). *Principles and Practice of Disinfection, Preservation and Sterilization*, 3rd edn. Oxford: Blackwell Scientific Publications.

13 Lowbury, E.J.L., Thom, B.T., Lilly, H.A., *et al*. (1970). Sources of infection with *Pseudomonas aeruginosa* in patients with tracheostomy. *J. Med. Microbiol.*, **3**, 39–56.

14 Maki, D.G., Rhame, F.S., Mackel, D.C. and Bennett, J.V. (1976). Nationwide epidemic of septicaemia caused by contaminated intravenous products. 1. Epidemiologic and clinical features. *Am. J. Med.*, **60**, 471–85.

15 Ayliffe, G.A.J., Babb, J.R. and Collins, B.J. (1976). Environmental hazards – real and imaginary. *Health Soc. Serv. J.*, (Suppl.), June, 3–4.

16 Williams, R.E.O., Blowers, R., Garrod, L.P. and Shooter, R.A. (1966). *Hospital Infection. Causes and Prevention*. London: Lloyd-Luke.

17 Macleod, J.W. (1958). The hospital urine bottle and bed pan as reservoirs of infection by *Pseudomonas pyocyanea*. *Lancet*, **1**, 394–7.

18 Spach, D., Silverstein, F.E. and Stamm, W.E. (1993). Transmission of infection by gastro-intestinal endoscopy and bronchoscopy. *Ann. Intern. Med.*, **118**, 117–28.

19 Ayliffe, G.A.J. (1999). Nosocomial infections associated with endoscopy. In *Hospital Epidemiology and Infection Control*, ed. C. Glen Mayhall, pp. 881–95. Baltimore: Williams and Wilkins.

20 Favero, M.S., Petersen, N.J., Carson, L.A., *et al*. (1975). Gram-negative water bacteria in haemodialysis systems. *Health. Lab. Sci.*, **12**, 321–34.

21 Skinner (1873). Anaesthetics and inhalers. *Br. Med. J.*, **1**, 353–4.

22 Magath, T.B. (1938). Method for preventing cross-infection with gas machines. *Anesth. Analg.*, **17**, 215–17.

23 Phillips, I. and Spencer, G. (1965). *Pseudomonas aeruginosa* cross-infection due to contaminated respiratory apparatus. *Lancet*, **2**, 1325–7.

24 Reinarz, J.A., Pierce, A.K., Mays, B.B. and Sanford, J.P. (1965). The potential role of inhalation equipment in nosocomial pulmonary infection. *J. Clin. Invest.*, **44**, 831–9.

25 Johanson, W.G., Pierce, A.K. and Sanford, J.P. (1969). Changing pharyngeal flora of hospitalized patients. Emergence of gram-negative bacilli. *N. Engl. J. Med.*, **281**, 1137–40.

26 Bray, J. (1945). Isolation of antigenically homogenous strains of *Bact coli neopolitanum* from summer diarrhoea of infants. *J. Pathol. Bacteriol.*, **57**, 239–47.

27 Rogers, K.B. (1963). Epidemiology of hospital coliform enteritis. In *Infection in Hospitals: Epidemiology and Control*, ed. R.E.O. Williams and R.A. Shooter, pp. 131–54. Oxford: Blackwell Scientific Publications.

28 Department of Health and Social Security (1986). *The Report of the Committee of Inquiry into an Outbreak of Food Poisoning at Stanley Royd Hospital.* London: HMSO.

29 Spink, W.W. (1978). *Infectious Diseases. Prevention and Treatment in the Nineteenth and Twentieth Centuries.* Folkestone: Dawson.

30 Taylor, J. (1963). Salmonella infections in hospitals. In *Infection in Hospitals: Epidemiology and Control*, ed. R.E.O. Williams and R.A. Shooter, pp. 145–54. Oxford: Blackwell Scientific Publications.

31 Datta, N. and Pridie, R.B. (1960). An outbreak of infection with *Salmonella typhimurium* in a general hospital. *J. Hyg. (Lond.).*, **58**, 229–41.

32 Bate, J.G. and James, U. (1958). *Salmonella typhimurium* dust-borne infection in a children's ward. *Lancet*, **2**, 713–15.

Chapter 14

1   Ministry of Health (1959). *Control of Staphylococcal Infections in Hospitals.* London: HMSO.

2   Altemeier, W.A. (1959). Report of the national conference on hospital-acquired staphylococcal disease. *Surgery*, **45**, 522–6.

3   Godber, G. (1963). *Prevention of Hospital Infection. The Personal Factor.* London: Royal Society of Health, 1–3.

4   Barnes, B.A., Behringer, G.E., Wheelock, F.C., *et al.* (1959). Surgical sepsis: an analysis of factors associated with sepsis in two operative procedures 1937–1957. *N. Engl. J. Med.*, **261**, 1351–7.

5   Barnes, B.A., Behringer, G.E. and Wheelock, F.C., *et al.* (1960). Surgical sepsis: report on subtotal gastrectomies. *J. Am. Med. Assoc.*, **173**, 1068–75.

6   Dineen, P. and Pearce, C. (1958). A ten-year study of wound infections. *Surg. Gynecol. Obstet.*, **106**, 453–8.

7   Jeffrey, J.S. and Sclaroff, S.A. (1958). Incidence of wound infection. *Lancet*, **1**, 365–8.

8   Clarke, S.K.R. (1957). Sepsis in surgical wounds with particular reference to *Staphylococcus aureus. Br. J. Surg.*, **44**, 592–6.

9   Williams, R.E.O., Blowers, R., Garrod, L.P. and Shooter, R.A. (1966). *Hospital Infection. Causes and Prevention.* London: Lloyd-Luke.

10 Hearn, G.W. (1987). *Dudley Road Hospital 1887–1987.* Birmingham: Postgraduate Centre.

11 Public Health Laboratory Service (1960). Incidence of surgical wound infection in England and Wales. *Lancet*, **2**, 659–63.

12 National Research Council (1964). Post-operative wound infections: the influence of ultra-violet irradiation of the operating room and of various other factors. *Ann. Surg.*, **160** (Suppl. 2), 1–191.

13 Ayliffe, G.A.J., Fraise, A.P., Geddes, A.M. and Mitchell, K. (2000). *Control of Hospital Infection. A Practical Handbook*, 4th edn. London: Arnold.

14 Lidwell, O.M. (1963). Methods of investigation and analysis of results. In *Infection in Hospitals. Epidemiology and Control*, ed. R.E.O. Williams and R.A. Shooter, pp. 43–6. Oxford: Blackwell Scientific Publications.

15 Cruse, P.J.E. and Foord, R. (1980). The epidemiology of wound infection. A 10-year prospective study of 62,939 wounds. *Surg. Clin. North Am.*, **60**, 27–40.

16 Bibby, B.A., Collins, B.J. and Ayliffe, G.A.J. (1986). A mathematical model for assessing post-operative wound infection. *J. Hosp. Infect.*, **8**, 31–9.

17 Simchen, E., Stein, H., Sacks, T.G., *et al.* (1984). Multivariate analysis of determinants of post-operative wound infection in orthopaedic patients *J. Hosp. Infect.*, **5**, 137–46.

18 Culver, D.H., Horan, T.C., Gaynes, R.P., *et al.* (1991). Surgical wound infection rates by wound class, operative procedure, and patient risk index. *Am. J. Med.*, **91**, (Suppl. 3B), 152S–157S.

19 Medical Research Council (1962). Design and ventilation of operating room suites for control of infection and for comfort. *Lancet*, **2**, 945–51.

20 Hart, D. (1960). Bactericidal ultraviolet irradiation in the operating room. *J. Am. Med. Assoc.*, **172**, 1019–28.

21 Charnley, J. and Eftekhar, M. (1969). Postoperative infection in total prosthetic replacement arthroplasty of the hip joint with special reference to the bacterial content of the air in the operating room. *Br. J. Surg.*, **56**, 641–9.

22 Lidwell, O.M., Lowbury, E.J.L., Whyte, W., *et al.* (1982). Effect of ultraclean air in operating rooms on deep sepsis in the joint after operation for total hip or knee replacement: a randomized study. *Br. Med. J.*, **285**, 10–14.

23 Babb, J.R., Lynam, P. and Ayliffe, G.A.J. (1995). Risk of airborne infection in an operating theatre containing four ultra clean air units. *J. Hosp. Infect.*, **31**, 159–68.

24 Meleney, F.L. (1948). *Treatise on Surgical Infections*. New York: Oxford University Press.

25 Walter, C.W. (1958). *The Aseptic Treatment of Wounds*. New York: Macmillan.

26 Altemeier, W.A., Burke, J.F., Pruitt, B.A. and Sandusky, W.R. (1984). *Manual on Control of Infection in Surgical Patients*. Philadelphia: Lippincott.

27 Medical Research Council (1968). Aseptic methods in the operating suite. *Lancet*, **1**, 705–9, 763–8, 831–9.

28 Tunevall, T.G. (1991). Post-operative wound infections and surgical masks: a controlled study. *World J. Surg.*, **15**, 383–8.

29 Belkin, N.L. (1997). The evolution of the surgical mask: filtering efficiency versus effectiveness. *Infect. Control Hosp. Epidemiol.*, **18**, 49–57.

30 Wypkema, W. and Alder, V.G. (1962). Hospital cross-infection and dirty walls. *Lancet*, **2**, 1066–8.

31 Ayliffe, G.A.J., Brightwell, K.M., Collins, B.J., *et al.* (1969). Varieties of practice in hospital wards. *Lancet*, **2**, 1117–20.

32 Centers for Disease Control (1970). *Isolation Techniques*. Washington, DC: US Government Printing Office.

33 Garner, J. (1996). Guideline for isolation precautions in hospitals. *Infect. Control Hosp. Epidemiol.*, **17**, 53–80.

34 Gillespie, W.A., Alder, V.G., Ayliffe, G.A.J., *et al.* (1961). Control of staphylococcal cross-infection in surgical wards. *Lancet*, **1**, 1299–1303.

35 Rountree, P.M., Loewenthal, J., Tedder, E., *et al.* (1962). Staphylococcal wound infection: the use of neomycin and chlorhexidine (Naseptin) nasal cream in its control. *Med. J. Aust.*, **2**, 367–70.

36 Henderson, R.J. and Williams, R.E.O. (1961). Nasal disinfection in prevention of post-operative staphylococcal infection of wounds. *Br. Med. J.*, **2**, 230–33.

37 Wenzel, R.P. and Perl, T.M. (1995). The significance of nasal carriage of *Staphylococcus aureus* and the incidence of postoperative wound infection. *J. Hosp. Infect.*, **31**, 13–24.

38 Solberg, C.O. (1965). A study of carriers of *Staphylococcus aureus*. *Acta. Med. Scand.*, **175** (Suppl. 436), 1–96.

39 McKissock, W., Wright, J. and Miles, A.A. (1941). The reduction of hospital infection of wounds. A controlled experiment. *Br. Med. J.*, **2**, 375–7.

40 Plueckhahn, V.D. and Banks, J. (1963). Antisepsis and staphylococcal disease in the newborn. *Med. J. Aust.*, **2**, 519–23.

41 Gezon, H.M., Thompson, D.J., Rogers, K.D., *et al.* (1964). Hexachlorophene bathing in early infancy. Effect on staphylococcal disease and infection. *N. Engl. J. Med.*, **270**, 379–86.

42 Simpson, K., Tozer, R.C. and Gillespie, W.A. (1960). Prevention of staphylococcal sepsis in a maternity hospital by means of hexachlorophene. *Br. Med. J.*, **1**, 315–17.

43 Dukes, C. (1928–29). Urinary infections after excision of rectum: their cause and prevention. *Proc. R. Soc. Med.*, **22**, 259–69.

44 Pyrah, L.H., Goldie, W., Parsons, F.M. and Raper, F. (1955). Control of *Pseudomonas pyocyanea* infection in a urological ward. *Lancet*, **2**, 314–17.

45 Miller, A., Gillespie, W.A., Linton, K.B., *et al.* (1958). Post-operative infection in urology. *Lancet*, **2**, 608–12.

46 Kunin, C.M. and McCormack, R.C. (1966). Prevention of catheter-induced urinary-tract infections by sterile closed drainage. *N. Engl. J. Med.*, **274**, 1155–61.

47 Slade, N. and Gillespie, W.A. (1985). *The Urinary Tract and the Catheter in Infection and Other Problems*. Chichester: John Wiley and Sons.

48 Fryklund, B., Haeggman, S. and Burman, L.G. (1997). Transmission of urinary bacterial strains between patients with indwelling catheters – nursing in the same and in separate rooms compared. *J. Hosp. Infect.*, **36**, 147–53.

49 Tablan, O.C., Anderson, L.J., Arden, N.H., *et al.* (1994). Guideline for prevention of nosocomial pneumonia. *Infect. Control Hosp. Epidemiol.*, **15**, 587–627.

50 Craven, D.I., Connolly, M.G., Lichtenberg, D.A., *et al.* (1982). Contamination of mechanical ventilators with tubing change every 24 or 48 hours. *N. Engl. J. Med.*, **306**, 1505–9.

51 Van Saene, H.K.F., Stoutenbeck, C.P. and Hart, C.A. (1991). Selective decontamination of the digestive tract (SSD) in intensive care patients: a critical evaluation of the clinical and epidemiological benefits. *J. Hosp. Infect.*, **18**, 261–77.

52 Knight, V. and Holzer, A.R. (1954). Studies on staphylococci from hospital patients. 1. Predominance of strains of group 3 phage patterns which are resistant to multiple antibiotics. *J. Clin. Invest.*, **33**, 1190–98.

53 McGowan, J.E. (1983). Antimicrobial resistance in hospital organisms and its relation to hospital use. *Rev. Infect. Dis.*, **5**, 1033–48.

54 Ayliffe, G.A.J., Brightwell, K.M., Collins, B.J., *et al.* (1977). Surveys of hospital infection in the Birmingham region. 1. Effect of age, sex, length of stay and antibiotic use on nasal carriage of tetracycline-resistant *Staphylococcus aureus* and on post-operative wound infection. *J. Hyg. (Lond.).*, **79**, 299–314.

55 Barber, M. and Garrod, L.P. (1963). *Antibiotic and Chemotherapy*. Edinburgh and London: Livingstone.

56 Barber, M., Dutton, A.A.C., Beard, M.A., *et al.* (1960). Reversal of antibiotic resistance in hospital staphylococcal infection. *Br. Med. J.*, **1**, 11–17.

57 Lowbury, E.J.L. (1957). Chemotherapy for *Staphylococcus aureus*. Combined use of novobiocin and erythromycin and other methods in the treatment of burns. *Lancet*, **2**, 305–10.

58 Price, D.J.E. and Sleigh, J.D. (1970). Control of infection due to *Klebsiella aerogenes* in a neurosurgical unit by withdrawal of all antibiotics. *Lancet*, **2**, 1213–15.

59 Lowbury, E.J.L. and Ayliffe, G.A.J. (1974). *Drug Resistance in Antimicrobial Therapy*, Springfield, IL: Charles C. Thomas.

60 Burke, J.F. (1961). The effective period of preventive antibiotic action in experimental incisions and dermal lesions. *Surgery*, **50**, 161–8.

61 Bernard, H.R. and Cole, W.R. (1964). The prophylaxis of surgical infection: the effect of prophylactic antimicrobial drugs on the incidence of infection following potentially contaminated operations. *Surgery*, **56**, 151–6.

62 Simchen, E., Shapiro, M., Michel, J. and Sacks, T.G. (1980). The successful use of antibiotic prophylaxis in selected high risk patients under non-trial everyday conditions. *J. Hosp. Infect.*, **1**, 211–20.

63 Colebrook, L. (1950). *A New Approach to the Treatment of Burns and Scalds*. London: Fine Technical Publications.

64 Lowbury, E.J.L. (1976). Prophylaxis and treatment for infection in burns. *Br. J. Hosp. Med.*, **15**, 566–72.

65 Newsom, S.W.B. (1999). Special problems in hospital antisepsis. In *Principles and Practice of Disinfection, Preservation and Sterilization*, ed. A.D. Russell, W.B. Hugo and G.A.J. Ayliffe, 3rd edn., pp. 416–37. Oxford: Blackwell Science.

66 Mayhall, C.G. (1999). Nosocomial burn wound infection. In *Hospital Epidemiology and Infection Control*, 2nd edn, ed. C. Glen Mayhall, pp. 275–86. Baltimore: Lippincott Williams and Wilkins.

67 Ayliffe, G.A.J. and Lawrence, J.C., eds. (1985). Symposium on infection control in burns. *J. Hosp. Infect.*, **6** (Suppl. B), 3–66.

Chapter 15

1 Benenson, A.S. (1995). *Control of Communicable Disease in Man*, 16th edn. New York: American Public Health Association.

2 La Force, F.M. (1997). The control of infections in hospitals: 1750–1950. In *Prevention and Control of Nosocomial Infections*, 3rd edn, ed. R.P. Wenzel, pp. 3–17. Baltimore: Lippincott Williams and Wilkins.

3 Watkins, A.G. and Lewis Faning, E. (1949). Incidence of cross-infection in children's wards. *Br. Med. J.*, **2**, 616–19.

4 Goodall, J.W.D. (1952). Cross-infection in hospital wards. Its incidence and prevention. *Lancet*, **1**, 807–12.

5 Gardner, A.M.N., Stamp, M., Bowgen, J.A. and Moore, B. (1962). The infection control sister. A new member of the infection control team in general hospitals. *Lancet*, **2**, 710–11.

6 Eikhoff, T.C., Brachman, P.S., Bennett, J.V. and Brown, J. (1969). Surveillance of nosocomial infections in community hospitals. 1. Surveillance methods, effectiveness and initial results. *J. Infect. Dis.*, **120**, 305–17.

7 Brachman, P.S. and Eikhoff, T.C., eds. (1971). *Proceedings of the International Conference on Nosocomial Infections, Centers for Disease Control, 1970.* Chicago: American Hospital Association.

8 Ayliffe, G.A.J. and Mitchell, K. (1993). Incidence of hospital acquired infection. *J. Hosp. Infect.*, **24**, 77–80.

9 National Nosocomial Surveillance System (1991). Nosocomial infection rates for inter-hospital comparisons: limitations and possible solutions. *Infect. Control Hosp. Epidemiol.*, **11**, 609–21.

10 Haley, R.W., Culver, D.H., White, J.W., *et al.* (1985). The efficacy of infection surveillance and control programs in preventing nosocomial infections in US hospitals. *Am. J. Epidemiol.*, **121**, 182–205.

11 McGowan, J.E. and Finland, M. (1974). Infection and antibiotic usage at Boston City Hospital: changes in prevalence during the decade 1964–1973. *J. Infect. Dis.*, **129**, 421–8.

12 Meers, P., Ayliffe, G.A.J., Emmerson, A.M., *et al.* (1981). Report on the national survey of infection in hospitals 1980. *J. Hosp. Infect.*, **2** (Suppl.), 1–51.

13 Mayon-White, R.T., Ducel, G., Kereselidze, T. and Tikhomirov, E. (1988). An international survey of the prevalence of hospital-acquired infection. *J. Hosp. Infect.*, **11** (Suppl. A), 43–8.

14 Emmerson, A.M. and Ayliffe, G.A.J., eds. (1996). *Surveillance of Nosocomial Infections.* London: Baillière Tindall.

15 Emmerson, A.M., Enstone, J.E. and Griffin, M., *et al.* (1996).The second national prevalence survey of infection in hospitals. Overview of the results. *J. Hosp. Infect.*, **32**, 175–90.

16 The French Prevalence Survey Study Group (2000). Prevalence of nosocomial infections in France: results of the nationwide survey in 1996. *J. Hosp. Infect.*, **46**, 186–93.

17 French, G.L. (1996). Repeated prevalence surveys. In *Surveillance of Nosocomial Infections*, ed. A.M. Emmerson and G.A.J. Ayliffe, pp. 178–95. London: Baillière Tindall.

18 Lowbury, E.J.L., Ayliffe, G.A.J., Geddes, A.M. and Williams, J.D. (1975). *Control of Hospital Infection. A Practical Handbook*, 1st edn. London: Chapman and Hall.

19 Kjaeldgaard, P., Cordtz, T., Sejberg, D., *et al.* (1989). The DANOP-DATA system: a low cost personal computer-based program for monitoring of wound infections in surgical wards. *J. Hosp. Infect.*, **13**, 273–9.

20 Worning, A.M. and Mertens, R. (1991). Developing quality of care through information systems. *J. Healthc. Mater. Manage.*, **9**, 74–6.

21 Mertens, R.A.F. (1996). Methodologies and results of national surveillance. In *Surveillance of Nosocomial Infections*, ed. A.M. Emmerson and G.A.J. Ayliffe, pp. 159–78. London: Baillière Tyndall.

22 Culver, D.H., Horan, T.C., Gaynes, R.P., *et al.* (1991). Surgical wound infection rates by wound class, operative procedure, and patient risk index. *Am. J. Med.*, **91** (Suppl. 3B), 152S–157S.

23 Wenzel, R.P. and Streed, S.A. (1989). Surveillance and use of computers in hospital infection control. *J. Hosp. Infect.*, **13**, 217–29.

24 Glenister, H.M., Taylor, L. and Bartlett, C.L.R., *et al.* (1993). An evaluation of surveillance method for detecting infections in hospital patients. *J. Hosp. Infect.*, **23**, 229–42.

25 Department of Health (1995). *Hospital Infection Control. Guidance on the Control of Infection in Hospitals.* London: Department of Health and HMSO.

26 Hughes, J.M. (1987). Nosocomial infection surveillance in the United States: historical perspective. *Infect. Control,* **8**, 450–553.

27 Colebrook, L. (1955). Infection acquired in hospital. *Lancet,* **2**, 885–90.

28 Williams, R.E.O., Blowers, R., Garrod, L.P. and Shooter, R.A. (1960). *Hospital Infection. Causes and Prevention.* London: Lloyd-Luke.

29 Bennett, J.V. and Brachman, P.S., eds. (1979). *Hospital Infections.* Boston: Little Brown.

30 Wise, R.I., Ossman, E.A. and Littlefield, D.R. (1989). Personal reflections on nosocomial staphylococcal infections and the development of hospital surveillance. *Rev. Infect. Dis.,* **11**, 1005–19.

31 United States Department of Health, Education and Welfare (1958). *Proceedings of the National Conference on Hospital-acquired Disease.* Washington, DC: National Academy of Sciences.

32 Jenner, E.A. and Wilson, J.A. (2000). Educating the infection control team – past, present and future. A British perspective. *J. Hosp. Infect.,* **46**, 96–105.

33 Goldman, D.A. (1986). Nosocomial infection control in the United States of America. *J. Hosp. Infect.,* **8**, 116–28.

34 Wenzel, R.P. (1987). Control of infection on the both sides of the Atlantic. *J. Hosp. Infect.,* **9**, 207–10.

35 Proceedings of the Second ICI/ Stuart Workshop (1986). Nosocomial infection. The irreducible minimum. *Infect. Control,* **7** (Suppl.), 91–152.

36 Garner, J.S. (1996). Guideline for isolation precautions in hospitals. *Infect. Control Hosp. Epidemiol.,* **17**, 53–80.

37 Hambraeus, A. and Walker, M. (2002). The International Federation of Infection Control. *Br. J. Infect. Control,* **3**(2), 18–19.

38 International Federation of Infection Control (1995). *Programme for Infection Control. Basic Concepts and Training.* UK: 3M Health Care.

Chapter 16

1 National Center for Infectious Diseases (1994). *Addressing Emerging Infectious Disease Threats. A Prevention Strategy for the United States.* Atlanta, GA: Centers for Disease Control.

2 World Health Organization (1997). *Infectious Diseases: Global Alert, Global Response.* Geneva: World Health Organization.

3 Spink, W.W. (1978). *Infectious Diseases. Prevention and Treatment in the Nineteenth and Twentieth Centuries.* Folkestone: Dawson.

4 Blumberg, B.S., Sutnick, A.I. and London, W.T. (1968). Hepatitis and leukaemia: their relation to the Australia antigen. *Bull. N.Y. Acad. Med.,* **44**, 1566–8.

5 Dane, D.S., Cameron, C.H. and Briggs, M. (1970). Virus-like particles in serum of patients with Australia-antigen-assciated hepatitis. *Lancet,* **1**, 695–8.

6 Krugman, S., Giles, J.P. and Hammond, J. (1967). Infectious hepatitis. Evidence for two distinctive clinical, epidemiolological and immunological types of infection. *J. Am. Med. Assoc.,* **200**, 365–73.

7 Thomas, D.L. (1999). Hepatitis viruses. In *Hospital Epidemiology and Infection Control,* ed. C. Glen Mayhall, 2nd edn, pp. 565–84. Baltimore: Lippincott Williams and Wilkins.

8 Zuckerman, A.J., Banatvala, J.E. and Pattison, J.R., eds. (1994). *Principles and Practice of Clinical Virology*, 3rd edn. Chichester and New York: John Wiley and Sons.

9 Barré-Sinoussi, F., Chermann, J.C., Rey, F., *et al.* (1983). Isolation of a T-lymphotropic retrovirus from a patient at risk for acquired immune deficiency syndrome (AIDS). *Science*, **220**, 868–70.

10 Gallo, R.C., Salahuddin, S.Z., Popovic, M., *et al.* (1984). Frequent detection and isolation of cytopathic retroviruses (HTLV-111) from patients with AIDS and at risk of AIDS. *Science*, **224**, 500–503.

11 Levy, J.A. (1993). Pathogenesis of human immunodeficiency virus. *Microbiol. Rev.*, **57**, 183–289.

12 Hughes, J.M., Garner, J.S., Marcus, R. and Jaffe, H.W. (1988). AIDS: epidemiological lessons from the health-care setting. *J. Hosp. Infect.*, **11** (Suppl. A), 209–17.

13 Garner, J.S. (1996). Guideline for isolation precautions in hospitals. *Infect. Control Hosp. Epidemiol.*, **17**, 53–80.

14 Sigurdsson, B. (1954). Rida, a chronic encephalitis of sheep. With general remarks on infections which develop slowly and some of their special characteristics. *Br. Vet. J.*, **110**, 341–54.

15 Hadlow, W.J. (1959). Scrapie and kuru. *Lancet*, **2**, 289–300.

16 Gajdusek, D.C., Gibbs, C.J., Jr and Alpers, M. (1966). Experimental transmission of a kuru-like syndrome to chimpanzees. *Nature*, **209**, 794–6.

17 Will, R.G., Ironside, J.W., Zeidler, M., *et al.* (1996). A new variant of Creutzfeldt–Jakob disease in the UK. *Lancet*, **347**, 921–5.

18 Prusiner, S.B. (1994). Human prion diseases. In *Principles and Practice of Clinical Virology*, ed. A.J Zuckerman, J.E. Banatvala and J.R. Pattison, 3rd edn, pp. 703–29. Chichester and New York: John Wiley and Sons.

19 Taylor, D.M. (1999). Transmissible degenerative encephalopathies: inactivation of the unconventional causal agents. In *Principles and Practice of Disinfection, Preservation and Sterilization*, ed. A.D. Russell, W.B. Hugo and G.A.J. Ayliffe, 3rd edn, pp. 222-36. Oxford: Blackwell Science.

20 Lloyd, G. Emergence and re-emergence of filoviruses. *Postgraduate Journal (Africa)*, **18**, 66–71.

21 Buckley, S.M. and Casals, J. (1970). Lassa fever: a new disease of man from West Africa. 3. Isolation and characterization of the virus. *Am. J. Trop. Med. Hyg.*, **19**, 680–91.

22 Advisory Committee on Dangerous Pathogens (1996). *Management and Control of Viral Haemorrhagic Fevers*. London: HMSO.

23 Holmes, G.P., McCormick, J.B., Trock, C.C., *et al.* (1990). Lassa fever in the United States: investigation of a case and new guidelines for management. *N. Engl. J. Med.*, **323**, 1120–23.

24 McDade, J., Shepard, C., Fraser, D., *et al.* (1977). Legionnaires' disease: isolation of a bacterium and demonstration of its role in other respiratory disease. *N. Engl. J. Med.*, **297**, 1197–203.

25 Edelstein, P.H. (1988). Nosocomial Legionnaires' disease: a global perspective. *J. Hosp. Infect.*, **11** (Suppl. A), 182–8.

26 Bartlett, L.C., Macrae, A.D. and Macfarlane, J.T. (1986). *Legionella Infections*. London: Edward Arnold.

27 Langenberg, W., Rauws, E.A., Oudbier, J.H., Tytgat, G.N.J. (1990). Patient to patient transfer of *Campylobacter pylori* infection by fiberoptic gastroduodenoscopy and biopsy. *J. Infect. Dis.*, **161**, 507–11.

28 Farber, J.M. and Peterkin, P.I. (1991). *Listeria monocytogenes*: a foodborne pathogen. *Microbiol. Rev.*, **55**, 476–511.

29 McLauchlin, J. (1990). Listeriosis in Britain 1967–1985: a summary of 722 cases during pregnancy and in the newborn. *Epidemiol. Infect.*, **104**, 181–9.

30 Lettau, L.A. (1991). Nosocomial transmission and infection control aspects of parasitic and endoparasitic disease. *Infect. Control Hosp. Epidemiol.*, **12**, 59–64.

31 Baxby, D., Hart, C.A. and Taylor, C. (1983). Human cryptosporidiosis: a possible cause of hospital cross-infection. *Br. Med. J.*, **287**, 1760–61.

32 Ayliffe, G.A.J. (1988). Equipment-related infection risks. *J. Hosp. Infect.*, **11** (Suppl. A), 279–84.

33 McGowan, J.E., Jr and Blumberg, H.M. (1995). Inner city tuberculosis in the USA. *J. Hosp. Infect.*, **30** (Suppl.), 282–95.

34 McEvoy, M. and Maguire, H. (1995). Tuberculosis in London: a review, and an account of the work of the London Consultants in Communicable Disease Control Group Working Party. *J. Hosp. Infect.*, **30** (Suppl.), 296–305.

35 Wallace, R.J. and Fraser, V. (1996). Non-tuberculous mycobacteria. In *Hospital Epidemiology and Infection Control*, ed. C. Glen. Mayhall, pp. 1224–37. Baltimore: Williams and Wilkins.

36 Pfaller, M.A. (1995). Epidemiology of candidiasis. *J. Hosp. Infect.*, **30** (Suppl.), 329–38.

37 Burnie, J.P. (1986). Candida and hands. *J. Hosp. Infect.*, **8**, 1–4.

38 Rhame, F.S. (1991). Prevention of nosocomial aspergillosis. *J. Hosp. Infect.*, **18** (Suppl. A), 466–72.

39 Walsh, T.J. and Dixon, D.M. (1989). Nosocomial aspergillosis: environmental microbiology, hospital epidemiology, diagnosis and treatment. *Eur. J. Epidemiol.*, **5**, 131–42.

40 Burdon, D.W. (1982). *Clostridium difficile*: the epidemiology and prevention of hospital acquired infection. *Infection*, **10**, 203–4.

41 Silva, J., Jr and Iezza, C. (1988). *Clostridium difficile* as a nosocomial pathogen. *J. Hosp. Infect.*, **11** (Suppl. A), 378–85.

42 Cartmill, T.D.I., Panigraphi, H., Worsley, M.A., *et al.* (1994). Management and control of a large outbreak of diarrhoea due to *Clostridium difficile*. *J. Hosp. Infect.*, **27**, 1–15.

43 Bergoyne-Berezin, E., Joly-Guillon, M.L. and Vieu, J.F. (1987). Epidemiology of nosocomial infections due to *Acinetobacter calcoaceticus*. *J. Hosp. Infect.*, **10**, 105–13.

44 French, G.L. and Phillips, I. (1999). Nosocomial infections and antimicrobial resistance. In *Hospital Epidemiology and Infection Control*, ed. C. Glen Mayhall, 2nd edn, pp. 1243–64. Baltimore: Lippincott Williams and Wilkins.

45 Livermore, D.M. (1998). Beta-lactamase-mediated resistance and opportunities for its control. *J. Antimicrob. Chemother.*, **41** (Suppl. D), 25–41.

46 Tomasz, A. (1997). Antibiotic resistance in *Streptococcus pneumoniae*. *Clin. Infect. Dis.*, **24** (Suppl. 1), S85–S88.

47 Murray, B.E. (1990). The life and times of the enterococcus. *Clin. Microbiol. Rev.*, **3**, 46–65.

48 Moellering, R.C. (1992). The enterococcus: a classic example of the impact of antimicrobial resistance on therapeutic options. *J. Antimicrob. Chemother.*, **28**, 1–12.

49 Uttley, A.H., Collins, C.H. and Naidoo, J. (1988). Vancomycin-resistant enterococci. *Lancet*, **1**, 57–8.

50 Wade, J.J. (1995). The emergence of *Enterococcus faecium* resistant to glycopeptides and other standard agents: a preliminary report. *J. Hosp. Infect.*, **30** (Suppl.), 483–93.

51 Hospital Infection Control Practices Committee (1995). Recommendations for preventing the spread of vancomycin resistance. *Infect. Control. Hosp. Epidemiol.*, **16**, 105–13.

52 Boyce, J.M., Mermel, L., Zervos, M., *et al.* (1995). Controlling vancomycin-resistant enterococci. *Infect. Control Hosp. Epidemiol.*, **16**, 634–7.

53 Noble, W.C. (1981). *Microbiology of Human Skin.* London: Lloyd-Luke.

54 Boyce, J.M. (1999). Coagulase-negative staphylococci. In *Hospital Epidemiology and Infection Control*, ed. C. Glen Mayhall, 2nd edn, pp. 365–83. Baltimore: Lippincott Williams and Wilkins.

55 Maki, D. (1992). Infections due to infusion therapy. In *Hospital Infections*, ed. J.V. Bennett and P.S. Brachman, 3rd edn, pp. 849–98. Boston: Little Brown.

56 Ayliffe, G.A.J., Lilly, H.A. and Lowbury, E.J.L. (1979). Decline of the hospital staphylococcus? Incidence of multi-resistant *Staphylococcus aureus* in three Birmingham hospitals. *Lancet*, **1**, 538–41.

57 Pavillard, R., Harvey, K., Douglas, D., *et al.* (1982). Epidemic of hospital-acquired infection due to methicillin-resistant *Staphylococcus aureus* in major Victorian hospitals. *Med. J. Aust.*, **1**, 451–4.

58 Pearman, J.W., Christiansen, K.J., Annear, D.I., *et al.* (1985). Control of methicillin-resistant *Staphylococcus aureus* (MRSA) in an Australian metropolitan teaching hospital complex. *Med. J. Aust.*, **142**, 103–8.

59 Keane, C.T. and Cafferky, M.T. (1984). Re-emergence of methicillin-resistant *Staphylococcus aureus* causing severe infection. *J. Infect.*, **9**, 6–16.

60 Duckworth, G.L., Lothian, J.L.F. and Williams, J.D. (1988). Methicillin-resistant *Staphylococcus aureus* in a London teaching hospital. *J. Hosp. Infect.*, **11**, 1–15.

61 Ayliffe, G.A.J. (1997). The progressive international spread of methicillin-resistant *Staphyloccus aureus*. *Clin. Infect. Dis.*, **24** (Suppl. 1), S74–S79.

62 Panlilio, A.L., Culver, D.H. and Gaynes, R.P. (1992). Methicillin-resistant *Staphylococcus aureus* in U.S. hospitals, 1975–1991. *Infect. Control Hosp. Epidemiol.*, **13**, 582–6.

63 Voss, A., Milatovic, D., Wallrauch-Schwarz, C., *et al.* (1994). Methicillin-resistant *Staphylococcus aureus* in Europe. *Eur. J. Clin. Microbiol. Infect. Dis.*, **13**, 50–55.

64 Fraise, A.M., Mitchell, K., O'Brien, S.J.O., *et al.* (1997). Methicillin-resistant *Staphylococcus aureus* (MRSA) in nursing homes in a major UK city: an anonymized point prevalence survey. *Epidemiol. Infect.*, **118**, 1–5.

65 Rosdahl, V.T. and Knudsen, A.M. (1991). The decline of methicillin-resistance among Danish staphylococcal strains. *Infect. Control Hosp. Epidemiol.*, **12**, 83–8.

66 Frenay, H.M., Schot, C.S., Van Leuven, W.J., *et al.* (1994). Methicillin-resistant staphylococcal infection. Infection spread between hospitals. *Br. Med. J.*, **308**, 58.

67 Wenzel, R.P., Reagan, D.R., Bertino, J.S., *et al.* (1998). Methicillin-resistant *Staphylococcus aureus* outbreak: a consensus panel's definition and guidelines. *Am. J. Infect. Control*, **26**, 102–10.

68 Boyce, J.M., Jackson, M.M. and Pugliese, G. (1995). Methicillin-resistant *Staphylococcus aureus*: a briefing for acute care hospitals and nursing facilities. *Infect. Control Hosp. Epidemiol.*, **15**, 105–15.

69 Report of a working party of the British Society for Antimicrobial Chemotherapy, the Hospital Infection Society and the Infection Control Nurses Association (1998). Revised guidelines for the control of methicillin-resistant *Staphylococcus aureus* in hospitals. *J. Hosp. Infect.*, **39**, 253–90.

70 Spicer, W.J. (1984). Three strategies in the control of staphylococci including methicillin-resistant *Staphylococcus aureus. J. Hosp. Infect.*, **5** (Suppl.), 45–9.

71 Ayliffe, G.A.J., Cookson, B.D., Ducel, G., *et al.* (1995). *World Health Scientific Working Group on the Global Control of MRSA*. Geneva: World Health Organization.

72 Arnold, M.S., Dempsey, J.M. and Fishman, M. (2002). The best hospital practices for controlling methicillin-resistant *Staphylococcus aureus*: on the cutting edge. *Infect. Control Hosp. Epidemiol.*, **23**, 69–76.

73 Pittet, D., Hugonnet, S., Harbarth, S., *et al.* (2000). Effectiveness of a hospital-wide programme to improve compliance with hand hygiene. *Lancet*, **356**, 1307–12.

74 Casewell, M.W. and Hill, R.L. (1986). Elimination of nasal carriage of *Staphylococcus aureus* with mupirocin ('pseudomonic acid'): a controlled trial. *J. Antimicrob. Chemother.*, **17**, 365–72.

75 Cookson, B.D. (1998). The emergence of mupirocin resistance: a challenge to infection control. *J. Antimicrob. Chemother.*, **41**, 11–18.

76 Hiramatsu, K., Hanaki, H., Ino, T., *et al.* (1997). Methicillin-resistant *Staphylococcus aureus* clinical strain with reduced vancomycin susceptibility. *J. Antimicrob. Chemother.*, **40**, 135–6.

Chapter 17

1 Selwyn, S. (1991). Hospital infection: the first 2500 years. *J. Hosp. Infect.*, **18** (Suppl. A), 5–64.

2 Rutkov, I.M. (1993). *Surgery. An Illustrated History*. St Louis: Mosby.

3 La Force, F.M. (1997). The control of infections in hospitals 1750–1850. In *Prevention and Control of Nosocomial Infections*, ed. R.P. Wenzel, 3rd edn, pp. 3–17. Baltimore: Lippincott Williams and Wilkins.

4 Public Health Laboratory Service (1997–8). *Surgical Site Infection. Analysis of a Year's Surveillance in English Hospitals*. London: Public Health Laboratory Service.

5 Mertens, R.A.F. (1996). Methodologies and results of national surveillance. In *Surveillance of Nosocomial Infections*, ed. A.M. Emmerson and G.A.J. Ayliffe, pp. 159–78. London: Baillière Tyndall.

6 Rennie, M.J. (1993). EPIC: infection in intensive care in Europe. Present status and future prospects. *Br. J. Intensive Care*, **3**, 27–36.

7 Garner, J.S. (1996). Guideline for isolation precautions in hospitals. *Infect. Control Hosp. Epidemiol.*, **17**, 53–80.

8 Pratt, R.J., Pellowe, C., Loveday, H.P., *et al.* (2001). The EPIC project: developing national evidence-based guidelines for preventing healthcare associated infections. *J. Hosp. Infect.*, **47** (Suppl.), S1–S82.

9 Wise, R., Hart, T., Cars, O., *et al.* (1998). Antimicrobial resistance. *Br. Med. J.*, **317**, 609–10.

10 Goldman, D.A., Weinstein, D., Wenzel, R.P., *et al.* (1996). Strategies to prevent and control the emergence and spread of antimicrobial-resistant microorganisms in hospitals: a challenge to hospital leadership. *J. Am. Med. Assoc.*, **275**, 234–40.

11 Pittet, D. (2002). Promotion of hand hygiene: magic, or scientific challenge? *Infect. Control Hosp. Epidemiol.*, **23**, 118–19.

12 Proceedings of the Second ICI/Stuart Workshop (1986). Nosocomial infection: the irreducible minimum. Proceedings of the Second Stuart Workshop (1986). *Infect. Control*, **7** (Suppl.), 95–152.

Bibliography

Altemeier, W.A., Burke, J.F., Pruitt, B.A. and Sandusky, W.R (1984). *Manual on Control of Infection in Surgical Patients.* Philadelphia: Lippincott.

Ayliffe, G.A.J., Babb, J.R. and Taylor, L.J. (1999). *Hospital-acquired Infection. Principles and Practice,* 3rd edn. Oxford: Butterworth Heinemann.

Ayliffe, G.A.J., Fraise, A.P., Geddes, A.M. and Mitchell, K. (2000). *Control of Hospital Infection. A Practical Handbook,* 4th edn. London, Arnold. (See also Lowbury, E.J.L., Ayliffe, G.A.J., Geddes, A.M. and Williams, J.D. (1975). 1st edn. London: Chapman and Hall.)

Bennett, J.V. and Brachman, P.S., eds. (1998). *Hospital Infections.* Philadelphia: Lippincott Williams and Wilkins.

Block, S.S. (2001). *Disinfection, Sterilization and Preservation,* 5th edn. Philadelphia: Lippincott Williams and Wilkins.

Bulloch, W. (1938). *The History of Bacteriology.* New York: Dover Publications.

Bynum, W.F and Nutton, V., eds. (1981). *Theories of Fever from Antiquity to the Enlightenment.* London: Wellcome Institute.

Chapin, C.V. (1910). *The Sources and Mode of Infection.* New York: John Wiley and Sons.

Collier, L.H., Balows, A. and Sussman, M., eds. (1997). *Topley and Wilson's Microbiology and Microbial Infections,* 9th edn. London: Arnold.

Creighton, C. (1891, 1894). *A History of Epidemics in Great Britain.* Cambridge: Cambridge University Press.

Donahue, M.P. (1996). *Nursing the Finest Art. An Illustrated History,* 2nd edn. St Louis and Baltimore: Mosby.

Elek, S.D. (1959). *Staphylococcus pyogenes and its Relation to Disease.* Edinburgh and London: Livingstone.

Gale, A.H. (1959). *Epidemic Diseases.* London: Penguin Books.

Garrison, F.H. (1929). *An Introduction to the History of Medicine.* Philadelphia and London: Saunders.

Godlee, R.J. (1917). *Lord Lister.* London: Macmillan.

Greenwood, D., Slack, R. and Petherer, J., eds. (1992). *Medical Microbiology: A Guide to Microbial Infection, Pathogenesis, Immunity, Laboratory Diagnosis and Control.* Edinburgh: Churchill Livingstone.

Loudon, I. (2000). *The Tragedy of Childbirth Fever.* Oxford: Oxford University Press.

Lowbury, E.J.L. and Ayliffe, G.A.J. (1974). *Drug Resistance in Antimicrobial Therapy.* Springfield IL: Charles C. Thomas.

Macdonald, A. and Smith, G., eds. (1981). *The Staphylococci. Proceedings of the Alexander Ogston Centennial Conference* Aberdeen: Aberdeen University Press.

Mayhall, C.G., ed. (1999). *Hospital Epidemiology and Infection Control,* 2nd edn. Baltimore: Williams and Wilkins.

Meleney, F.M. (1948). *Treatise on Surgical Infections.* New York: Oxford University Press.

Murchison, C. (1873). *A Treatise on Continued Fevers of Great Britain.* London: Lloyd-Luke.

O'Grady, F.W., Lambert, H.P., Finch, R.G. and Greenwood, D. (1997). *Antibiotic and Chemotherapy. Anti-infective Agents and their Use in Therapy,* 7th edn. Edinburgh: Churchill Livingstone. (See also Barber, M. and Garrod L.P. (1963), 1st edn.)

Porter, R. (1997). *The Greatest Benefit to Mankind. A Medical History of Humanity from Antiquity to the Present.* London: Harper Collins.

Poynter, F.N.L., ed. (1981). *The Evolution of Hospitals in Britain.* London: Pitman.

Russell, A.D., Hugo, W.B. and Ayliffe, G.A.J. (1999). *Principles and Practice of Disinfection, Preservation and Sterilization,* 3rd edn. Oxford: Blackwell Science.

Rutkov, I.M. (1993). *Surgery. An Illustrated History.* St Louis: Mosby.

Schimmelbusch, C. (1893). *The Aseptic Treatment of Wounds.* Transl. 1894 A.T. Rake. London: H.K. Lewis.

Sim, A.J.W. and Jeffries, D.J., eds. (1990). *AIDS and Surgery.* Oxford: Blackwell Scientific Publications.

Spink, W.W. (1978). *Infectious Diseases. Prevention and Treatment in the Nineteenth and Twentieth Centuries.* Folkestone: Dawson.

Thompson, J.D. and Goldin, G. (1975). *The Hospital: A Social and Architectural History.* New Haven and London: Yale University Press.

Walter, C. (1948). *The Aseptic Treatment of Wounds.* New York: Macmillan.

Wangensteen, O.H. and Wangensteen, S.D. (1978). *The Rise of Surgery from Empiric Craft to Scientific Discipline.* Minnesota: University of Minnesota Press.

Watson-Cheyne, W. (1882). *Antiseptic Surgery: Its Principles, Practice, History and Results.* London: Smith and Elder.

Wenzel, R.P. (1997). *Prevention and Control of Nosocomial Infections,* 3rd edn. Baltimore: Lippincott Williams and Wilkins.

Williams, R.E.O. and Shooter, R.A., eds. (1963). *Infection in Hospitals: Epidemiology and Control.* Oxford: Blackwell Scientific Publications.

Williams, R.E.O., Blowers, R., Garrod, L.P. and Shooter, R.A. (1966). *Hospital Infection. Causes and Prevention.* London: Lloyd-Luke.

Winslow, C.E.A. (1944). *The Conquest of Epidemic Disease. A Chapter in the History of Ideas.* Princeton, NJ: Princeton University Press.

Woodham-Smith, C. (1951). *Florence Nightingale.* New York: McGraw-Hill.

Woodward, J. (1974). *To Do the Sick No Harm. A Study of the British Voluntary Hospital System to 1875.* London: Routledge and Kegan.

Zinsser, H. (1935). *Rats, Lice and History.* Boston: Little Brown.

Zuckerman, A.J., Banatvala, J.E. and Pattison, J.R., eds. (1994). *Principles and Practice of Clinical Virology,* 3rd edn. Chichester and New York: John Wiley and Sons.

Index

Numbers in italics refer to *tables* and *figures*.